A.D.A.M. Student Atlas of Anatomy

This is the second edition of a volume renowned for its innovative approach to understanding the human body. It features full-color art throughout, using a three-dimensional approach to anatomic structure. The *A.D.A.M. Student Atlas of Anatomy* is an invaluable learning and review tool developed for medical, allied health, and human biology undergraduate and graduate students.

This new edition emphasizes surface anatomy and features unique additional views (posterior, medial, lateral) of important structures. It has extensive coverage of those areas, such as the perineum, head, and neck, that are often difficult for students to understand and appreciate.

Todd R. Olson is Professor of Anatomy and Structural Biology and Director of Clinical and Developmental Anatomy at the Albert Einstein College of Medicine, New York.

Wojciech Pawlina is Professor and Chair of the Department of Anatomy at the Mayo Medical School, College of Medicine, Mayo Clinic, Rochester, Minnesota.

A.D.A.M. Student Atlas of Anatomy

2nd Edition

Todd R. Olson, Ph.D.

Professor
Department of Anatomy & Structural Biology
Albert Einstein College of Medicine
Yeshiva University
Bronx, New York

Wojciech Pawlina, M.D.

Professor and Chair
Department of Anatomy
Mayo Medical School
College of Medicine, Mayo Clinic
Rochester, Minnesota

Illustrative Art
A.D.A.M.®, Inc.
Atlanta, Georgia

Cadaver Photographs
The Bassett Collection
Stanford University
School of Medicine
Stanford, California

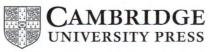

CAMBRIDGE
UNIVERSITY PRESS

CAMBRIDGE UNIVERSITY PRESS
Cambridge, New York, Melbourne, Madrid, Cape Town, Singapore, São Paolo, Delhi

Cambridge University Press
32 Avenue of the Americas, New York, NY 10013-2473, USA

www.cambridge.org
Information on this title: www.cambridge.org/9780521887564

First published 2008

Printed in Hong Kong by Golden Cup

A catalog record for this publication is available from the British Library.

Library of Congress Cataloging in Publication Data

Olson, Todd R.
   A.D.A.M. student atlas of anatomy / Todd R. Olson, Wojciech Pawlina.
– 2nd ed.
      p. ; cm.
   Includes bibliographical references and index.
   ISBN 978-0-521-88756-4 (hardback) – ISBN 978-0-521-71005-3
(paperback) 1. Human anatomy – Atlases.   I. Pawlina, Wojciech.
II. Title.   III. Title: Student atlas of anatomy.   IV. Title: ADAM student
atlas of anatomy.
   [DNLM: 1. Anatomy – Atlases. QS 17 O52a 2007]

   QM25.O47 2007
   611.0022′2–dc22   2007034103

ISBN 978-0-521-88756-4 hardback
ISBN 978-0-521-71005-3 paperback

To my mother and father
for the greatest of all contributions
to my existence, optimism, and ability to dream
and to my teachers, colleagues, and students
for their encouragement and contributions
to the realization of this dream.

Todd R. Olson

To my father, Dr. Kazimierz Pawlina,
who was my first anatomy teacher and
my inspiration to pursue an academic career.

Wojciech Pawlina

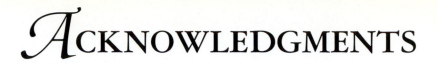 ACKNOWLEDGMENTS

I (TRO) must express my appreciation and gratitude to Prof. Wojciech Pawlina, M.D., for joining me as a co-author on this edition. Wojciech provided substantial help in the production of this work, and his presence as a co-author is a much-deserved recognition of the hours of work and creative input he contributed to the production of both editions of this atlas. We (TRO & WP) wish also to acknowledge the insightful changes introduced by Prof. Herbert Lippert in the German edition—some of which have been incorporated here—and the helpful comments of Prof. Christian Fontaine, who produced the French translation of the first edition. We also wish to acknowledge and express our gratitude to our colleagues, **Dr. Nirusha Lachman** at the Mayo Clinic and **Dr. Sherry A. Downie** at Albert Einstein, for their invaluable help, suggestions, and support in the production of this new edition.

The second edition of the *A.D.A.M. Student Atlas of Anatomy* is truly the product of a major collaborative effort. The authors wish to extend our appreciation to all individuals who worked on this project and, in particular, to six people whose contribution to this edition were most noteworthy. At Cambridge University Press, **Marc Strauss,** who had the determination and skill to assemble the talent needed to undertake the production of a second edition of this work, and **Nat Russo,** who had the conviction to push for its publication. At A.D.A.M., **Meredith Nienkamp** for her work in championing the second edition and **Lisa Higginbotham,** who worked tirelessly to produce the new artwork for this edition. **Robert A. Chase** at Stanford University School of Medicine for allowing us to include photographs from the David L. Bassett anatomical collection. And **Matthew Byrd** and his superb team at Aptara, Inc., for their excellent work in laying out and producing this book. The dedication to every detail of Matt's team elevated the content and quality of this edition well beyond what was originally perceived by the authors. Thank you!

The talent, dedication, and professionalism of all those at A.D.A.M. who were responsible for the artwork—both in this work and in the A.D.A.M. Interactive Anatomy products—are clearly visible on every page of this atlas. Their efforts and commitment to making this book a learning resource will benefit students everywhere.

A.D.A.M. Anatomical Illustration Team:
Meredith Nienkamp, VP of Production/Medical Illustrator
Mike Gleason, Medical Illustrator
Lisa Higginbotham, Medical Illustrator
Dan Johnson, Medical Illustrator
Kyle McNeir, VP of Production & Internet Design/Medical Illustrator

Prior edition contributions made by:
Mary Beth Clough, Medical Illustrator
Ron Collins, Medical Illustrator
Eric D. Grafman, Medical Illustrator
Lynda Leigh Levy, Medical Illustrator
Virginia Sue Mabry, Illustrator
Dee Mustafa-Bowne, Illustrator
Ed M. Stewart, Medical Illustrator
Gregory M. Swayne, Medical Illustrator
Lelayne Weiss, Illustrator

The authors and A.D.A.M., Inc., wish to thank all of the individuals at Cambridge University Press whose expertise, enthusiasm, and commitment to quality have been at the heart of this project from the beginning: Marc Strauss, Nat Russo, Cathy Felgar, Jennifer Bossert, and Carlos Aguirre. In particular, we wish to thank Marc Strauss for the kindness, patience within limits, and the good humor he displayed in performing his role as the drill sergeant for this entire effort. Finally, we wish to extend our appreciation to Lisa Adamitis, who designed the cover.

Todd R. Olson
Wojciech Pawlina
A.D.A.M., Inc.

PREFACE

Although our knowledge of human anatomy has changed relatively little in the past hundred years, the teaching of anatomy in all health science professions has changed profoundly. During most of the 20th century, gross human anatomy was the principle course in the first year of medical school. Today, one hundred years later, the importance of anatomy within the curriculum has been reduced in pedagogic and temporal significance to the degree that first-year medical students spend two to three times more time studying cellular, subcellular, molecular, and biochemical processes than they do the gross structure of the human body. The major reason for this de-emphasis has been the spectacular development of bioscience technology and the resultant explosion in clinically relevant knowledge that has been incorporated into basic medical education.

Anatomists successfully responded to the challenges created by this reduction in curricular importance and time in three ways. First, and most significantly, we have largely reduced the body of knowledge covered in our courses to those aspects of anatomy that are clinically relevant and therefore of greatest potential value to the student's future clinical practice. Second, we have sifted the body of anatomical knowledge to winnow out the specialist details that must now be taught in postgraduate programs, leaving the anatomical essentials that are fundamental to the basic clinical education of every health sciences and medical student. And third, we have expanded our teaching into the later years of the medical curriculum, introduced specialty and subspecialty focused elective courses for students prior to graduation, and greatly expanded our participation in graduate and continuing education courses. The vertical expansion of anatomical education into these new venues, beyond the traditional first-year course, has allowed a more effective and focused delivery of appropriate anatomical detail to students and graduated physicians who have a direct and specific need to know this information.

All three of these new pedagogic frontiers are critical components in the anatomical education of our future healthcare professionals. The purpose of this work is to focus on the initial phase of this educational process in which it is increasingly necessary to distill the voluminous details present in gross anatomy to their fundamental essentials. While there are an ever-growing number of gross anatomy textbooks that have adopted an "essentials" perspective, we have long thought it remarkable that no one has successfully incorporated this perspective into an anatomy atlas for beginning students. This all changed ten years ago when the first edition of the *A.D.A.M. Student Atlas of Anatomy* was published. From its inception in 1994, we have viewed the *A.D.A.M. Student Atlas* as, first and foremost, a visual guide and interactive learning resource to be used along with a clinical anatomy textbook. In the organization and content of the *A.D.A.M. Student Atlas*, our goal has been and remains to emphasize those parts of the body and structures that are fundamental to the clinical education of every medical and health sciences student.

To accomplish our goal, we decided to include more images of fewer structures and, in particular, more images of those parts of the body that present the beginning student with the greatest difficulties to comprehend and appreciate. We expect and fully hope that most students who use this book will soon become aware of both this distinctive emphasis and limited scope, as well as their own need to consult a more comprehensive atlas as their study of human anatomy matures. *Our primary design concept in support of our goal was neither to duplicate the efforts seen in existing comprehensive atlases, which fully display every named feature in the human body, nor to create an atlas to accompany and guide dissection.*

Nowhere in the *A.D.A.M. Student Atlas* is the emphasis on essentials of the most difficult regions of the body more evident than in Chapter 4 ("Pelvis and Perineum"), which is substantially longer than normally found in traditional atlases. There were two reasons why this chapter was created in this expanded form: First, there is a clear need to know the basic anatomy of the pelvis and perineum in the major clerkship of obstetrics and gynecology, and it is only slightly less important in urology; second, experience indicates that this region is possibly the most difficult for first time students to understand. The pelvis and perineum present unique problems of spatial and surface relationships, which are compounded by the fact that dissection of the pelvis only partially reveals its contents *in situ* and the perineum dissection is difficult and time-consuming, even for an experienced dissector working on an ideal specimen. In contrast to Chapter 4, the preceding chapter on the abdominal contents and their peritoneal relationships is relatively short because the beginning student generally finds them easier to dissect and identify their important anatomical structures and relationships.

All of the atlas's chapters, except the cranial nerves, are topographically/regionally arranged and organized to begin with surface anatomy and to end with the traditional sequences of superficial-to-deep images that the student will see when dissecting. Another innovation that we have included in the *A.D.A.M. Student*

Atlas is the lengthy systemic sections found at the beginning of the chapters on the trunk, limbs, and head and neck. Systemic descriptions were not included in Chapters 2 and 3, the thoracic and abdominal contents, respectively, because the systemic anatomy of the body walls of these regions is covered extensively in Chapter 1 on the trunk, and the distribution and pattern of deeper neurovasculature structures can be clearly appreciated in the sequence of dissection images within each of these two chapters.

While it is ultimately the objective in teaching patient-oriented anatomy to provide the student with an understanding of the composite anatomy of all or selected regions of the body, experience has convinced us that many, or even most, students initially find it easier to organize information by systems. The addition of these extensive systemic sections should not only make the *A.D.A.M. Student Atlas* a more useful book for beginning students but also make it a valuable resource for allied health students whose courses are usually systemically taught but who have never had access to a regional atlas that also emphasized this arrangement.

Another distinctive innovation of the *A.D.A.M. Student Atlas* is the placement of photographs of dissected or osteological specimens adjacent to newly rendered A.D.A.M. images. The rationale for this arrangement and the way we have chosen to label them is based upon the experience we have had with many first year medical students who purchase an expensive photographic atlas that is then used for a short period of time prior to laboratory practical exams. These atlases are helpful because students can test their knowledge on the pictures, which more closely approximate what they will see on the practical exam.

In structuring the *A.D.A.M. Student Atlas*, we have selected and arranged the cadaveric photographs to provide beginning students with an overview of the more important dissections that she/he will see in the lab. Also, by placing them adjacent to similar A.D.A.M. images, the student gains the benefit of seeing a detailed artistic image (as opposed to a highly simplified schematic drawing) that enhances and highlights what is most important in this view.

While an appreciation of both cross-sectional and radiographic anatomy is important in many areas of basic clinical work, it was impossible, within the scope of this atlas, to incorporate more than a limited number into each chapter. The cross-sections and radiographs that do appear have been included because they either best display the distribution of prominent structures, e.g., peritoneum, or provide another means of visualizing the relationships within a region. The limited use of these important visual methods and modalities reflects the physical restrictions of the book and does not imply that they are unimportant or should not be part of a course in clinical anatomy.

TRO & WP

CONTENTS

saphenous vein, and cutaneous nerves of the lower limb much easier. The extensive use of these multiple views is one of the most striking and valuable characteristics of the *A.D.A.M. Student Atlas of Anatomy*.

Illustrations and Cadaver Photographs

The two figures here in Plate 1.48 illustrate how A.D.A.M. illustrations have been paired with photographs taken from Stanford University's Bassett Collection and intended use in the atlas.

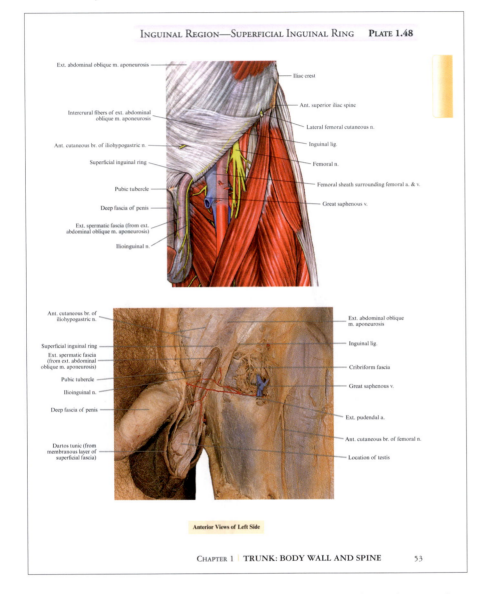

INGUINAL REGION—SUPERFICIAL INGUINAL RING   PLATE 1.48

Ext. abdominal oblique m. aponeurosis

Intercrural fibers of ext. abdominal oblique m. aponeurosis

Ant. cutaneous br. of iliohypogastric n.

Superficial inguinal ring

Pubic tubercle

Deep fascia of penis

Ext. spermatic fascia (from ext. abdominal oblique m. aponeurosis)

Ilioinguinal n.

Iliac crest

Ant. superior iliac spine

Lateral femoral cutaneous n.

Inguinal lig.

Femoral n.

Femoral sheath surrounding femoral a. & v.

Great saphenous v.

Ant. cutaneous br. of iliohypogastric n.

Superficial inguinal ring

Ext. spermatic fascia (from ext. abdominal oblique m. aponeurosis)

Pubic tubercle

Ilioinguinal n.

Deep fascia of penis

Dartos tunic (from membranous layer of superficial fascia)

Ext. abdominal oblique m. aponeurosis

Inguinal lig.

Cribriform fascia

Great saphenous v.

Ext. pudendal a.

Ant. cutaneous br. of femoral n.

Location of testis

Anterior Views of Left Side

CHAPTER 1 | **TRUNK: BODY WALL AND SPINE**   53

In structuring the *A.D.A.M. Student Atlas*, we have selected and arranged the cadaveric photographs to provide an overview of the more important dissections. By associating these photographs with adjacent A.D.A.M. images that depict similar but not identical anatomy, the student gains the benefit of seeing a detailed artistic image (as opposed to a highly simplified schematic drawing) to enhance and highlight what is most important to be seen in the photograph of the dissected specimen.

Joint Motion and Segmentary Nerve Supply

Motions in a single plane at each joint are typically initiated by motor neurons found in four successive spinal cord segments and their spinal nerves. The cranial pair of neurons innervate the muscles that produce movement in one direction and the caudal two innervate the muscles that produce the opposite motion. An appreciation of the actions, especially in the limbs, and their innervation is basic clinical knowledge that has practical value to a wide variety of health care professionals. The atlas includes tables that list the muscles and the nerve(s) that innervate them. The segmentary origin of each nerve is also listed. In those cases where a specific segmentary level is primarily associated with the supply of the muscle, the level is printed in **BOLD**. In addition, information about segmentary innervation is provided in illustrations showing how different spinal levels control antagonistic movements in the upper and lower limb.

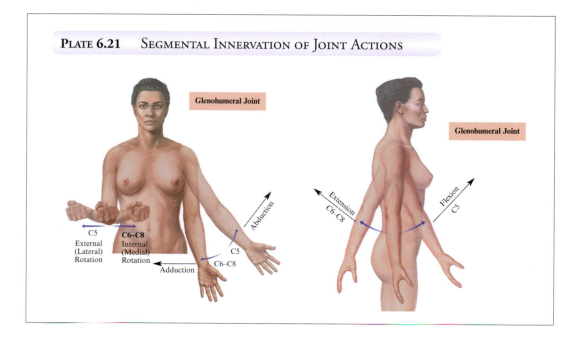

PLATE 6.21   SEGMENTAL INNERVATION OF JOINT ACTIONS

Anatomical Terminology

The anglicized and classical terminology used in the *A.D.A.M Student Atlas* follows the recent edition of the Terminologica *Anatomica*. In some case, the use of square [ ] and parentheses ( ) has formal meaning in the internationally recognized code of anatomical nomenclature.

> **[Square] brackets** signify:
> 1. An officially recognized alternative name or synonym.
>> Fibularis [Peroneus] longus m.
>> L. vagus n. [CN X], where CN refers to a cranial nerve
>> L. gastro-omental [gastroepiploic] v.
>
> 2. An equivalent anatomical name for this structure.
>> Subcostal n. [T12], where T12 = 12th thoracic spinal n.
>> C1 [Atlas]

> **(Round) brackets** identify:
> 1. An official name of *inconsistent* structures.
>> (Accessory parotid gland)
>> (Frontal suture)
>
> 2. Eponyms and alternative names that are not officially recognized as appropriate in contemporary usage.
>> Omental foramen (f. of Winslow)
>> L. colic (splenic) flexure
>> Costoaxillary (ext. mammary) v.
>> Hepatopancreatic ampulla (of Vater)

3. Additional components of a name that are usually omitted that have been added for clarification or that are supplemental to the name.

> Greater tuberosity (of humerus)
> Acromion (process of scapula)
> Posterior basal bronchopulmonary segment (S10)

4. Motor and sensory segmental and spinal nerve levels of a peripheral nerve.

> Femoral n. (L2-L4)
> Lat. femoral cutaneous n. (L2,L3)
> Middle cluneal nn. (dorsal rami of S1-S3)

For TWO adjacent spinal nn., they are separated by a comma; however, when more than two spinal nn. are involved, only the cranial and caudal-most are listed, separated by a hyphen.

5. Conditions specific or unique to the image or dissection.

> L. rectus abdominis m. (reflected medially)
> R. primary bronchus (pulled to L.)

Hyphenated names. Hyphens appear in a name to:
1. More specifically identify a constituent part of a larger complex structure.

> Triceps brachii m. - long head
> Pectoralis major m. - sternal head

2. Separate the parts of compound name where the same vowel is found at the end of the first name and beginning of the second.

> Gastro-omental [gastroepiploic] v.
> Atlanto-occipital joint

Abbreviations

The following abbreviations are used in the atlas. **Bold** entries are abbreviated everywhere they appear, other entries are sometimes abbreviated in order to save space.

&	**= and**	inf.	= inferior	nn.	= nerves
a.	**= artery**	int.	= internal	port.	= portion
aa.	**= arteries**	**L.**	**= Left**	post.	= posterior
ant.	= anterior	lat.	= lateral	proc.	= process
asc.	= ascending	**lig.**	**= ligament**	pt.	= part
br.	**= branch**	**ligg.**	**= ligaments**	**R.**	**= Right**
brr.	**= branches**	**m.**	**= muscle**	sup.	= superior
comm.	**= communicating**	**mm.**	**= muscles**	trib.	= tributary
desc.	= descending	med.	= medial	**v.**	**= vein**
ext.	= external	**n.**	**= nerve**	**vv.**	**= veins**

Another system of abbreviation is typically used when segmental structures (i.e., vertebrae, spinal or intercostal nerves, ribs) are superimposed on or immediately adjacent to the structure. Thus, **C6** on or next to a vertebra identifies the sixth cervical vertebrae; the "C" distinguishes the vertebral type and the number its segmental location. Abbreviations used in this way are:

> C = Cervical
> Cc = Coccygeal
> L = Lumbar
> R = Rib
> S = Sacral
> T = Thoracic

1

TRUNK: BODY WALL AND SPINE

SURFACE ANATOMY

SKELETON

JOINTS &
LIGAMENTS

MUSCLES

VASCULATURE

NERVES

SPINAL CORD &
VERTEBRAL CANAL

ANTERIOR BODY WALL
& MAMMARY GLAND

LATERAL BODY WALL

INGUINAL REGION

SUPERFICIAL BACK

DEEP BACK

SUBOCCIPITAL REGION

PLATE 1.1   SURFACE ANATOMY

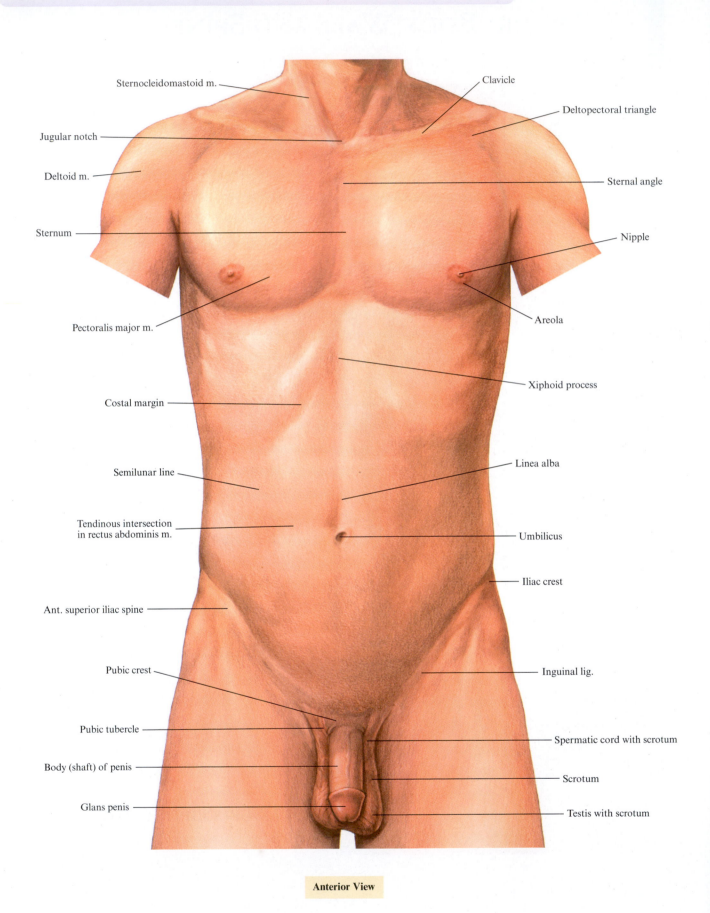

Sternocleidomastoid m.

Clavicle

Deltopectoral triangle

Jugular notch

Deltoid m.

Sternal angle

Sternum

Nipple

Pectoralis major m.

Areola

Xiphoid process

Costal margin

Linea alba

Semilunar line

Tendinous intersection in rectus abdominis m.

Umbilicus

Iliac crest

Ant. superior iliac spine

Inguinal lig.

Pubic crest

Pubic tubercle

Spermatic cord with scrotum

Body (shaft) of penis

Scrotum

Glans penis

Testis with scrotum

Anterior View

A.D.A.M. | Student Atlas of Anatomy

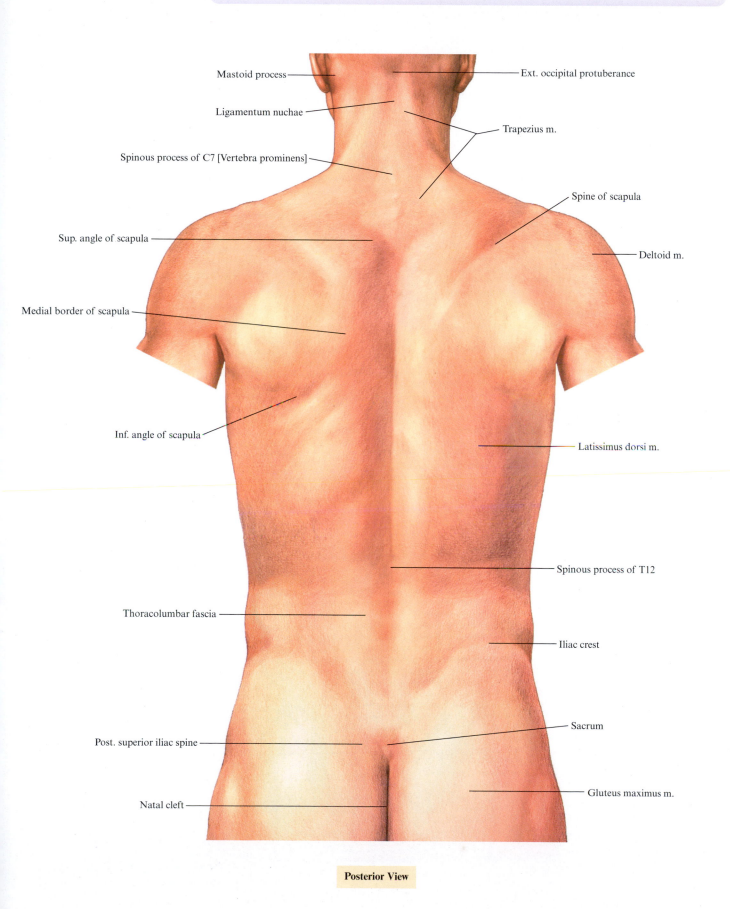

Mastoid process

Ext. occipital protuberance

Ligamentum nuchae

Trapezius m.

Spinous process of C7 [Vertebra prominens]

Spine of scapula

Sup. angle of scapula

Deltoid m.

Medial border of scapula

Inf. angle of scapula

Latissimus dorsi m.

Spinous process of T12

Thoracolumbar fascia

Iliac crest

Sacrum

Post. superior iliac spine

Gluteus maximus m.

Natal cleft

Posterior View

PLATE 1.3   SKELETON—MUSCLE ATTACHMENTS

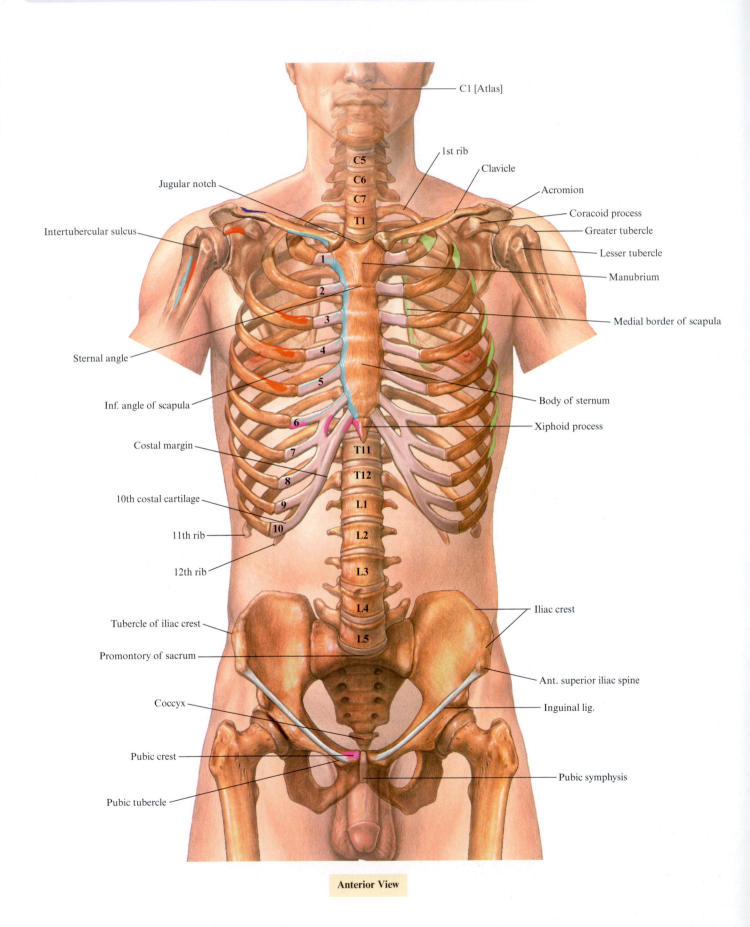

C1 [Atlas]

1st rib

Clavicle

Jugular notch

Acromion

Coracoid process

Greater tubercle

Intertubercular sulcus

Lesser tubercle

Manubrium

Medial border of scapula

Sternal angle

Body of sternum

Inf. angle of scapula

Xiphoid process

Costal margin

10th costal cartilage

11th rib

12th rib

Tubercle of iliac crest

Iliac crest

Promontory of sacrum

Ant. superior iliac spine

Coccyx

Inguinal lig.

Pubic crest

Pubic symphysis

Pubic tubercle

C5
C6
C7
T1

1
2
3
4
5
6
7
8
9
10

T11
T12
L1
L2
L3
L4
L5

Anterior View

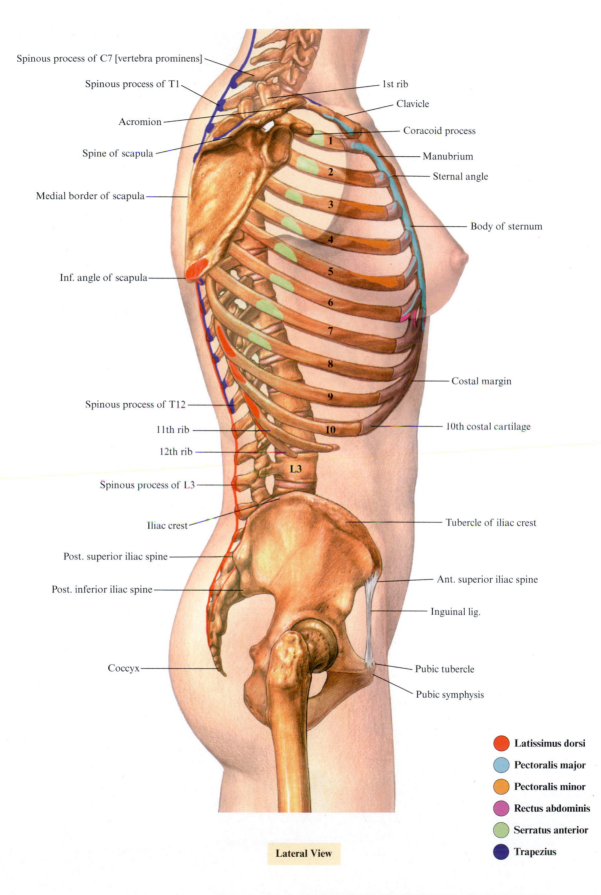

Spinous process of C7 [vertebra prominens]

Spinous process of T1

Acromion

Spine of scapula

Medial border of scapula

Inf. angle of scapula

Spinous process of T12

11th rib

12th rib

Spinous process of L3

Iliac crest

Post. superior iliac spine

Post. inferior iliac spine

Coccyx

1st rib

Clavicle

Coracoid process

Manubrium

Sternal angle

Body of sternum

Costal margin

10th costal cartilage

Tubercle of iliac crest

Ant. superior iliac spine

Inguinal lig.

Pubic tubercle

Pubic symphysis

L3

Lateral View

● **Latissimus dorsi**
● **Pectoralis major**
● **Pectoralis minor**
● **Rectus abdominis**
● **Serratus anterior**
● **Trapezius**

CHAPTER 1 │ **TRUNK: BODY WALL AND SPINE** 5

PLATE 1.5   SKELETON—MUSCLE ATTACHMENTS

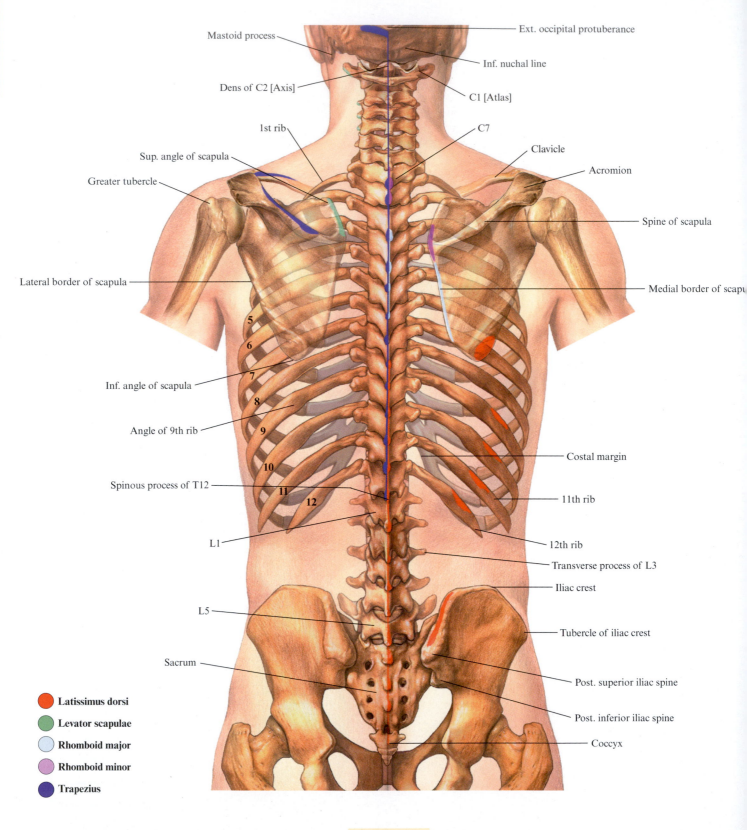

Mastoid process

Dens of C2 [Axis]

1st rib

Sup. angle of scapula

Greater tubercle

Lateral border of scapula

5
6
7
8
9
10
11
12

Inf. angle of scapula

Angle of 9th rib

Spinous process of T12

L1

L5

Sacrum

Ext. occipital protuberance

Inf. nuchal line

C1 [Atlas]

C7

Clavicle

Acromion

Spine of scapula

Medial border of scapu[la]

Costal margin

11th rib

12th rib

Transverse process of L3

Iliac crest

Tubercle of iliac crest

Post. superior iliac spine

Post. inferior iliac spine

Coccyx

● **Latissimus dorsi**

● **Levator scapulae**

● **Rhomboid major**

● **Rhomboid minor**

● **Trapezius**

Posterior View

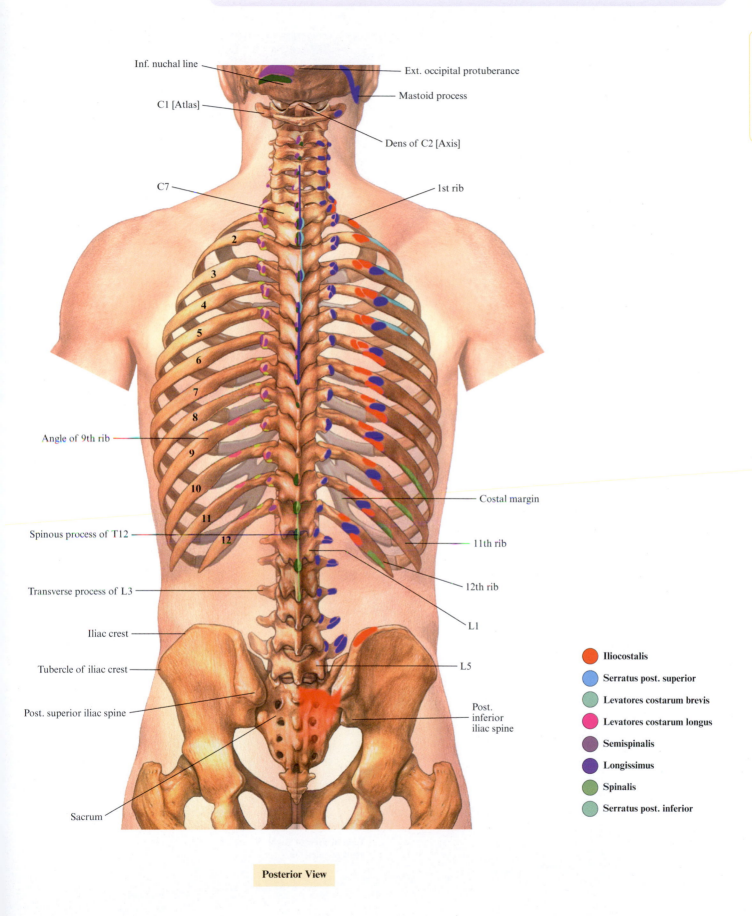

Inf. nuchal line

Ext. occipital protuberance

C1 [Atlas]

Mastoid process

Dens of C2 [Axis]

C7

1st rib

2

3

4

5

6

7

8

Angle of 9th rib

9

10

11

Costal margin

Spinous process of T12

12

11th rib

12th rib

Transverse process of L3

L1

Iliac crest

L5

Tubercle of iliac crest

Post. superior iliac spine

Post. inferior iliac spine

Sacrum

Iliocostalis

Serratus post. superior

Levatores costarum brevis

Levatores costarum longus

Semispinalis

Longissimus

Spinalis

Serratus post. inferior

Posterior View

CHAPTER 1 | **TRUNK: BODY WALL AND SPINE**

7

PLATE 1.7   SKELETON—SPINE

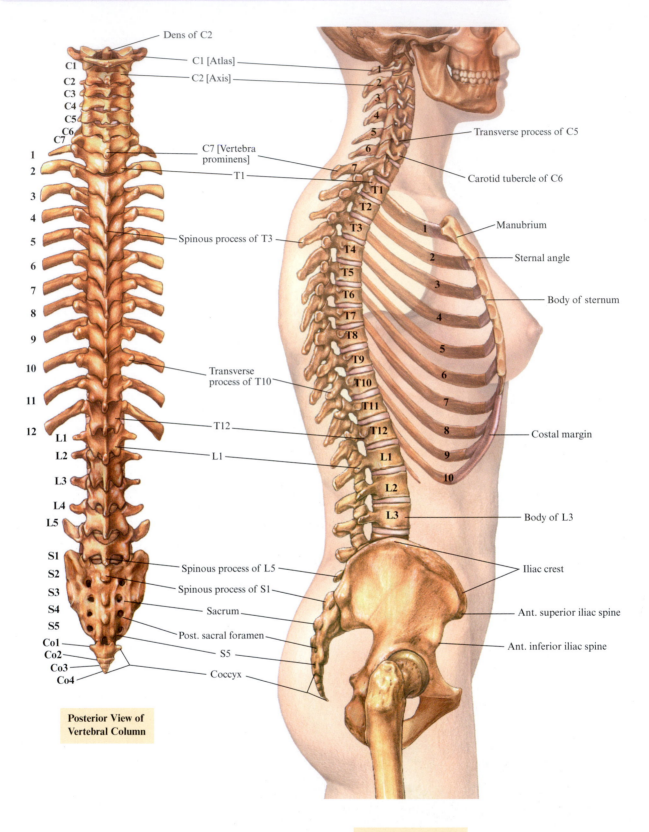

Dens of C2

C1 [Atlas]

C2 [Axis]

C1
C2
C3
C4
C5
C6
C7

1
2
3
4
5
6
7
8
9
10
11
12

L1
L2
L3
L4
L5

S1
S2
S3
S4
S5

Co1
Co2
Co3
Co4

C7 [Vertebra prominens]

T1

Spinous process of T3

Transverse process of T10

T12

L1

Spinous process of L5

Spinous process of S1

Sacrum

Post. sacral foramen

S5

Coccyx

Posterior View of Vertebral Column

1
2
3
4
5
6
7
T1
T2
T3
T4
T5
T6
T7
T8
T9
T10
T11
T12
L1
L2
L3

1
2
3
4
5
6
7
8
9
10

Transverse process of C5

Carotid tubercle of C6

Manubrium

Sternal angle

Body of sternum

Costal margin

Body of L3

Iliac crest

Ant. superior iliac spine

Ant. inferior iliac spine

Lateral View of Right Half of Skeleton

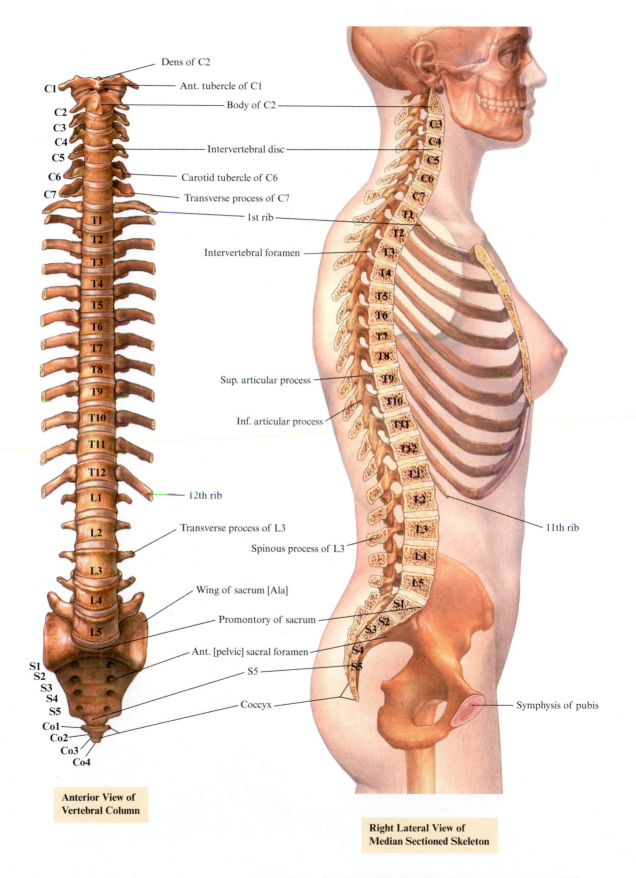

Anterior View of Vertebral Column

Dens of C2
Ant. tubercle of C1
Body of C2
Intervertebral disc
Carotid tubercle of C6
Transverse process of C7
1st rib
Intervertebral foramen
Sup. articular process
Inf. articular process
12th rib
Transverse process of L3
Spinous process of L3
Wing of sacrum [Ala]
Promontory of sacrum
Ant. [pelvic] sacral foramen
S5
Coccyx
11th rib
Symphysis of pubis

C1
C2
C3
C4
C5
C6
C7
T1
T2
T3
T4
T5
T6
T7
T8
T9
T10
T11
T12
L1
L2
L3
L4
L5
S1
S2
S3
S4
S5
Co1
Co2
Co3
Co4

C3
C4
C5
C6
C7
T1
T2
T3
T4
T5
T6
T7
T8
T9
T10
T11
T12
L1
L2
L3
L4
L5
S1
S2
S3
S4
S5

Right Lateral View of Median Sectioned Skeleton

CHAPTER 1 | **TRUNK: BODY WALL AND SPINE**

9

PLATE 1.9   CERVICAL VERTEBRAE

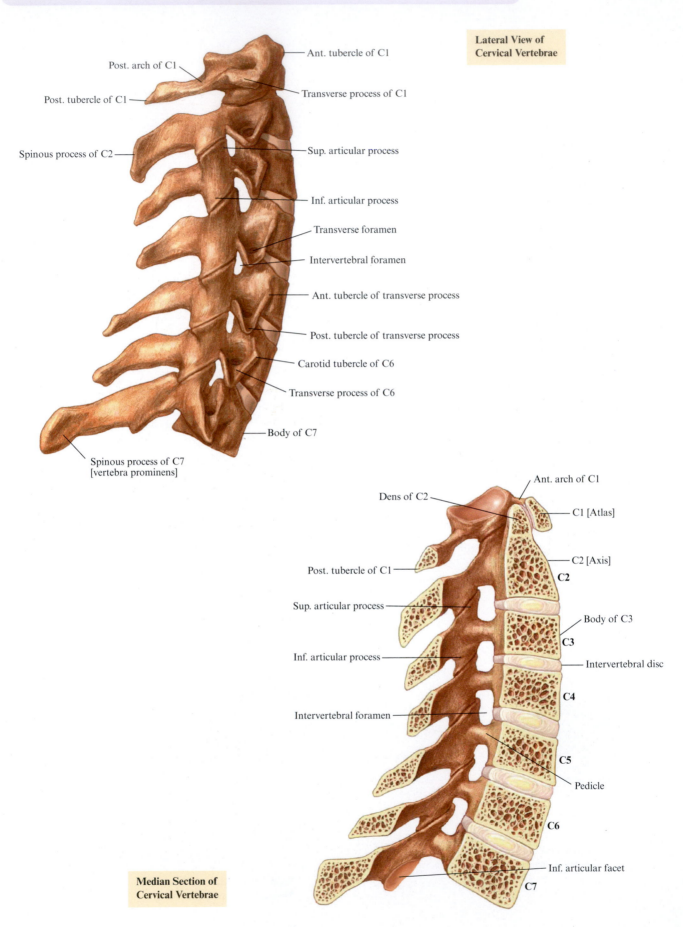

Lateral View of Cervical Vertebrae

Post. arch of C1

Ant. tubercle of C1

Post. tubercle of C1

Transverse process of C1

Spinous process of C2

Sup. articular process

Inf. articular process

Transverse foramen

Intervertebral foramen

Ant. tubercle of transverse process

Post. tubercle of transverse process

Carotid tubercle of C6

Transverse process of C6

Body of C7

Spinous process of C7 [vertebra prominens]

Median Section of Cervical Vertebrae

Dens of C2

Ant. arch of C1

C1 [Atlas]

Post. tubercle of C1

C2 [Axis]

C2

Sup. articular process

Body of C3

C3

Inf. articular process

Intervertebral disc

C4

Intervertebral foramen

C5

Pedicle

C6

Inf. articular facet

C7

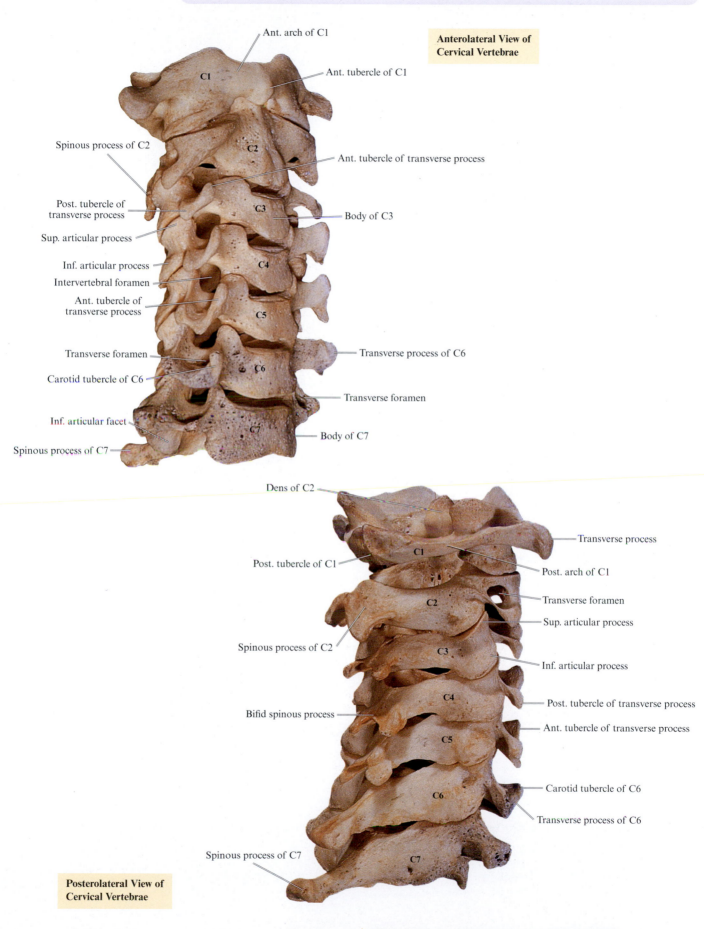

Anterolateral View of Cervical Vertebrae

Ant. arch of C1

C1

Ant. tubercle of C1

Spinous process of C2

C2

Ant. tubercle of transverse process

Post. tubercle of transverse process

C3

Body of C3

Sup. articular process

Inf. articular process

C4

Intervertebral foramen

Ant. tubercle of transverse process

C5

Transverse foramen

Transverse process of C6

Carotid tubercle of C6

C6

Transverse foramen

Inf. articular facet

C7

Body of C7

Spinous process of C7

Dens of C2

Transverse process

Post. tubercle of C1

C1

Post. arch of C1

Transverse foramen

C2

Sup. articular process

Spinous process of C2

C3

Inf. articular process

C4

Post. tubercle of transverse process

Bifid spinous process

Ant. tubercle of transverse process

C5

Carotid tubercle of C6

C6

Transverse process of C6

Spinous process of C7

C7

Posterolateral View of Cervical Vertebrae

PLATE 1.11   THORACIC VERTEBRAE

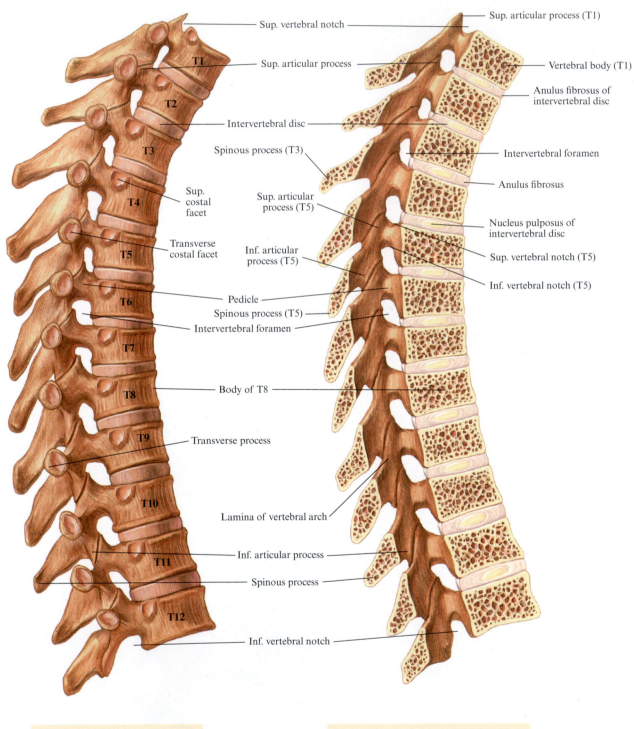

Sup. vertebral notch

Sup. articular process (T1)

T1

Sup. articular process

Vertebral body (T1)

T2

Anulus fibrosus of
intervertebral disc

Intervertebral disc

T3

Spinous process (T3)

Intervertebral foramen

Anulus fibrosus

T4

Sup.
costal
facet

Sup. articular
process (T5)

Nucleus pulposus of
intervertebral disc

T5

Transverse
costal facet

Inf. articular
process (T5)

Sup. vertebral notch (T5)

Inf. vertebral notch (T5)

T6

Pedicle

Spinous process (T5)

Intervertebral foramen

T7

T8

Body of T8

T9

Transverse process

T10

Lamina of vertebral arch

T11

Inf. articular process

Spinous process

T12

Inf. vertebral notch

Lateral View of Thoracic Vertebrae

Midsagittal Section of Thoracic Vertebrae

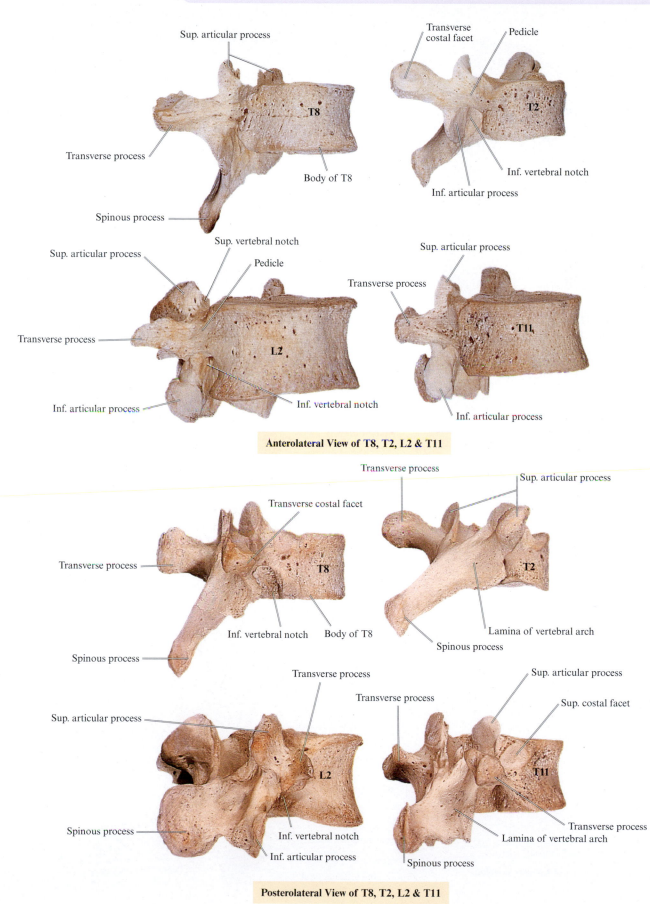

Sup. articular process

Transverse
costal facet

Pedicle

T8

T2

Transverse process

Body of T8

Inf. vertebral notch

Spinous process

Inf. articular process

Sup. vertebral notch

Sup. articular process

Sup. articular process

Pedicle

Transverse process

Transverse process

L2

T11

Inf. articular process

Inf. vertebral notch

Inf. articular process

Anterolateral View of T8, T2, L2 & T11

Transverse process

Sup. articular process

Transverse costal facet

Transverse process

Sup. articular process

T8

T2

Inf. vertebral notch

Body of T8

Lamina of vertebral arch

Spinous process

Spinous process

Transverse process

Sup. articular process

Transverse process

Sup. costal facet

Sup. articular process

L2

T11

Spinous process

Inf. vertebral notch

Transverse process

Inf. articular process

Lamina of vertebral arch

Spinous process

Posterolateral View of T8, T2, L2 & T11

CHAPTER 1 | **TRUNK: BODY WALL AND SPINE**   13

PLATE 1.13   LUMBAR VERTEBRAE

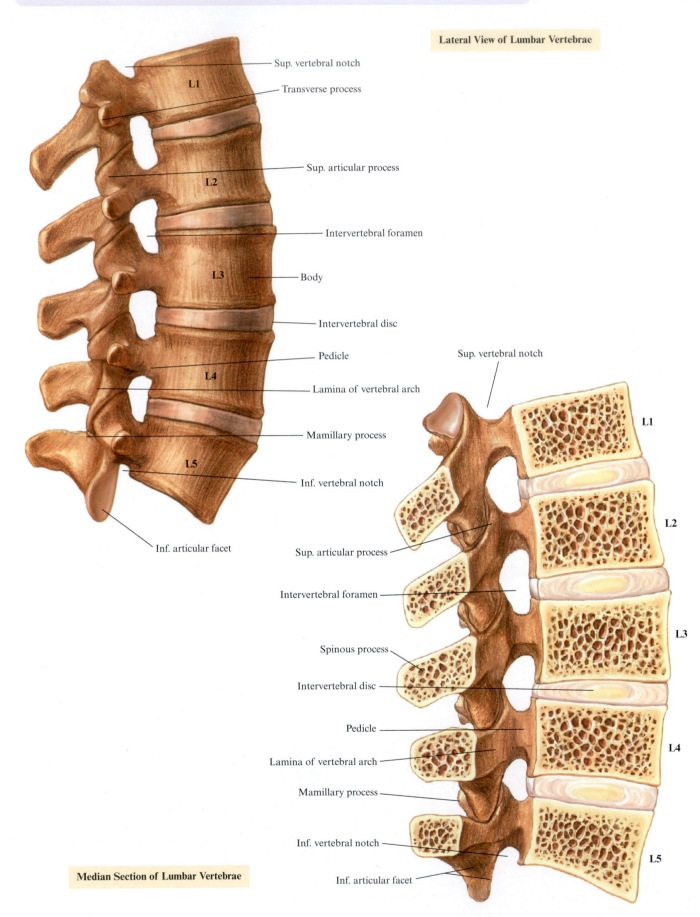

Lateral View of Lumbar Vertebrae

Sup. vertebral notch

L1

Transverse process

Sup. articular process

L2

Intervertebral foramen

L3

Body

Intervertebral disc

Pedicle

L4

Lamina of vertebral arch

Mamillary process

L5

Inf. vertebral notch

Inf. articular facet

Sup. vertebral notch

L1

L2

Sup. articular process

Intervertebral foramen

L3

Spinous process

Intervertebral disc

Pedicle

L4

Lamina of vertebral arch

Mamillary process

Inf. vertebral notch

L5

Inf. articular facet

Median Section of Lumbar Vertebrae

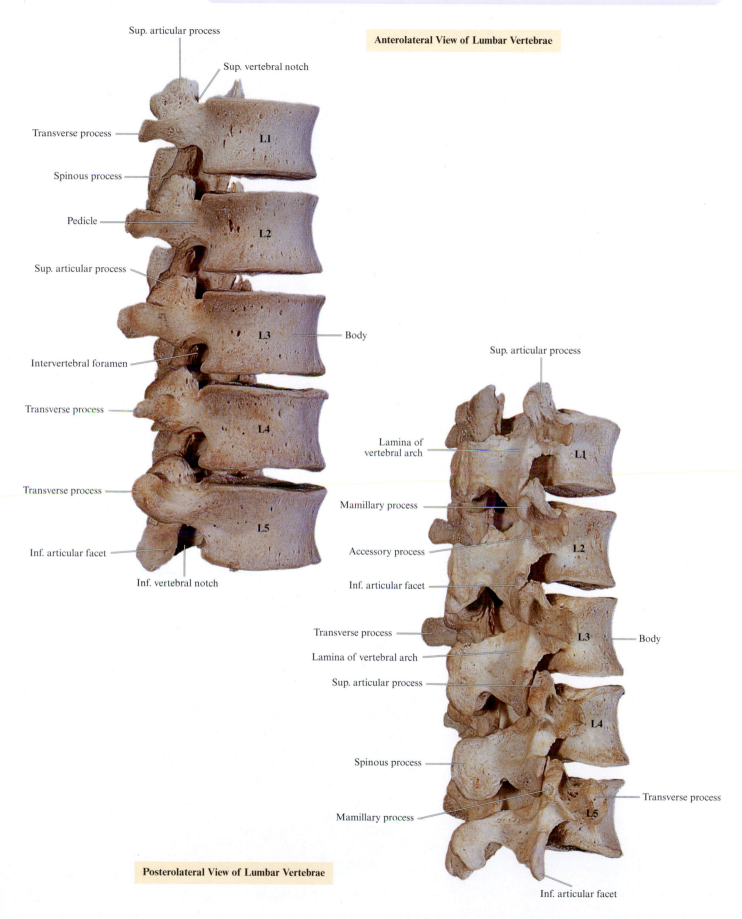

Anterolateral View of Lumbar Vertebrae

Sup. articular process

Sup. vertebral notch

Transverse process

L1

Spinous process

Pedicle

L2

Sup. articular process

L3

Body

Intervertebral foramen

Sup. articular process

Transverse process

L4

Lamina of
vertebral arch

L1

Transverse process

Mamillary process

L2

L5

Accessory process

Inf. articular facet

Inf. articular facet

Transverse process

L3

Body

Inf. vertebral notch

Lamina of vertebral arch

Sup. articular process

L4

Spinous process

Posterolateral View of Lumbar Vertebrae

Transverse process

L5

Mamillary process

Inf. articular facet

PLATE 1.15   SACRUM

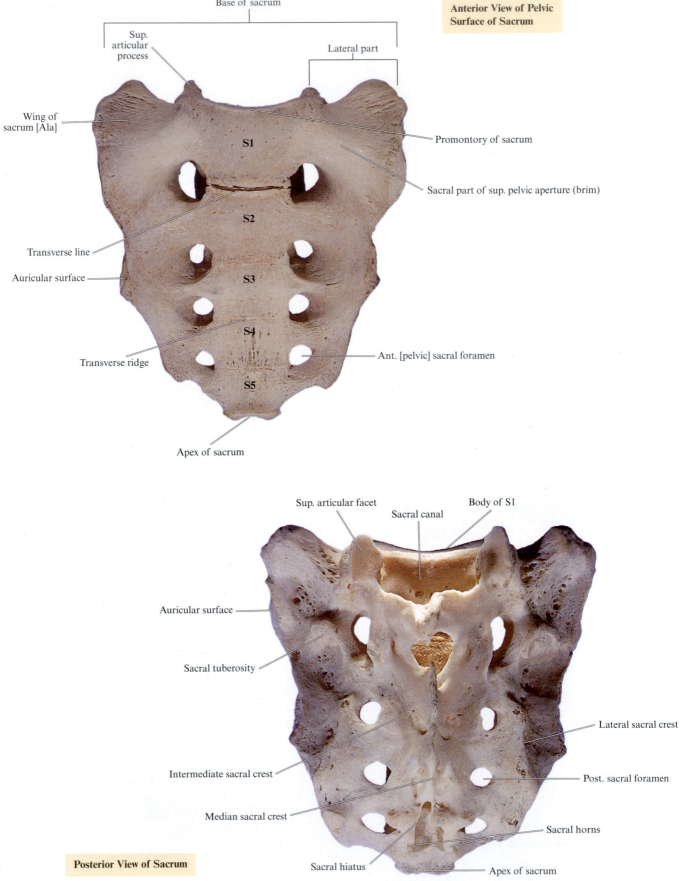

Base of sacrum

Sup. articular process

Lateral part

Anterior View of Pelvic Surface of Sacrum

Wing of sacrum [Ala]

Promontory of sacrum

S1

Sacral part of sup. pelvic aperture (brim)

Transverse line

S2

Auricular surface

S3

Transverse ridge

S4

Ant. [pelvic] sacral foramen

S5

Apex of sacrum

Sup. articular facet

Sacral canal

Body of S1

Auricular surface

Sacral tuberosity

Lateral sacral crest

Intermediate sacral crest

Post. sacral foramen

Median sacral crest

Sacral horns

Posterior View of Sacrum

Sacral hiatus

Apex of sacrum

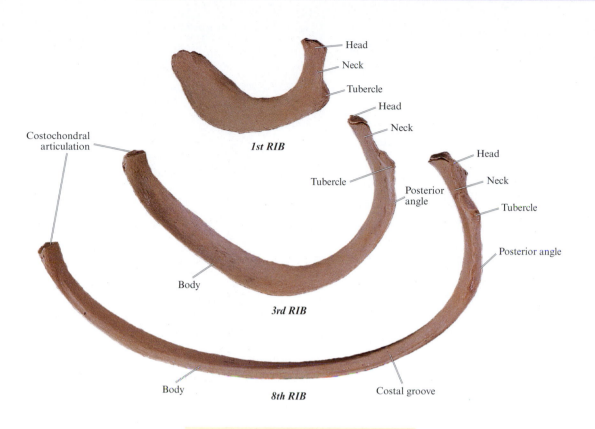

Inferior View of Right Ribs 1, 3 & 8 (Right Side)

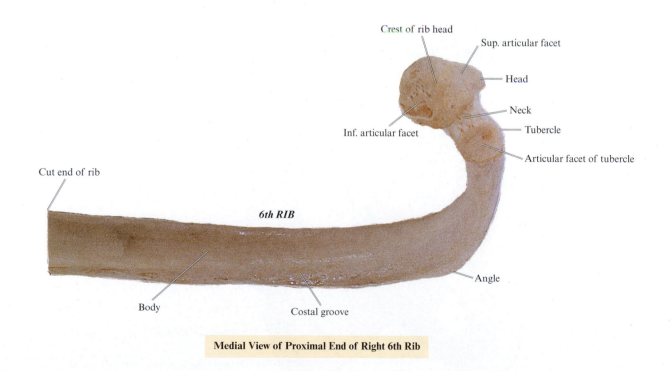

Medial View of Proximal End of Right 6th Rib

PLATE 1.17   JOINTS & LIGAMENTS

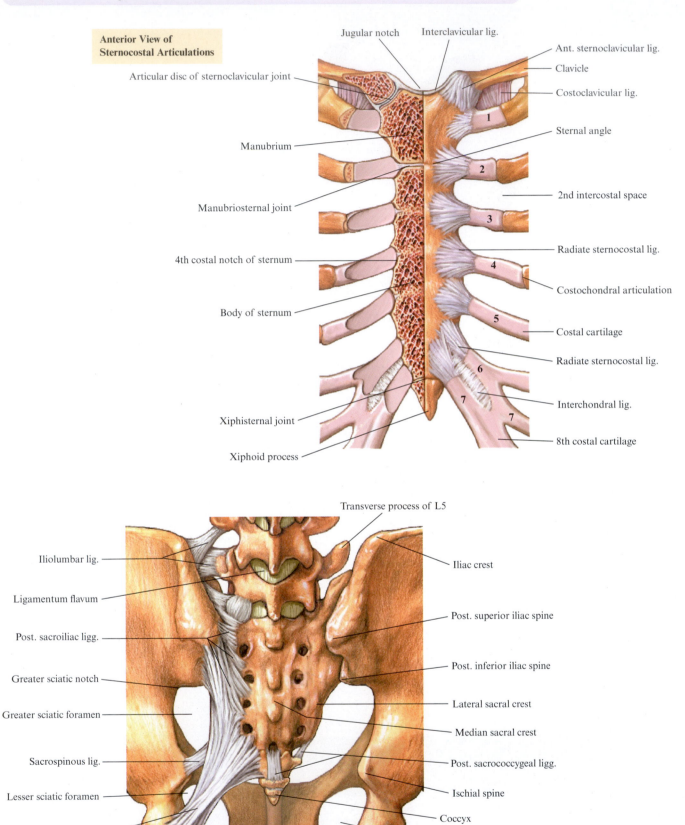

Anterior View of Sternocostal Articulations

Jugular notch

Interclavicular lig.

Articular disc of sternoclavicular joint

Ant. sternoclavicular lig.

Clavicle

Costoclavicular lig.

Manubrium

Sternal angle

Manubriosternal joint

2nd intercostal space

4th costal notch of sternum

Radiate sternocostal lig.

Costochondral articulation

Body of sternum

Costal cartilage

Radiate sternocostal lig.

Interchondral lig.

Xiphisternal joint

8th costal cartilage

Xiphoid process

Transverse process of L5

Iliolumbar lig.

Iliac crest

Ligamentum flavum

Post. sacroiliac ligg.

Post. superior iliac spine

Greater sciatic notch

Post. inferior iliac spine

Greater sciatic foramen

Lateral sacral crest

Median sacral crest

Sacrospinous lig.

Post. sacrococcygeal ligg.

Lesser sciatic foramen

Ischial spine

Sacrotuberous lig.

Coccyx

Obturator foramen

Ischial tuberosity

Posterior View of Pelvic Ligaments

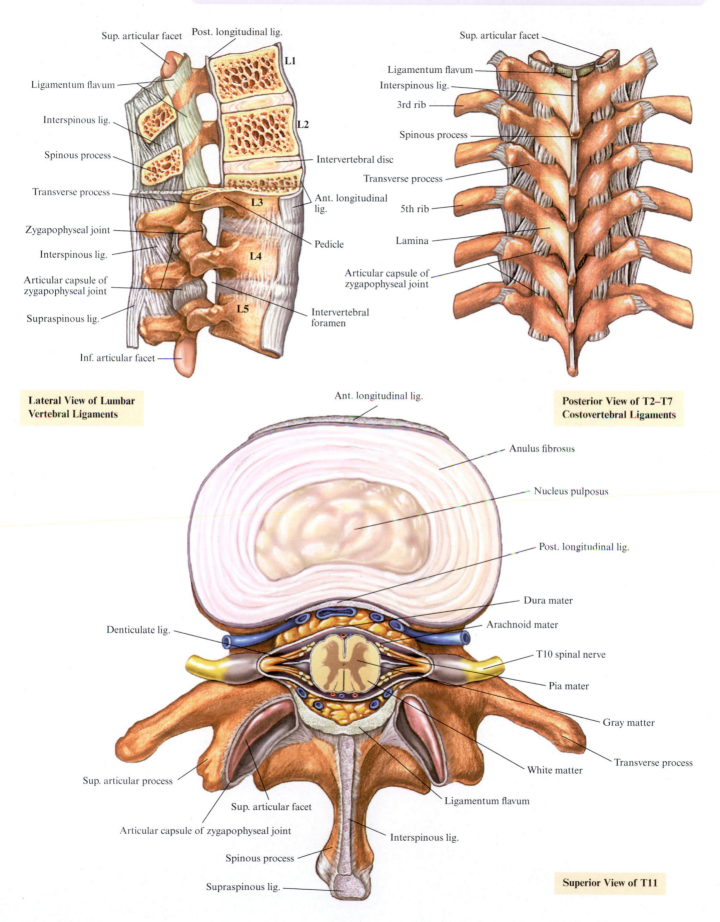

Sup. articular facet
Post. longitudinal lig.
L1
Ligamentum flavum
Interspinous lig.
L2
Spinous process
Intervertebral disc
Transverse process
Ant. longitudinal lig.
L3
Zygapophyseal joint
Pedicle
Interspinous lig.
L4
Articular capsule of zygapophyseal joint
Supraspinous lig.
L5
Intervertebral foramen
Inf. articular facet

Lateral View of Lumbar Vertebral Ligaments

Sup. articular facet
Ligamentum flavum
Interspinous lig.
3rd rib
Spinous process
Transverse process
5th rib
Lamina
Articular capsule of zygapophyseal joint

Posterior View of T2–T7 Costovertebral Ligaments

Ant. longitudinal lig.
Anulus fibrosus
Nucleus pulposus
Post. longitudinal lig.
Denticulate lig.
Dura mater
Arachnoid mater
T10 spinal nerve
Pia mater
Gray matter
Transverse process
White matter
Sup. articular process
Sup. articular facet
Ligamentum flavum
Articular capsule of zygapophyseal joint
Interspinous lig.
Spinous process
Supraspinous lig.

Superior View of T11

TABLE 1.1   MUSCLES—THORACIC WALL

Muscle	Superior or Medial Attachment	Inferior or Lateral Attachment	Innervation	Action(s)
External intercostal		Sup. border of rib bounding intercostal space caudally, muscular from costal tubercle to end of rib with membranous connection to sternum		
Internal intercostal	Inf. border of rib that bounds intercostal space cranially	Sup. border of rib bounding intercostal space caudally, muscular from angle to sternum	1st to 11th intercostal nn. & subcostal n.	Elevate ribs in inspiration
Innermost intercostal		Separated from int. intercostal mm. only by neurovascular bundle		
Subcostal	Inf. border lateral to angle of rib that bounds intercostal space cranially	Int. surface near angle of rib that bounds intercostal space caudally, best developed between ribs 6 & 12, may cross 2 intercostal spaces		Depress ribs in expiration
Transversus thoracis	Int. surface of body & xiphoid of sternum	Inf. border of 2nd to 6th costal cartilages	2nd to 6th intercostal nn.	Depress costal cartilages in expiration
Levatores costarum L. c. brevis m. L. c. longus m.	Transverse processes of C7 to T11	Between tubercle & angle on ext. surface of rib caudal to vertebral attachment	Dorsal primary rami of C8 & T1 to T11 spinal nn.	Elevate ribs in inspiration; laterally flex spine
Serratus posterior superior	Inf. part of ligamentum nuchae & spinous process from C7 to T2/T3	Sup. border of 2nd to 5th ribs just lateral to angles	2nd to 5th intercostal nn.	Elevate ribs in inspiration
Serratus posterior inferior	Spinous processes & thoracolumbar fascia from T11/T12 to L3	Inf. border of 9th/10th to 12th ribs just lateral to angles	9th to 11th intercostal nn. & subcostal n.	Depress ribs in expiration

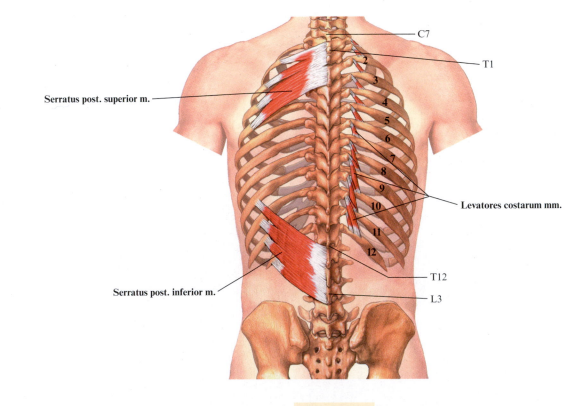

Posterior View

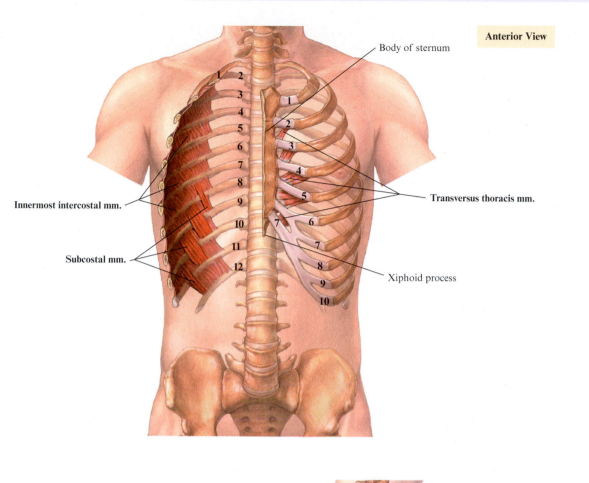

Anterior View

Body of sternum

Innermost intercostal mm.

Subcostal mm.

Transversus thoracis mm.

Xiphoid process

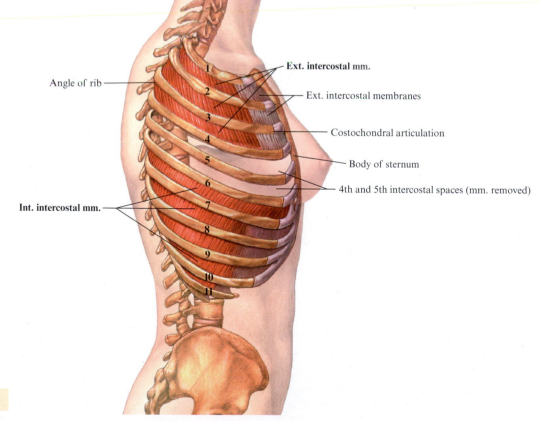

Lateral View

Angle of rib

Int. intercostal mm.

Ext. intercostal mm.

Ext. intercostal membranes

Costochondral articulation

Body of sternum

4th and 5th intercostal spaces (mm. removed)

TABLE 1.2   MUSCLES—ABDOMINAL WALL

Muscle	Lateral or Superior Attachment	Medial or Inferior Attachment	Innervation	Action(s)
External oblique	Ext. surfaces of 5th to 12th ribs	Linea alba, pubic tubercle & ant. half of iliac crest	Inf. six thoracic nn. & subcostal n.	Compress & support abdominal viscera; flex & rotate tunk
Internal oblique	Thoracolumbar fascia, ant. two-thirds of iliac crest & lateral half of inguinal lig.	Inf. borders of 10th to 12th ribs, linea alba & pubis via the conjoint tendon	Ventral rami of T6 to L1	
Transversus abdominis	Int. surfaces of 7th to 12th costal cartilages, thoracolumbar fascia, iliac crest & lateral third of inguinal lig.	Linea alba with aponeurosis of int. oblique, pubic crest & pecten pubis via conjoint tendon		Compress & support abdominal viscera
Rectus abdominis	Xiphoid process & 5th to 7th costal cartilages	Pubic symphysis & pubic crest	Ventral rami of inf. six thoracic nn.	Flex trunk & compress abdominal viscera
Quadratus lumborum	Medial half of inf. border of 12th rib & tips of lumbar transverse processes	Iliolumbar lig. & int. lip of iliac crest	Ventral rami of T12 & L1 to L4	Extend & laterally fixes the vertebral column; flex 12th rib during inspiration
Cremaster	Inf. edge of int. abdominal oblique, inguinal lig., pubic tubercle & pubic crest	Invest spermatic cord and testis	Genital br. of genitofemoral n. (L1 & L2)	Retract testis

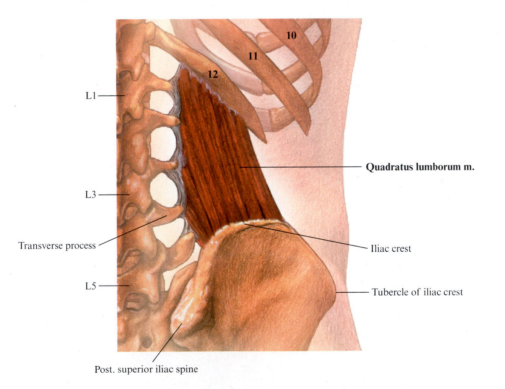

Posterior View

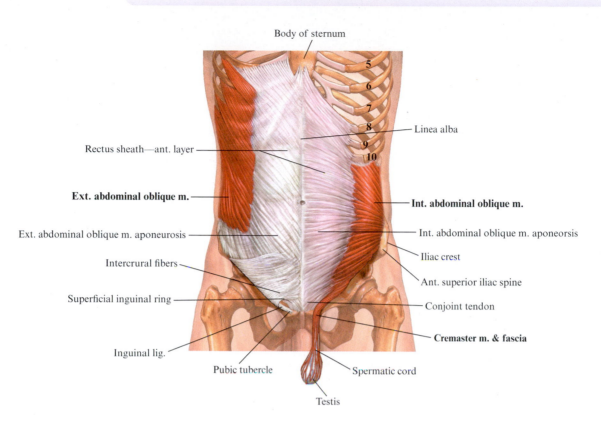

Body of sternum

5
6
7
8
9
10

Linea alba

Rectus sheath—ant. layer

Ext. abdominal oblique m.

Ext. abdominal oblique m. aponeurosis

Intercrural fibers

Superficial inguinal ring

Inguinal lig.

Pubic tubercle

Testis

Int. abdominal oblique m.

Int. abdominal oblique m. aponeorsis

Iliac crest

Ant. superior iliac spine

Conjoint tendon

Cremaster m. & fascia

Spermatic cord

Anterior Views

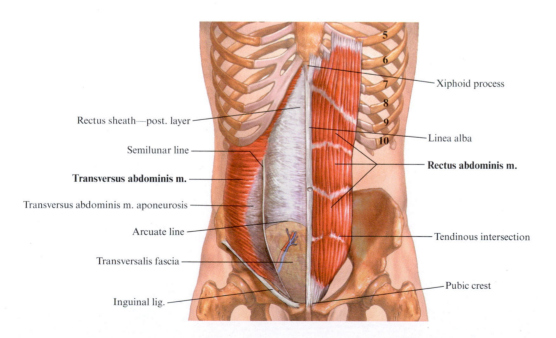

5
6
7
8
9
10

Xiphoid process

Rectus sheath—post. layer

Semilunar line

Transversus abdominis m.

Transversus abdominis m. aponeurosis

Arcuate line

Transversalis fascia

Inguinal lig.

Linea alba

Rectus abdominis m.

Tendinous intersection

Pubic crest

TABLE 1.3   INTRINSIC MUSCLES OF THE BACK

Intrinsic Muscles of the Back[a]

Muscle	Inferior or Medial Attachment	Superior or Lateral Attachment	Innervation	Action(s)
SUPERFICIAL LAYER—SPINOTRANSVERSE GROUP				
Splenius capitis	Inf. half of ligamentum nuchae, spinous processes of C7 to T3/T4	Mastoid process, lateral third of the sup. nuchal line	Dorsal primary rami of middle cervical spinal nn.	Unilaterally, rotate & laterally flex neck to same side, bilaterally, extend the neck & head
Splenius cervicis	Spinous processes of T3/T4 to T6	Post. tubercles of transverse processes of C1 to C3	Dorsal primary rami of lower cervical spinal nn.	
INTERMEDIATE LAYER—ERECTOR SPINAE GROUP				
Iliocostalis m. *I. cervicis* *I. thoracis* *I. lumborum*	Sacrum, medial part of iliac crest, 12th to 3rd ribs	Angles of all ribs, transverse processes of C7 to C4	Dorsal primary rami of all cervical, thoracic & lumbar spinal nn.	Unilaterally, flex vertebral column to same side; bilaterally, extend vertebral column; important in maintaining erect posture while standing or walking
Longissimus m. *L. capitis* *L. cervicis* *L. thoracis*	Sacrum, transverse processes of all vertebrae from L5 to C7, transverse & articular processes of C6 to C4	Transverse processes of all vertebrae from T12 to C2, angles of all ribs, mastoid process		
Spinalis m. *S. capitis* *S. cervicis* *S. thoracis*	Spinous processes of L2/L3 to T11, ligamentum nuchae & spinous processes of T2 to C7, transverse processes of C7/C6 to C2, articular processes of C6 to C4	Spinous processes from T9/T8 to C7/C6, spinous processes of C3/C4 & C2, occipital bone between sup. & inf. nuchal lines with semispinalis m.		
DEEP LAYER—TRANSVERSOSPINAL GROUP				
Semispinalis m. *S. capitis* *S. cervicis* *S. thoracis*	Transverse processes of all vertebrae from T10 to C3, articular processes of C6 to C4	Spinous processes from T4 to C2, occipital bone between sup. & inf. nuchal lines; usually includes spinalis capitis m.	Dorsal primary rami of T6 T1, all cervical spinal nn.	Unilaterally, lateral flex and/or rotate vertebral column & head to opposite side; bilaterally, extend vertebral column & head
Multifidus	All lamina from S4 to C2 transverse processes L5 to T1, articular processes C7 to C3	Spinous process of all vertebrae; spans 1 to 3 vertebrae	Dorsal primary rami of T6 to C1 spinal nn.	Unilaterally, lateral flex and/or rotate vertebral column to opposite side; bilaterally, extend or stabilize vertebral column
Rotatores	Transverse processes of all vertebrae L5 to T2	Lamina & roots of spinous process of next vertebra superiorly; best developed in thoracic region	Dorsal primary rami of L4 to T1 spinal nn.	

[a]The most superficial layer also includes the trapezius, latissimus dorsi, levator scapulae & rhomboid muscles which move the upper limb. The intermediate layer is formed by the serratus posterior muscles. The muscles of both of these layers are considered extrinsic to the back. The intrinsic muscles of the back form the deepest three muscle layers of the back.

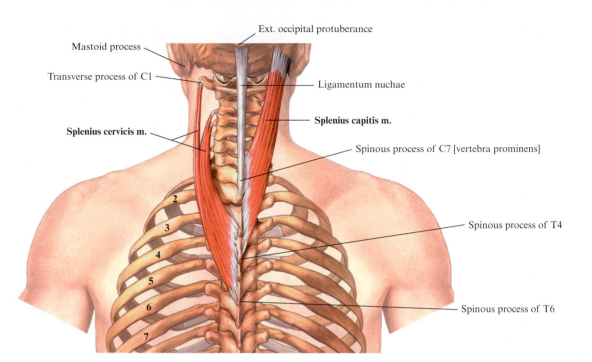

Ext. occipital protuberance

Mastoid process

Transverse process of C1

Ligamentum nuchae

Splenius cervicis m.

Splenius capitis m.

Spinous process of C7 [vertebra prominens]

Spinous process of T4

Spinous process of T6

Posterior Views

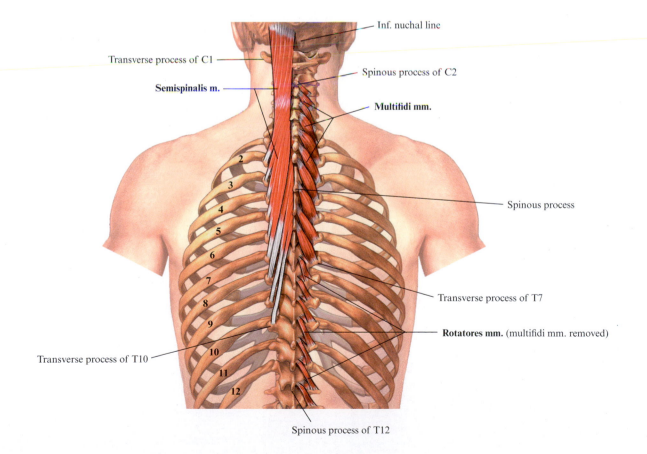

Inf. nuchal line

Transverse process of C1

Spinous process of C2

Semispinalis m.

Multifidi mm.

Spinous process

Transverse process of T7

Transverse process of T10

Rotatores mm. (multifidi mm. removed)

Spinous process of T12

PLATE 1.22 MUSCLES—ERECTOR SPINAE

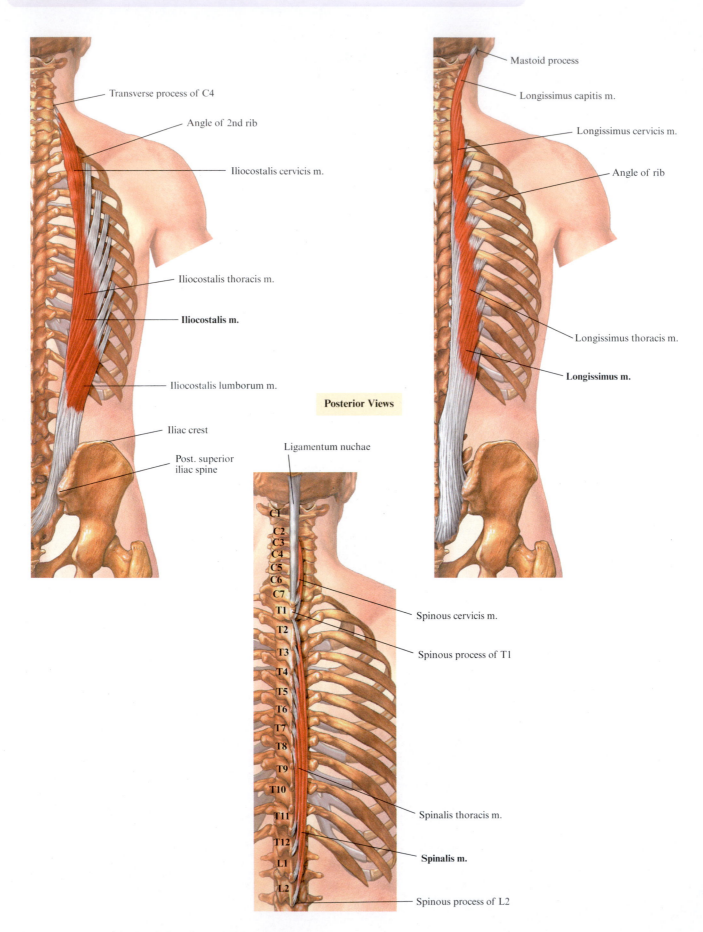

Transverse process of C4

Angle of 2nd rib

Iliocostalis cervicis m.

Iliocostalis thoracis m.

Iliocostalis m.

Iliocostalis lumborum m.

Iliac crest

Post. superior
iliac spine

Mastoid process

Longissimus capitis m.

Longissimus cervicis m.

Angle of rib

Longissimus thoracis m.

Longissimus m.

Posterior Views

Ligamentum nuchae

C1
C2
C3
C4
C5
C6
C7
T1
T2
T3
T4
T5
T6
T7
T8
T9
T10
T11
T12
L1
L2

Spinous cervicis m.

Spinous process of T1

Spinalis thoracis m.

Spinalis m.

Spinous process of L2

Muscle	Inferior or Medial Attachment	Superior or Lateral Attachment	Innervation	Action(s)
DEEP LAYER—SUBOCCIPITAL GROUP				
Rectus capitis posterior major	Spinous process of C2	Lateral part of inf. nuchal line	Dorsal primary ramus of C1 [suboccipital] n.	Unilaterally, rotate head to same side; bilaterally, extend head at atlanto-occipital joint
Rectus capitis posterior minor	Post. tubercle of C1	Medial part of inf. nuchal line		
Obliquus capitis superior	Transverse process of C1	Sup. to inf. nuchal line		Unilaterally, rotate C1 & head to same side around odontoid process; bilaterally, extend head at atlanto-axial joint
Obliquus capitis inferior	Spinous process of C2	Transverse process of C1		

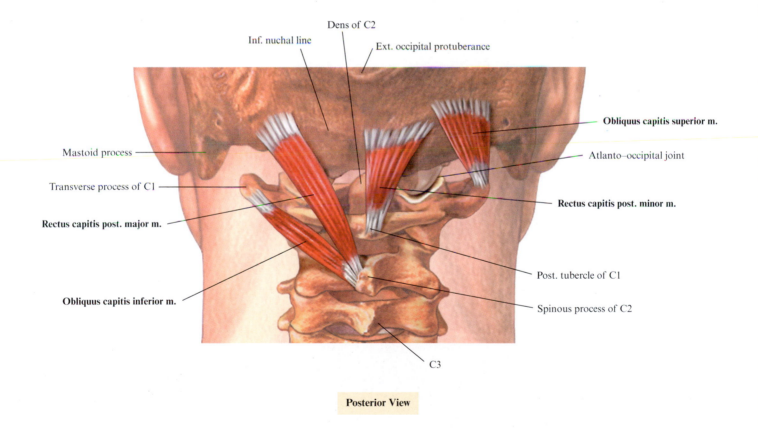

Posterior View

PLATE 1.23   **VASCULATURE—ARTERIES**

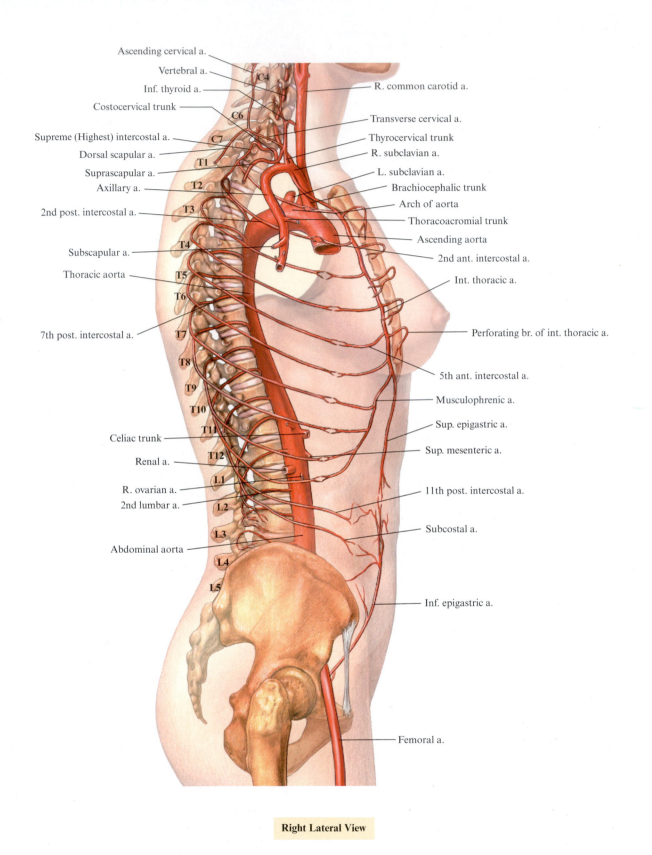

Ascending cervical a.
Vertebral a.
Inf. thyroid a.
Costocervical trunk
Supreme (Highest) intercostal a.
Dorsal scapular a.
Suprascapular a.
Axillary a.
2nd post. intercostal a.
Subscapular a.
Thoracic aorta
7th post. intercostal a.
Celiac trunk
Renal a.
R. ovarian a.
2nd lumbar a.
Abdominal aorta

C4
C6
C7
T1
T2
T3
T4
T5
T6
T7
T8
T9
T10
T11
T12
L1
L2
L3
L4
L5

R. common carotid a.
Transverse cervical a.
Thyrocervical trunk
R. subclavian a.
L. subclavian a.
Brachiocephalic trunk
Arch of aorta
Thoracoacromial trunk
Ascending aorta
2nd ant. intercostal a.
Int. thoracic a.
Perforating br. of int. thoracic a.
5th ant. intercostal a.
Musculophrenic a.
Sup. epigastric a.
Sup. mesenteric a.
11th post. intercostal a.
Subcostal a.
Inf. epigastric a.
Femoral a.

Right Lateral View

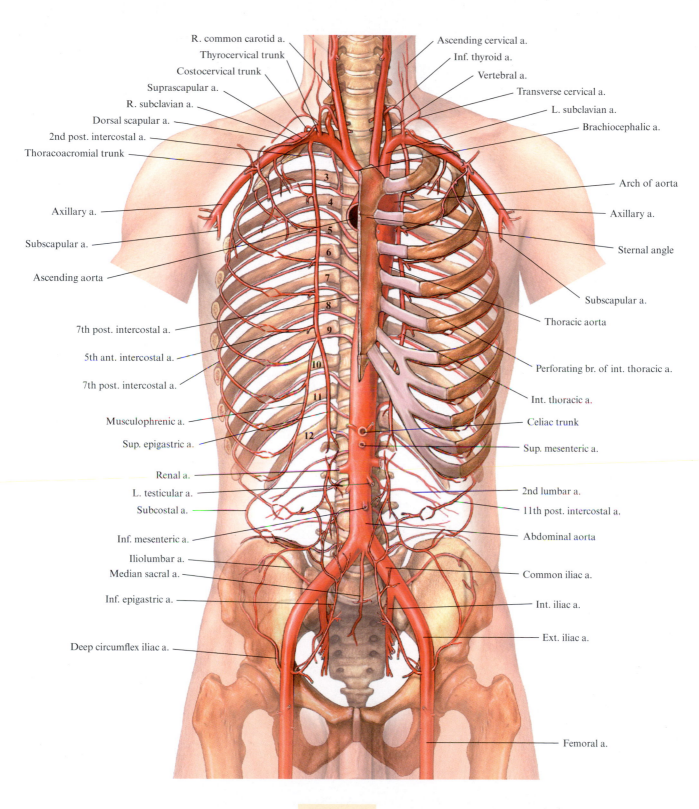

R. common carotid a.
Thyrocervical trunk
Costocervical trunk
Suprascapular a.
R. subclavian a.
Dorsal scapular a.
2nd post. intercostal a.
Thoracoacromial trunk

Ascending cervical a.
Inf. thyroid a.
Vertebral a.
Transverse cervical a.
L. subclavian a.
Brachiocephalic a.

Axillary a.

Arch of aorta
Axillary a.
Sternal angle

Subscapular a.

Ascending aorta

Subscapular a.
Thoracic aorta

7th post. intercostal a.
5th ant. intercostal a.
7th post. intercostal a.

Perforating br. of int. thoracic a.
Int. thoracic a.

Musculophrenic a.
Sup. epigastric a.

Celiac trunk
Sup. mesenteric a.

Renal a.
L. testicular a.
Subcostal a.

2nd lumbar a.
11th post. intercostal a.
Abdominal aorta

Inf. mesenteric a.
Iliolumbar a.
Median sacral a.
Inf. epigastric a.

Common iliac a.
Int. iliac a.
Ext. iliac a.

Deep circumflex iliac a.

Femoral a.

3
4
5
6
7
8
9
10
11
12

Anterior View

CHAPTER 1 | **TRUNK: BODY WALL AND SPINE**   29

PLATE 1.25 VASCULATURE—VEINS

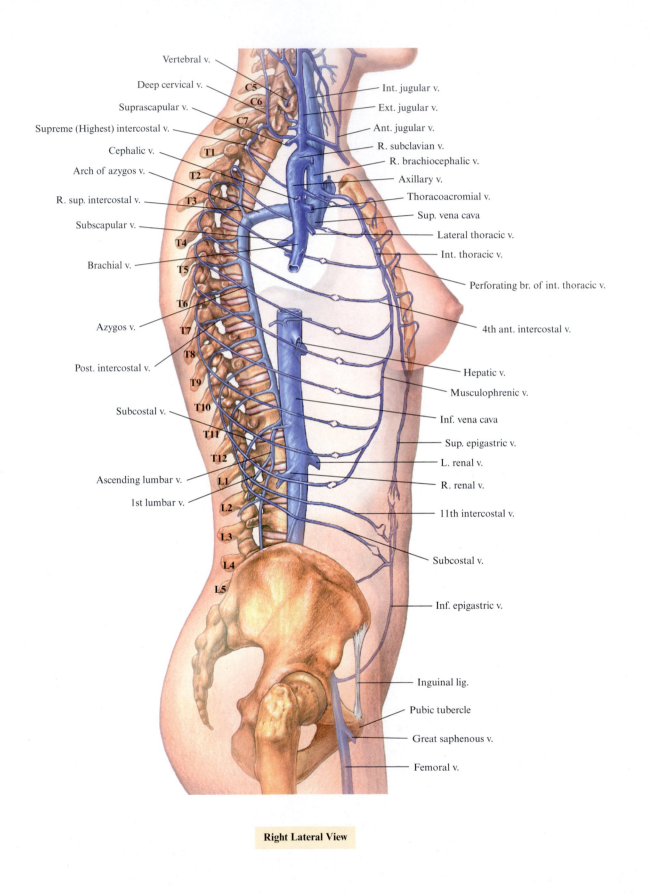

Vertebral v.
Deep cervical v.
Suprascapular v.
Supreme (Highest) intercostal v.
Cephalic v.
Arch of azygos v.
R. sup. intercostal v.
Subscapular v.
Brachial v.
Azygos v.
Post. intercostal v.
Subcostal v.
Ascending lumbar v.
1st lumbar v.

C5
C6
C7
T1
T2
T3
T4
T5
T6
T7
T8
T9
T10
T11
T12
L1
L2
L3
L4
L5

Int. jugular v.
Ext. jugular v.
Ant. jugular v.
R. subclavian v.
R. brachiocephalic v.
Axillary v.
Thoracoacromial v.
Sup. vena cava
Lateral thoracic v.
Int. thoracic v.
Perforating br. of int. thoracic v.
4th ant. intercostal v.
Hepatic v.
Musculophrenic v.
Inf. vena cava
Sup. epigastric v.
L. renal v.
R. renal v.
11th intercostal v.
Subcostal v.
Inf. epigastric v.
Inguinal lig.
Pubic tubercle
Great saphenous v.
Femoral v.

Right Lateral View

A.D.A.M. | Student Atlas of Anatomy

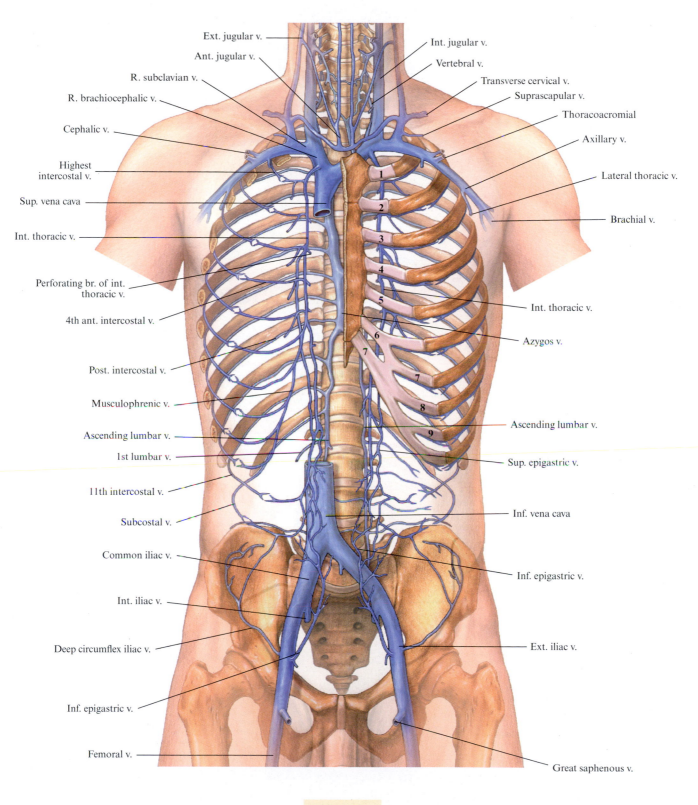

Ext. jugular v.

Ant. jugular v.

R. subclavian v.

R. brachiocephalic v.

Cephalic v.

Highest intercostal v.

Sup. vena cava

Int. thoracic v.

Perforating br. of int. thoracic v.

4th ant. intercostal v.

Post. intercostal v.

Musculophrenic v.

Ascending lumbar v.

1st lumbar v.

11th intercostal v.

Subcostal v.

Common iliac v.

Int. iliac v.

Deep circumflex iliac v.

Inf. epigastric v.

Femoral v.

Int. jugular v.

Vertebral v.

Transverse cervical v.

Suprascapular v.

Thoracoacromial

Axillary v.

Lateral thoracic v.

Brachial v.

Int. thoracic v.

Azygos v.

Ascending lumbar v.

Sup. epigastric v.

Inf. vena cava

Inf. epigastric v.

Ext. iliac v.

Great saphenous v.

Anterior View

PLATE 1.27   AZYGOS, HEMIAZYGOS & LUMBAR VEINS

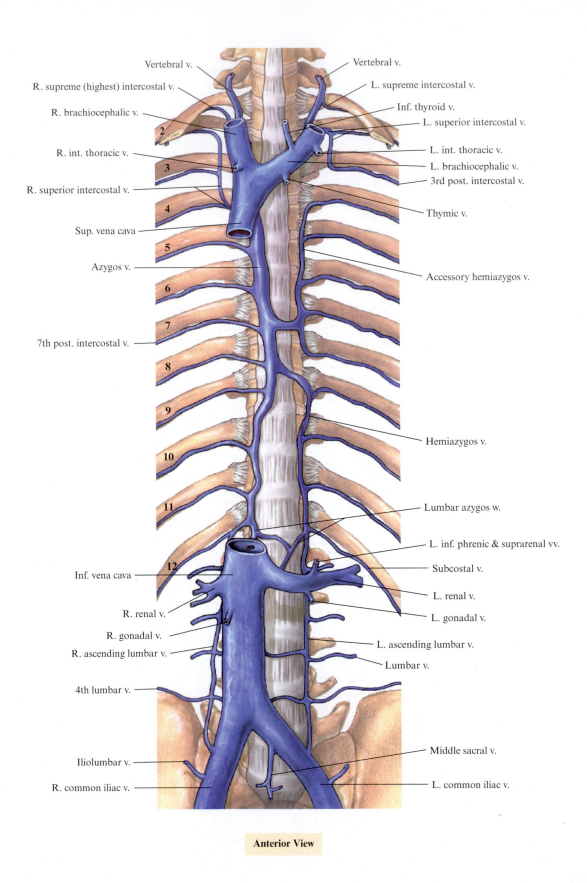

Vertebral v.

Vertebral v.

R. supreme (highest) intercostal v.

L. supreme intercostal v.

R. brachiocephalic v.

Inf. thyroid v.

L. superior intercostal v.

R. int. thoracic v.

L. int. thoracic v.

L. brachiocephalic v.

R. superior intercostal v.

3rd post. intercostal v.

Thymic v.

Sup. vena cava

Azygos v.

Accessory hemiazygos v.

7th post. intercostal v.

Hemiazygos v.

Lumbar azygos vv.

L. inf. phrenic & suprarenal vv.

Inf. vena cava

Subcostal v.

L. renal v.

R. renal v.

L. gonadal v.

R. gonadal v.

R. ascending lumbar v.

L. ascending lumbar v.

Lumbar v.

4th lumbar v.

Iliolumbar v.

Middle sacral v.

R. common iliac v.

L. common iliac v.

Anterior View

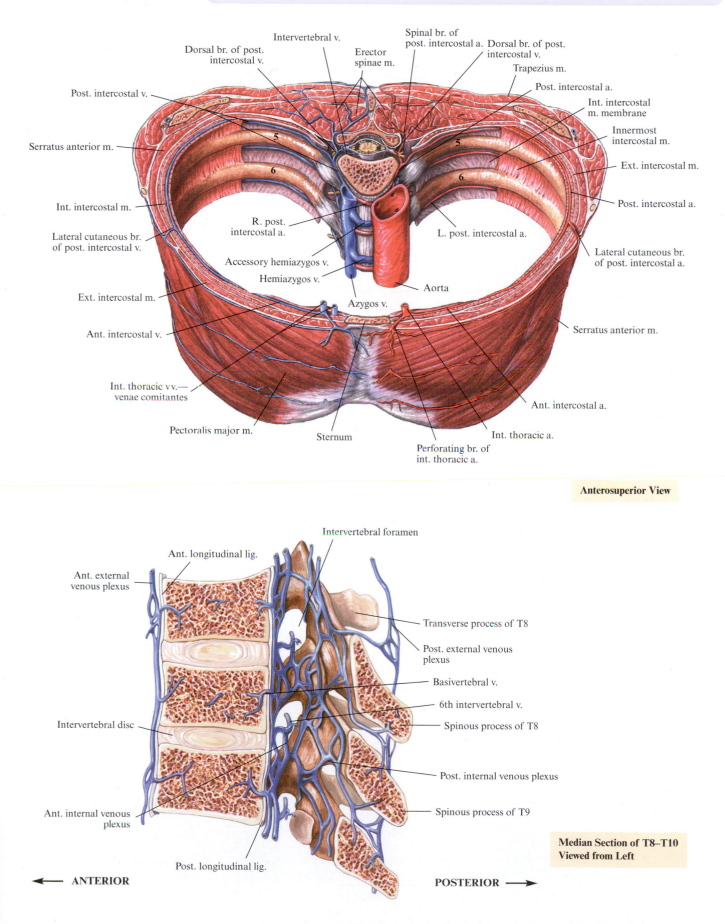

Intervertebral v.

Dorsal br. of post.
intercostal v.

Spinal br. of
post. intercostal a.

Dorsal br. of post.
intercostal v.

Erector
spinae m.

Trapezius m.

Post. intercostal v.

Post. intercostal a.

Int. intercostal
m. membrane

Serratus anterior m.

Innermost
intercostal m.

Ext. intercostal m.

Int. intercostal m.

Post. intercostal a.

Lateral cutaneous br.
of post. intercostal v.

R. post.
intercostal a.

L. post. intercostal a.

Accessory hemiazygos v.

Lateral cutaneous br.
of post. intercostal a.

Hemiazygos v.

Ext. intercostal m.

Aorta

Ant. intercostal v.

Azygos v.

Serratus anterior m.

Int. thoracic vv.—
venae comitantes

Ant. intercostal a.

Pectoralis major m.

Sternum

Int. thoracic a.

Perforating br. of
int. thoracic a.

Anterosuperior View

Intervertebral foramen

Ant. longitudinal lig.

Ant. external
venous plexus

Transverse process of T8

Post. external venous
plexus

Basivertebral v.

6th intervertebral v.

Intervertebral disc

Spinous process of T8

Intervertebral disc

Post. internal venous plexus

Ant. internal venous
plexus

Spinous process of T9

**Median Section of T8–T10
Viewed from Left**

Post. longitudinal lig.

← **ANTERIOR**

POSTERIOR →

PLATE 1.29   SPINAL CORD VASCULATURE

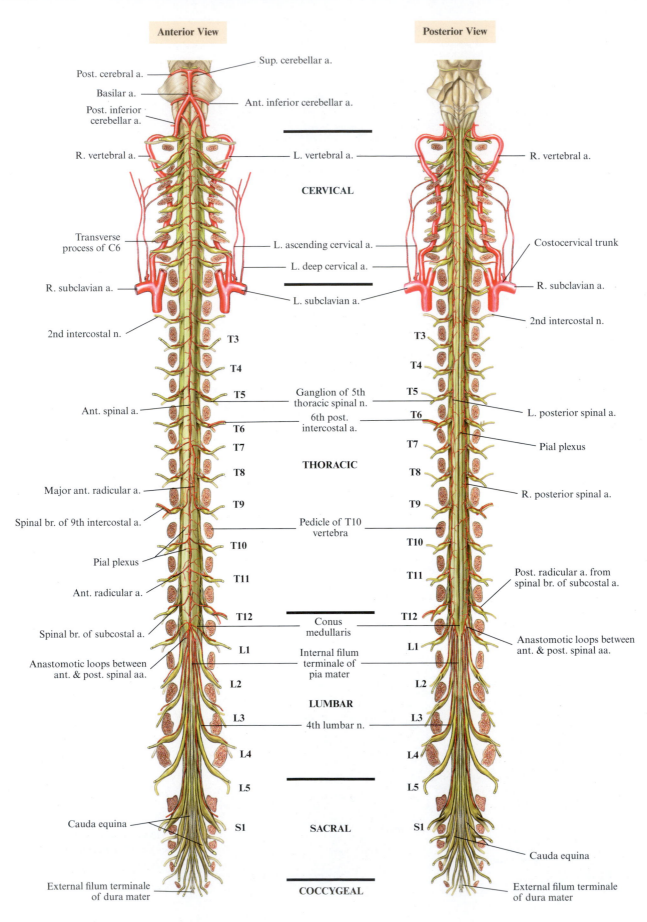

Anterior View

Post. cerebral a.
Basilar a.
Post. inferior cerebellar a.
R. vertebral a.

Transverse process of C6
R. subclavian a.
2nd intercostal n.

Ant. spinal a.

Major ant. radicular a.
Spinal br. of 9th intercostal a.

Pial plexus
Ant. radicular a.

Spinal br. of subcostal a.
Anastomotic loops between ant. & post. spinal aa.

Cauda equina

External filum terminale of dura mater

Sup. cerebellar a.

Ant. inferior cerebellar a.

L. vertebral a.

CERVICAL

L. ascending cervical a.
L. deep cervical a.

L. subclavian a.

T3
T4
T5
Ganglion of 5th thoracic spinal n.
6th post. intercostal a.
T6
T7
THORACIC
T8
T9

Pedicle of T10 vertebra
T10
T11

T12
Conus medullaris
L1
Internal filum terminale of pia mater
L2
LUMBAR
L3   4th lumbar n.
L4
L5
S1   **SACRAL**

COCCYGEAL

Posterior View

R. vertebral a.

Costocervical trunk
R. subclavian a.
2nd intercostal n.

T3
T4
T5
L. posterior spinal a.
T6
Pial plexus
T7
T8
R. posterior spinal a.
T9
T10
T11
Post. radicular a. from spinal br. of subcostal a.
T12
Anastomotic loops between ant. & post. spinal aa.
L1
L2
L3
L4
L5
S1

Cauda equina

External filum terminale of dura mater

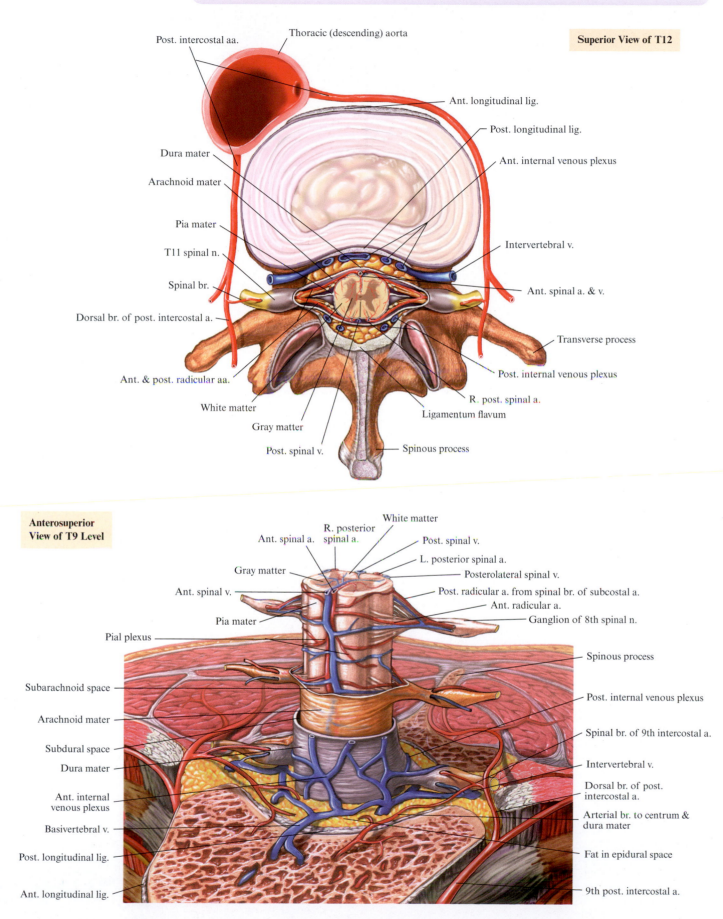

Superior View of T12

Post. intercostal aa.

Thoracic (descending) aorta

Ant. longitudinal lig.

Post. longitudinal lig.

Dura mater

Ant. internal venous plexus

Arachnoid mater

Pia mater

Intervertebral v.

T11 spinal n.

Spinal br.

Ant. spinal a. & v.

Dorsal br. of post. intercostal a.

Transverse process

Post. internal venous plexus

Ant. & post. radicular aa.

R. post. spinal a.

White matter

Ligamentum flavum

Gray matter

Post. spinal v.

Spinous process

Anterosuperior View of T9 Level

White matter

R. posterior spinal a.

Ant. spinal a.

Post. spinal v.

Gray matter

L. posterior spinal a.

Posterolateral spinal v.

Ant. spinal v.

Post. radicular a. from spinal br. of subcostal a.

Pia mater

Ant. radicular a.

Ganglion of 8th spinal n.

Pial plexus

Spinous process

Subarachnoid space

Post. internal venous plexus

Arachnoid mater

Spinal br. of 9th intercostal a.

Subdural space

Intervertebral v.

Dura mater

Dorsal br. of post. intercostal a.

Ant. internal venous plexus

Arterial br. to centrum & dura mater

Basivertebral v.

Fat in epidural space

Post. longitudinal lig.

Ant. longitudinal lig.

9th post. intercostal a.

PLATE 1.31   DERMATOMES & CUTANEOUS INNERVATION

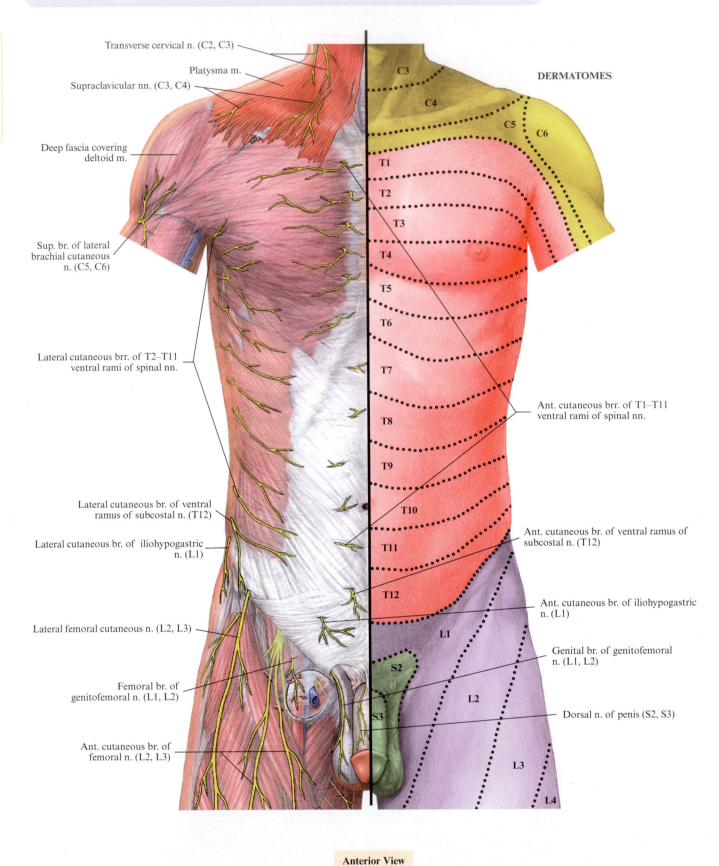

Transverse cervical n. (C2, C3)

Platysma m.

Supraclavicular nn. (C3, C4)

Deep fascia covering deltoid m.

Sup. br. of lateral brachial cutaneous n. (C5, C6)

Lateral cutaneous brr. of T2–T11 ventral rami of spinal nn.

Lateral cutaneous br. of ventral ramus of subcostal n. (T12)

Lateral cutaneous br. of iliohypogastric n. (L1)

Lateral femoral cutaneous n. (L2, L3)

Femoral br. of genitofemoral n. (L1, L2)

Ant. cutaneous br. of femoral n. (L2, L3)

DERMATOMES

C3

C4

C5   C6

T1

T2

T3

T4

T5

T6

T7

T8

T9

T10

T11

T12

L1

S2

S3

L2

L3

L4

Ant. cutaneous brr. of T1–T11 ventral rami of spinal nn.

Ant. cutaneous br. of ventral ramus of subcostal n. (T12)

Ant. cutaneous br. of iliohypogastric n. (L1)

Genital br. of genitofemoral n. (L1, L2)

Dorsal n. of penis (S2, S3)

Anterior View

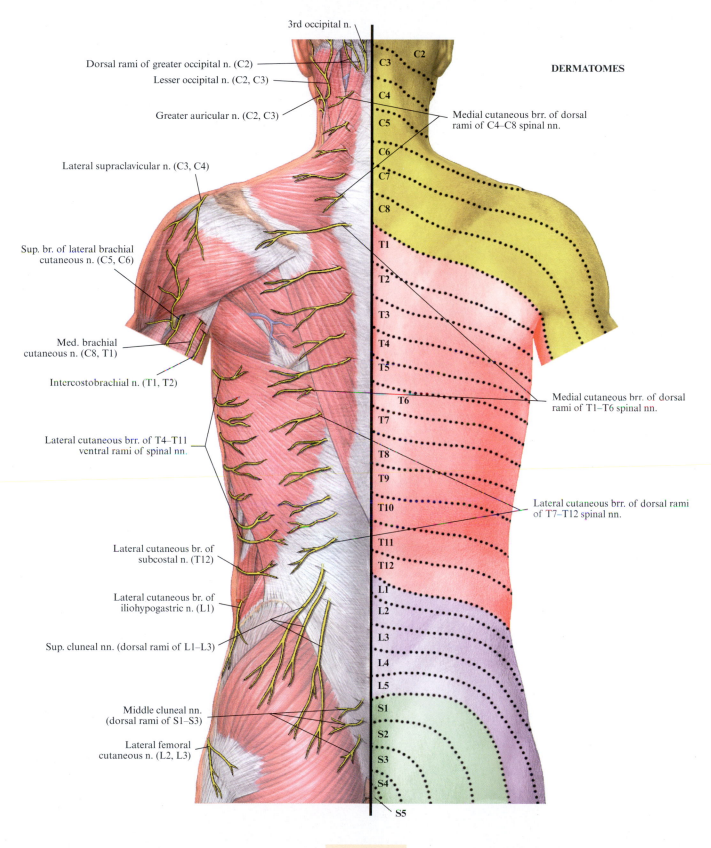

3rd occipital n.

Dorsal rami of greater occipital n. (C2)

Lesser occipital n. (C2, C3)

Greater auricular n. (C2, C3)

Lateral supraclavicular n. (C3, C4)

Sup. br. of lateral brachial cutaneous n. (C5, C6)

Med. brachial cutaneous n. (C8, T1)

Intercostobrachial n. (T1, T2)

Lateral cutaneous brr. of T4–T11 ventral rami of spinal nn.

Lateral cutaneous br. of subcostal n. (T12)

Lateral cutaneous br. of iliohypogastric n. (L1)

Sup. cluneal nn. (dorsal rami of L1–L3)

Middle cluneal nn. (dorsal rami of S1–S3)

Lateral femoral cutaneous n. (L2, L3)

DERMATOMES

Medial cutaneous brr. of dorsal rami of C4–C8 spinal nn.

Medial cutaneous brr. of dorsal rami of T1–T6 spinal nn.

Lateral cutaneous brr. of dorsal rami of T7–T12 spinal nn.

C2, C3, C4, C5, C6, C7, C8, T1, T2, T3, T4, T5, T6, T7, T8, T9, T10, T11, T12, L1, L2, L3, L4, L5, S1, S2, S3, S4, S5

Posterior View

PLATE **1.33** NERVES

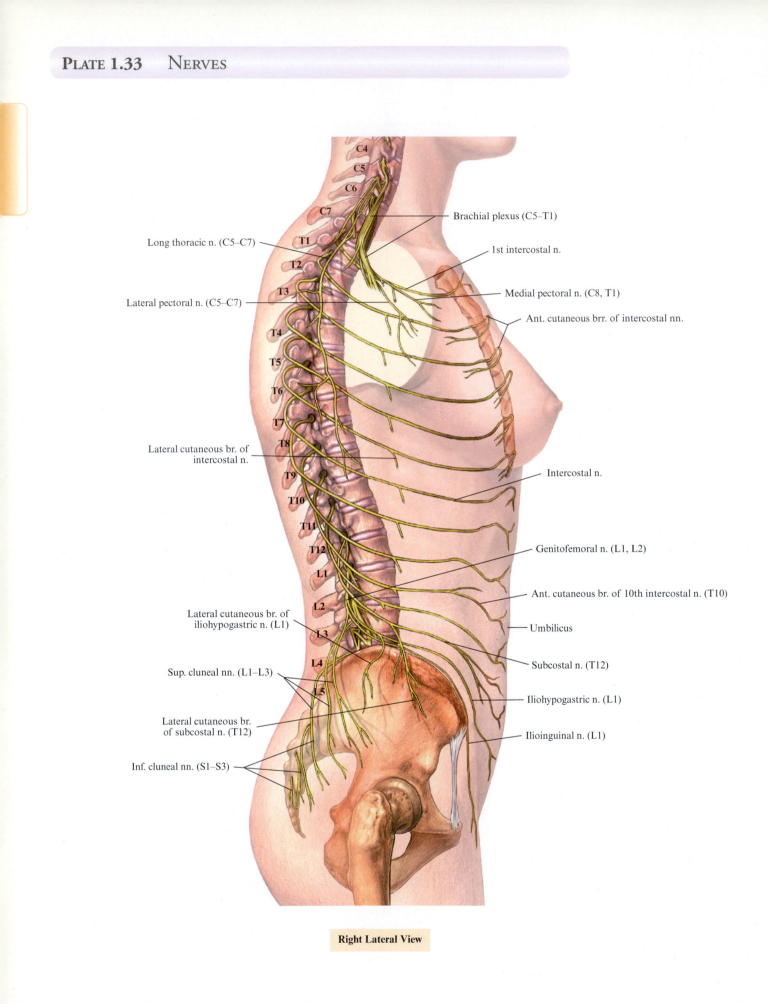

C4
C5
C6
C7
T1
T2
T3
T4
T5
T6
T7
T8
T9
T10
T11
T12
L1
L2
L3
L4
L5

Long thoracic n. (C5–C7)

Lateral pectoral n. (C5–C7)

Lateral cutaneous br. of
intercostal n.

Lateral cutaneous br. of
iliohypogastric n. (L1)

Sup. cluneal nn. (L1–L3)

Lateral cutaneous br.
of subcostal n. (T12)

Inf. cluneal nn. (S1–S3)

Brachial plexus (C5–T1)

1st intercostal n.

Medial pectoral n. (C8, T1)

Ant. cutaneous brr. of intercostal nn.

Intercostal n.

Genitofemoral n. (L1, L2)

Ant. cutaneous br. of 10th intercostal n. (T10)

Umbilicus

Subcostal n. (T12)

Iliohypogastric n. (L1)

Ilioinguinal n. (L1)

Right Lateral View

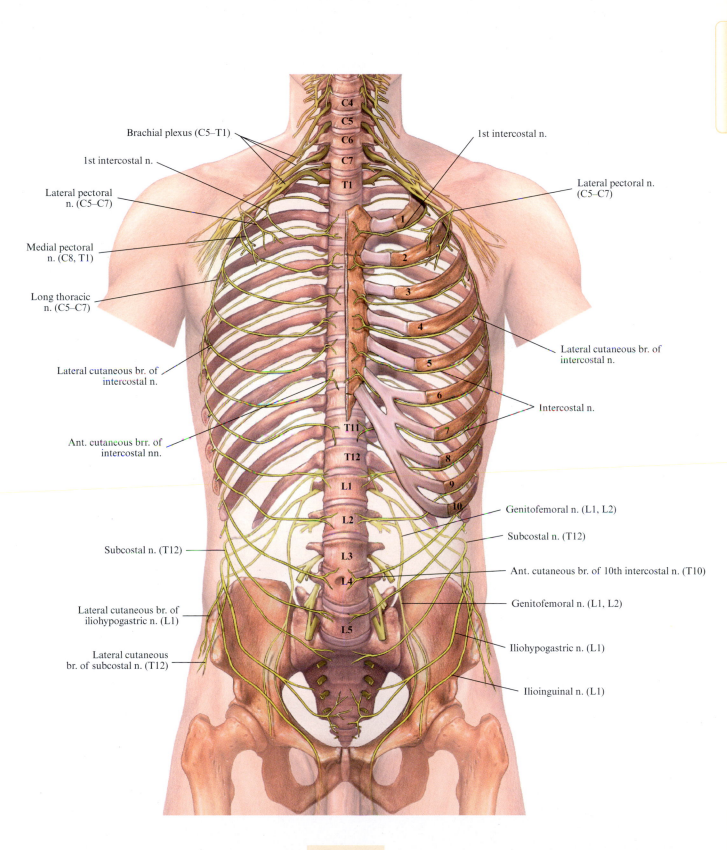

Brachial plexus (C5–T1)

1st intercostal n.

Lateral pectoral n. (C5–C7)

Medial pectoral n. (C8, T1)

Long thoracic n. (C5–C7)

Lateral cutaneous br. of intercostal n.

Ant. cutaneous brr. of intercostal nn.

Subcostal n. (T12)

Lateral cutaneous br. of iliohypogastric n. (L1)

Lateral cutaneous br. of subcostal n. (T12)

1st intercostal n.

Lateral pectoral n. (C5–C7)

Lateral cutaneous br. of intercostal n.

Intercostal n.

Genitofemoral n. (L1, L2)

Subcostal n. (T12)

Ant. cutaneous br. of 10th intercostal n. (T10)

Genitofemoral n. (L1, L2)

Iliohypogastric n. (L1)

Ilioinguinal n. (L1)

C4
C5
C6
C7
T1

T11
T12
L1
L2
L3
L4
L5

1
2
3
4
5
6
7
8
9
10

Anterior View

Chapter 1 | **TRUNK: BODY WALL AND SPINE**

PLATE 1.35   INTERCOSTAL NERVES

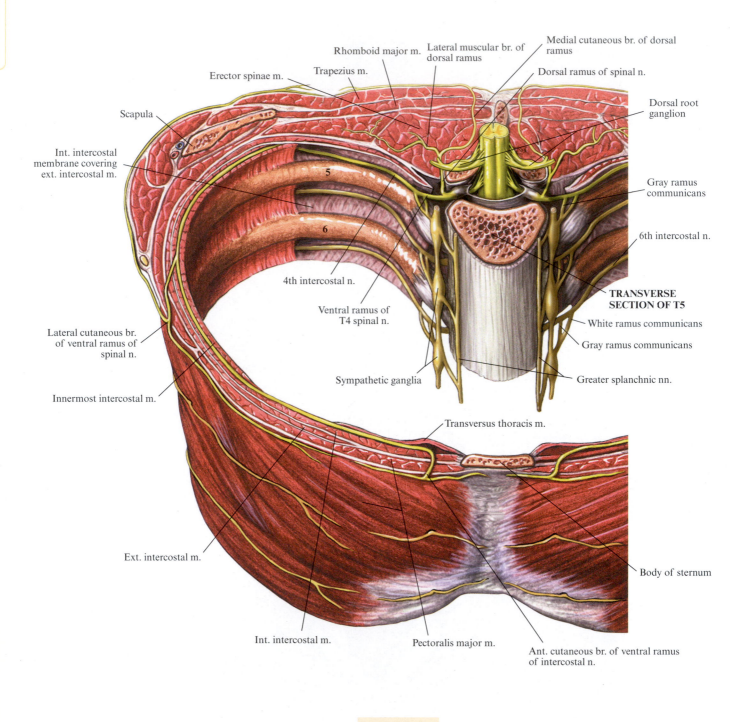

Rhomboid major m.

Lateral muscular br. of
dorsal ramus

Medial cutaneous br. of dorsal
ramus

Erector spinae m.

Trapezius m.

Dorsal ramus of spinal n.

Scapula

Dorsal root
ganglion

Int. intercostal
membrane covering
ext. intercostal m.

5

Gray ramus
communicans

6

6th intercostal n.

4th intercostal n.

**TRANSVERSE
SECTION OF T5**

Ventral ramus of
T4 spinal n.

White ramus communicans

Lateral cutaneous br.
of ventral ramus of
spinal n.

Gray ramus communicans

Sympathetic ganglia

Greater splanchnic nn.

Innermost intercostal m.

Transversus thoracis m.

Ext. intercostal m.

Body of sternum

Int. intercostal m.

Pectoralis major m.

Ant. cutaneous br. of ventral ramus
of intercostal n.

Anterosuperior

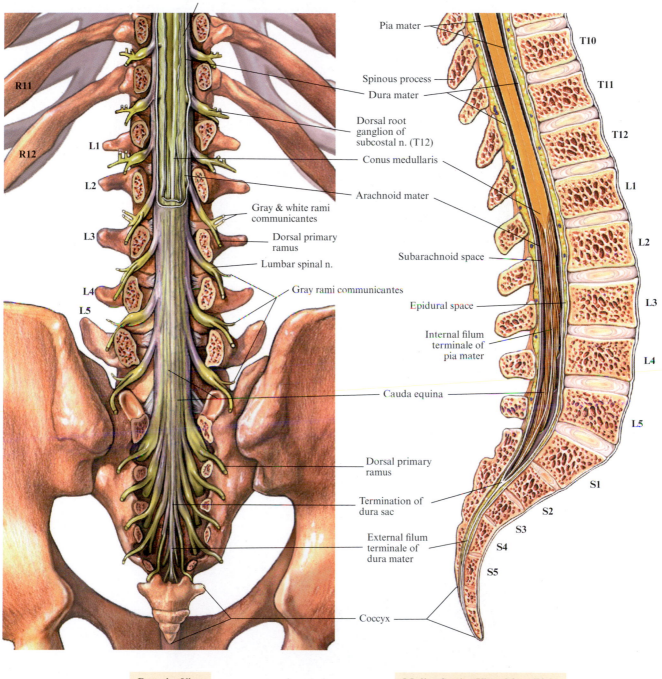

Arachnoid mater

Pia mater

Spinous process

Dura mater

Dorsal root ganglion of subcostal n. (T12)

Conus medullaris

Arachnoid mater

Gray & white rami communicantes

Dorsal primary ramus

Lumbar spinal n.

Gray rami communicantes

Subarachnoid space

Epidural space

Internal filum terminale of pia mater

Cauda equina

Dorsal primary ramus

Termination of dura sac

External filum terminale of dura mater

Coccyx

R11

R12

L1

L2

L3

L4

L5

T10

T11

T12

L1

L2

L3

L4

L5

S1

S2

S3

S4

S5

Posterior View

Median Section Viewed from Right

PLATE 1.37   ANTERIOR BODY WALL—SUPERFICIAL

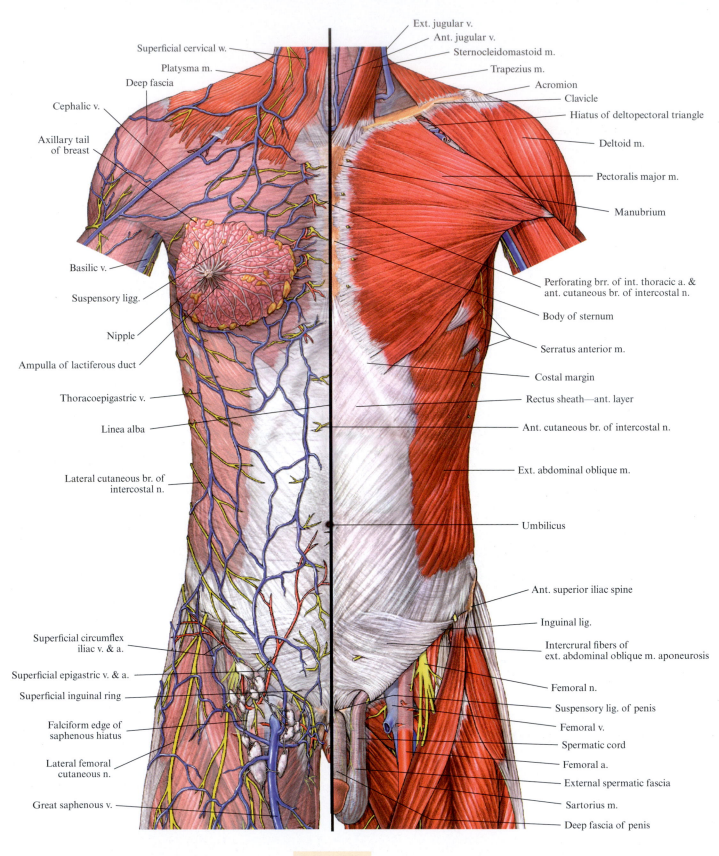

Superficial cervical w.

Platysma m.

Deep fascia

Cephalic v.

Axillary tail of breast

Basilic v.

Suspensory ligg.

Nipple

Ampulla of lactiferous duct

Thoracoepigastric v.

Linea alba

Lateral cutaneous br. of intercostal n.

Superficial circumflex iliac v. & a.

Superficial epigastric v. & a.

Superficial inguinal ring

Falciform edge of saphenous hiatus

Lateral femoral cutaneous n.

Great saphenous v.

Ext. jugular v.

Ant. jugular v.

Sternocleidomastoid m.

Trapezius m.

Acromion

Clavicle

Hiatus of deltopectoral triangle

Deltoid m.

Pectoralis major m.

Manubrium

Perforating brr. of int. thoracic a. & ant. cutaneous br. of intercostal n.

Body of sternum

Serratus anterior m.

Costal margin

Rectus sheath—ant. layer

Ant. cutaneous br. of intercostal n.

Ext. abdominal oblique m.

Umbilicus

Ant. superior iliac spine

Inguinal lig.

Intercrural fibers of ext. abdominal oblique m. aponeurosis

Femoral n.

Suspensory lig. of penis

Femoral v.

Spermatic cord

Femoral a.

External spermatic fascia

Sartorius m.

Deep fascia of penis

Anterior View

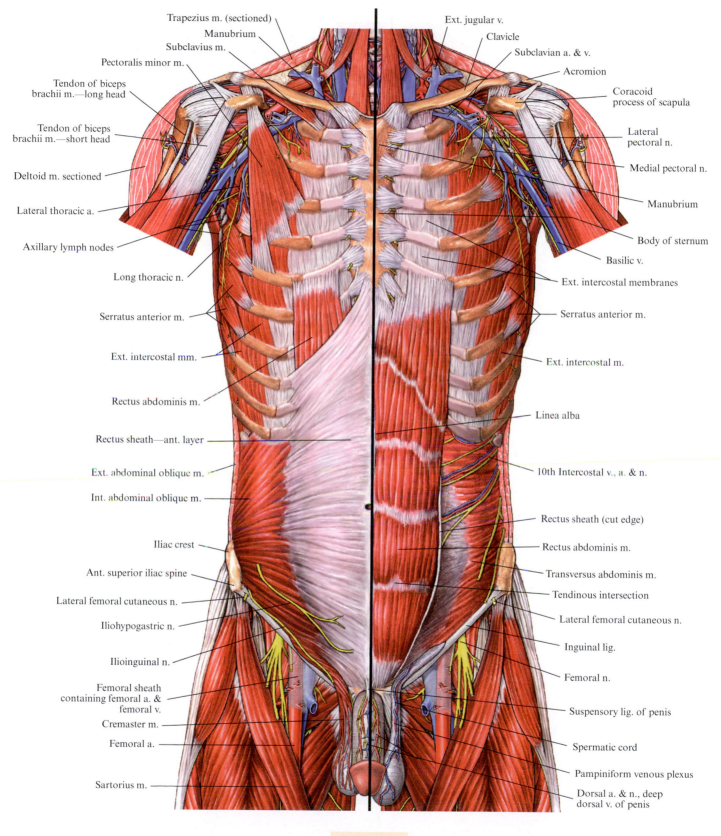

Trapezius m. (sectioned)
Manubrium
Subclavius m.
Pectoralis minor m.
Tendon of biceps brachii m.—long head
Tendon of biceps brachii m.—short head
Deltoid m. sectioned
Lateral thoracic a.
Axillary lymph nodes
Long thoracic n.
Serratus anterior m.
Ext. intercostal mm.
Rectus abdominis m.
Rectus sheath—ant. layer
Ext. abdominal oblique m.
Int. abdominal oblique m.
Iliac crest
Ant. superior iliac spine
Lateral femoral cutaneous n.
Iliohypogastric n.
Ilioinguinal n.
Femoral sheath containing femoral a. & femoral v.
Cremaster m.
Femoral a.
Sartorius m.

Ext. jugular v.
Clavicle
Subclavian a. & v.
Acromion
Coracoid process of scapula
Lateral pectoral n.
Medial pectoral n.
Manubrium
Body of sternum
Basilic v.
Ext. intercostal membranes
Serratus anterior m.
Ext. intercostal m.
Linea alba
10th Intercostal v., a. & n.
Rectus sheath (cut edge)
Rectus abdominis m.
Transversus abdominis m.
Tendinous intersection
Lateral femoral cutaneous n.
Inguinal lig.
Femoral n.
Suspensory lig. of penis
Spermatic cord
Pampiniform venous plexus
Dorsal a. & n., deep dorsal v. of penis

Anterior View

PLATE 1.41   ANTERIOR BODY WALL—MAMMARY GLAND

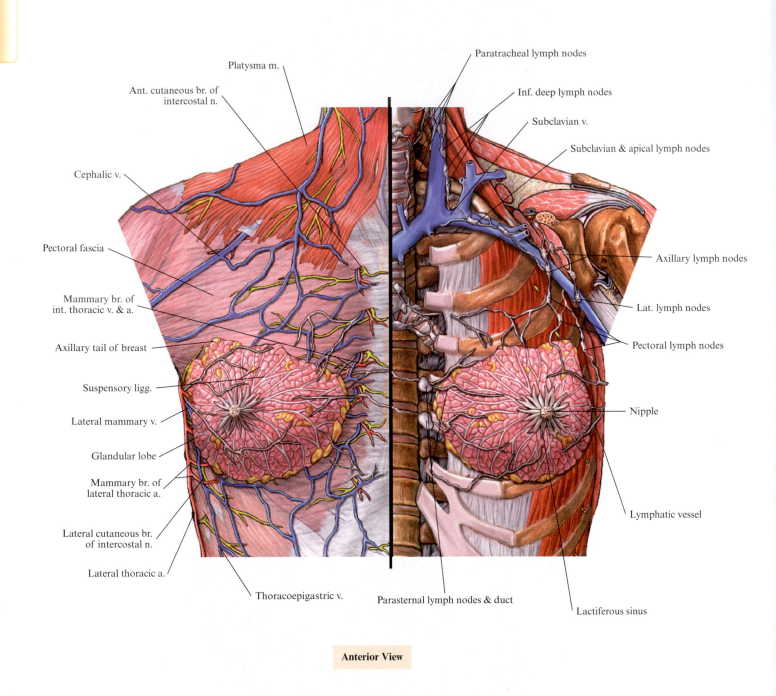

Platysma m.

Ant. cutaneous br. of
intercostal n.

Cephalic v.

Pectoral fascia

Mammary br. of
int. thoracic v. & a.

Axillary tail of breast

Suspensory ligg.

Lateral mammary v.

Glandular lobe

Mammary br. of
lateral thoracic a.

Lateral cutaneous br.
of intercostal n.

Lateral thoracic a.

Thoracoepigastric v.

Paratracheal lymph nodes

Inf. deep lymph nodes

Subclavian v.

Subclavian & apical lymph nodes

Axillary lymph nodes

Lat. lymph nodes

Pectoral lymph nodes

Nipple

Lymphatic vessel

Lactiferous sinus

Parasternal lymph nodes & duct

Anterior View

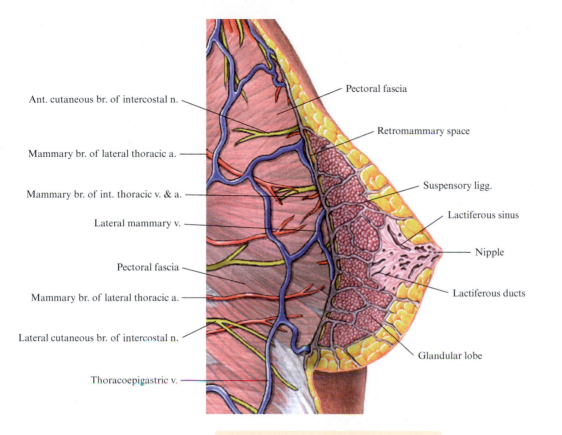

Ant. cutaneous br. of intercostal n.

Mammary br. of lateral thoracic a.

Mammary br. of int. thoracic v. & a.

Lateral mammary v.

Pectoral fascia

Mammary br. of lateral thoracic a.

Lateral cutaneous br. of intercostal n.

Thoracoepigastric v.

Pectoral fascia

Retromammary space

Suspensory ligg.

Lactiferous sinus

Nipple

Lactiferous ducts

Glandular lobe

Right Lateral View of Median Sectioned Breast

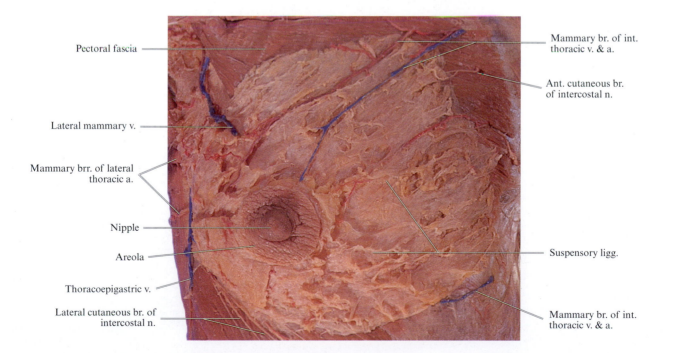

Pectoral fascia

Lateral mammary v.

Mammary brr. of lateral thoracic a.

Nipple

Areola

Thoracoepigastric v.

Lateral cutaneous br. of intercostal n.

Mammary br. of int. thoracic v. & a.

Ant. cutaneous br. of intercostal n.

Suspensory ligg.

Mammary br. of int. thoracic v. & a.

Anterior View of Right Breast

PLATE 1.43 ANTERIOR BODY WALL—INTERNAL SURFACE

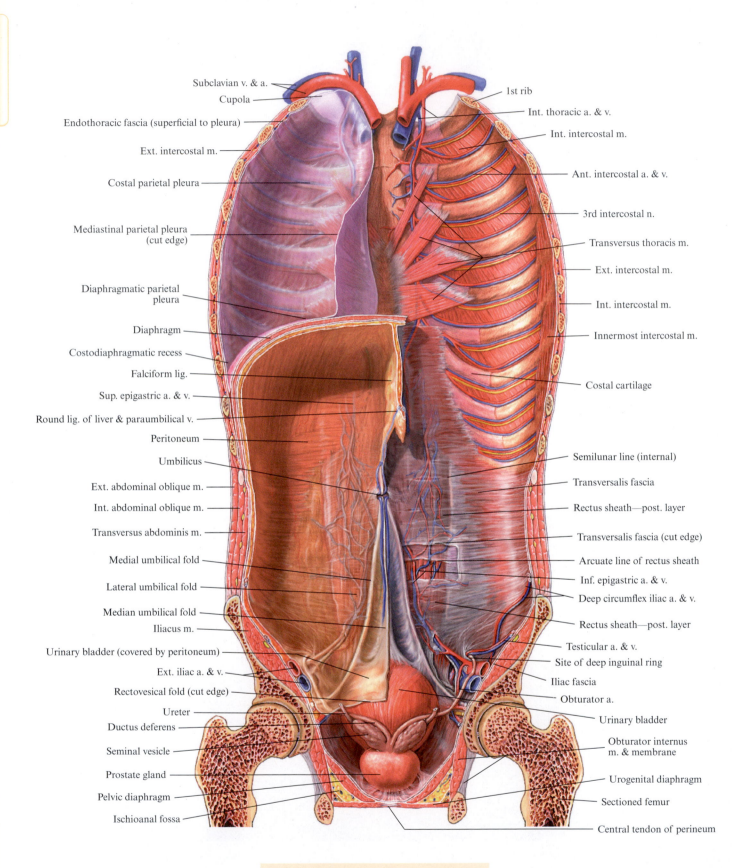

Subclavian v. & a.
Cupola
Endothoracic fascia (superficial to pleura)
Ext. intercostal m.
Costal parietal pleura
Mediastinal parietal pleura (cut edge)
Diaphragmatic parietal pleura
Diaphragm
Costodiaphragmatic recess
Falciform lig.
Sup. epigastric a. & v.
Round lig. of liver & paraumbilical v.
Peritoneum
Umbilicus
Ext. abdominal oblique m.
Int. abdominal oblique m.
Transversus abdominis m.
Medial umbilical fold
Lateral umbilical fold
Median umbilical fold
Iliacus m.
Urinary bladder (covered by peritoneum)
Ext. iliac a. & v.
Rectovesical fold (cut edge)
Ureter
Ductus deferens
Seminal vesicle
Prostate gland
Pelvic diaphragm
Ischioanal fossa

1st rib
Int. thoracic a. & v.
Int. intercostal m.
Ant. intercostal a. & v.
3rd intercostal n.
Transversus thoracis m.
Ext. intercostal m.
Int. intercostal m.
Innermost intercostal m.
Costal cartilage
Semilunar line (internal)
Transversalis fascia
Rectus sheath—post. layer
Transversalis fascia (cut edge)
Arcuate line of rectus sheath
Inf. epigastric a. & v.
Deep circumflex iliac a. & v.
Rectus sheath—post. layer
Testicular a. & v.
Site of deep inguinal ring
Iliac fascia
Obturator a.
Urinary bladder
Obturator internus m. & membrane
Sectioned femur
Urogenital diaphragm
Central tendon of perineum

Posterior (Internal) View of Anterior Body Wall

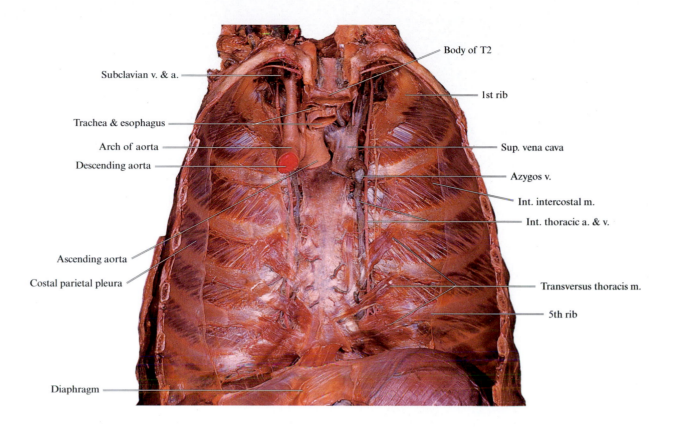

Subclavian v. & a.

Trachea & esophagus

Arch of aorta

Descending aorta

Ascending aorta

Costal parietal pleura

Diaphragm

Body of T2

1st rib

Sup. vena cava

Azygos v.

Int. intercostal m.

Int. thoracic a. & v.

Transversus thoracis m.

5th rib

Posterior (Internal) View of Anterior Thoracic Wall

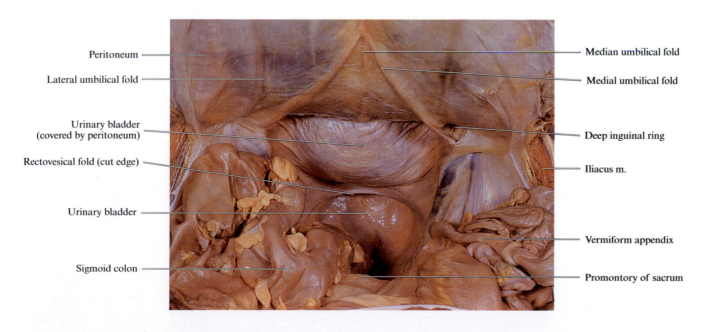

Peritoneum

Lateral umbilical fold

Urinary bladder
(covered by peritoneum)

Rectovesical fold (cut edge)

Urinary bladder

Sigmoid colon

Median umbilical fold

Medial umbilical fold

Deep inguinal ring

Iliacus m.

Vermiform appendix

Promontory of sacrum

Posterosuperior View of Anterior Abdominal Wall & Pelvic Contents

CHAPTER 1 | **TRUNK: BODY WALL AND SPINE**   49

PLATE 1.45   LATERAL BODY WALL—SUPERFICIAL

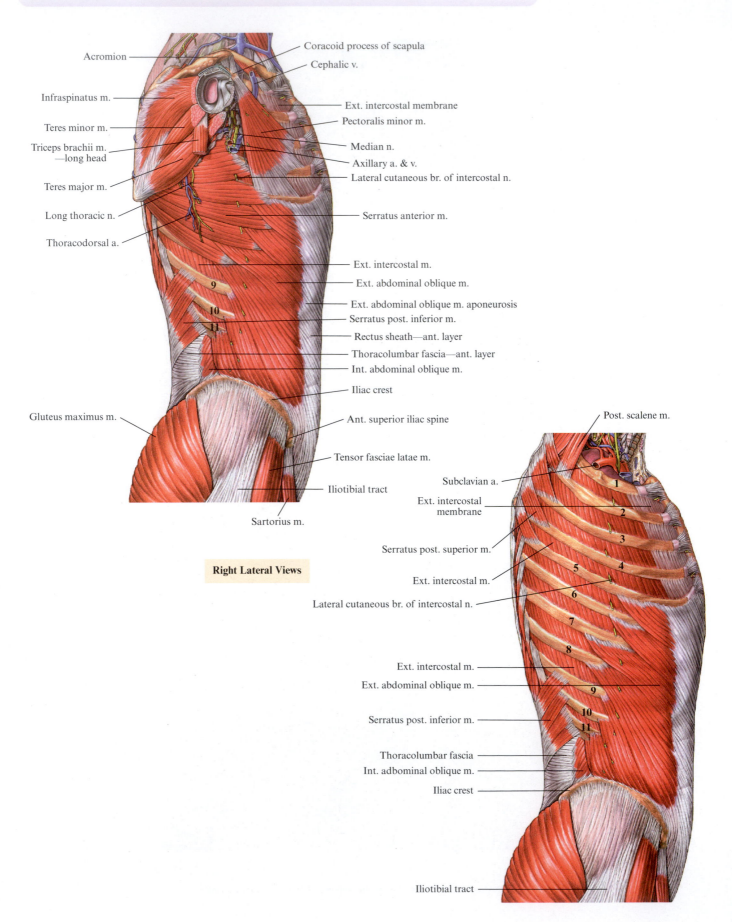

Acromion

Infraspinatus m.

Teres minor m.

Triceps brachii m.
—long head

Teres major m.

Long thoracic n.

Thoracodorsal a.

Coracoid process of scapula

Cephalic v.

Ext. intercostal membrane

Pectoralis minor m.

Median n.

Axillary a. & v.

Lateral cutaneous br. of intercostal n.

Serratus anterior m.

Ext. intercostal m.

Ext. abdominal oblique m.

9

10

11

Ext. abdominal oblique m. aponeurosis

Serratus post. inferior m.

Rectus sheath—ant. layer

Thoracolumbar fascia—ant. layer

Int. abdominal oblique m.

Iliac crest

Gluteus maximus m.

Ant. superior iliac spine

Tensor fasciae latae m.

Iliotibial tract

Sartorius m.

Right Lateral Views

Post. scalene m.

Subclavian a.

Ext. intercostal
membrane

Serratus post. superior m.

Ext. intercostal m.

Lateral cutaneous br. of intercostal n.

Ext. intercostal m.

Ext. abdominal oblique m.

Serratus post. inferior m.

Thoracolumbar fascia

Int. adbominal oblique m.

Iliac crest

Iliotibial tract

1

2

3

4

5

6

7

8

9

10

11

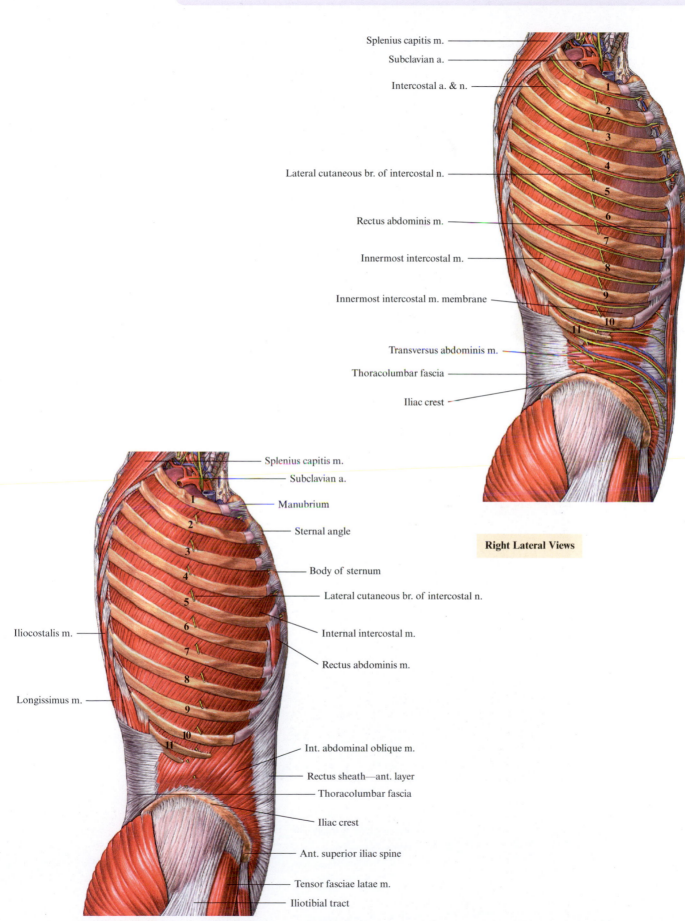

Splenius capitis m.

Subclavian a.

Intercostal a. & n.

Lateral cutaneous br. of intercostal n.

Rectus abdominis m.

Innermost intercostal m.

Innermost intercostal m. membrane

Transversus abdominis m.

Thoracolumbar fascia

Iliac crest

Right Lateral Views

Splenius capitis m.

Subclavian a.

Manubrium

Sternal angle

Body of sternum

Lateral cutaneous br. of intercostal n.

Internal intercostal m.

Rectus abdominis m.

Iliocostalis m.

Longissimus m.

Int. abdominal oblique m.

Rectus sheath—ant. layer

Thoracolumbar fascia

Iliac crest

Ant. superior iliac spine

Tensor fasciae latae m.

Iliotibial tract

PLATE 1.47   **INGUINAL REGION—SUPERFICIAL FASCIA**

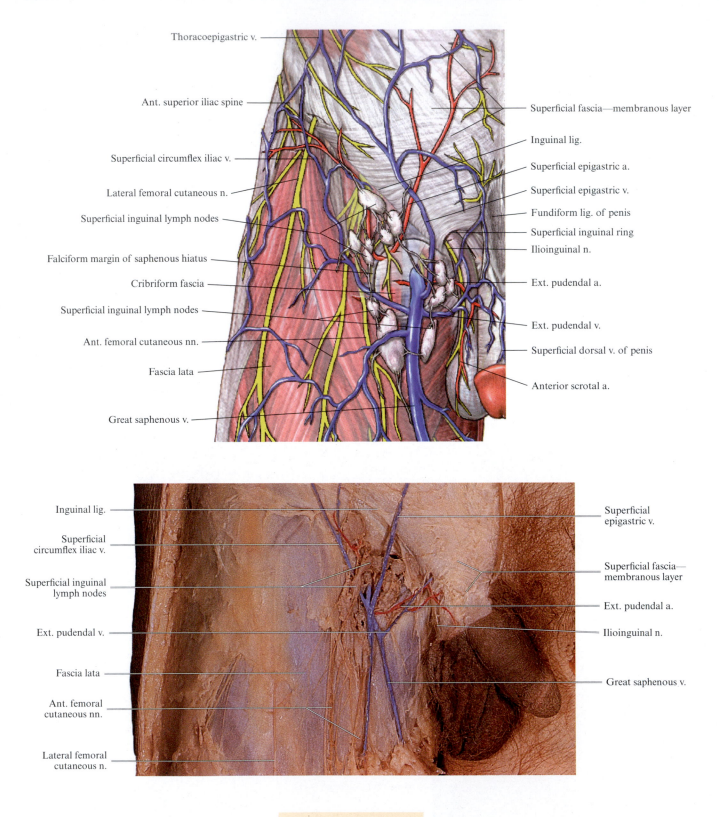

Thoracoepigastric v.

Ant. superior iliac spine

Superficial circumflex iliac v.

Lateral femoral cutaneous n.

Superficial inguinal lymph nodes

Falciform margin of saphenous hiatus

Cribriform fascia

Superficial inguinal lymph nodes

Ant. femoral cutaneous nn.

Fascia lata

Great saphenous v.

Superficial fascia—membranous layer

Inguinal lig.

Superficial epigastric a.

Superficial epigastric v.

Fundiform lig. of penis

Superficial inguinal ring

Ilioinguinal n.

Ext. pudendal a.

Ext. pudendal v.

Superficial dorsal v. of penis

Anterior scrotal a.

Inguinal lig.

Superficial circumflex iliac v.

Superficial inguinal lymph nodes

Ext. pudendal v.

Fascia lata

Ant. femoral cutaneous nn.

Lateral femoral cutaneous n.

Superficial epigastric v.

Superficial fascia— membranous layer

Ext. pudendal a.

Ilioinguinal n.

Great saphenous v.

Anterior Views of Right Side

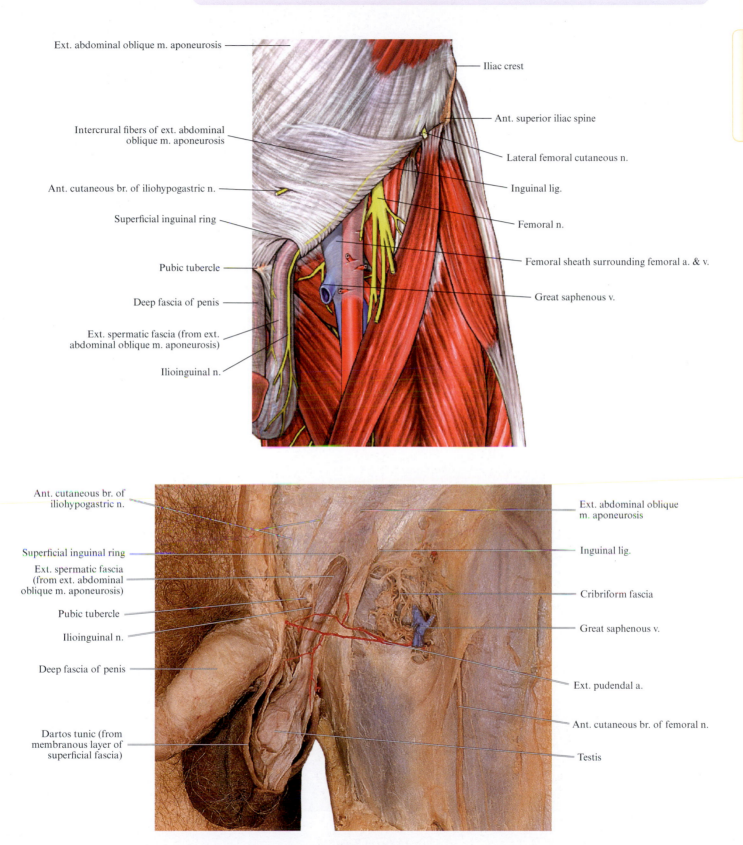

Ext. abdominal oblique m. aponeurosis

Intercrural fibers of ext. abdominal oblique m. aponeurosis

Ant. cutaneous br. of iliohypogastric n.

Superficial inguinal ring

Pubic tubercle

Deep fascia of penis

Ext. spermatic fascia (from ext. abdominal oblique m. aponeurosis)

Ilioinguinal n.

Iliac crest

Ant. superior iliac spine

Lateral femoral cutaneous n.

Inguinal lig.

Femoral n.

Femoral sheath surrounding femoral a. & v.

Great saphenous v.

Ant. cutaneous br. of iliohypogastric n.

Superficial inguinal ring

Ext. spermatic fascia (from ext. abdominal oblique m. aponeurosis)

Pubic tubercle

Ilioinguinal n.

Deep fascia of penis

Dartos tunic (from membranous layer of superficial fascia)

Ext. abdominal oblique m. aponeurosis

Inguinal lig.

Cribriform fascia

Great saphenous v.

Ext. pudendal a.

Ant. cutaneous br. of femoral n.

Testis

Anterior Views of Left Side

PLATE 1.49   INGUINAL REGION—EXTERNAL SPERMATIC FASCIA

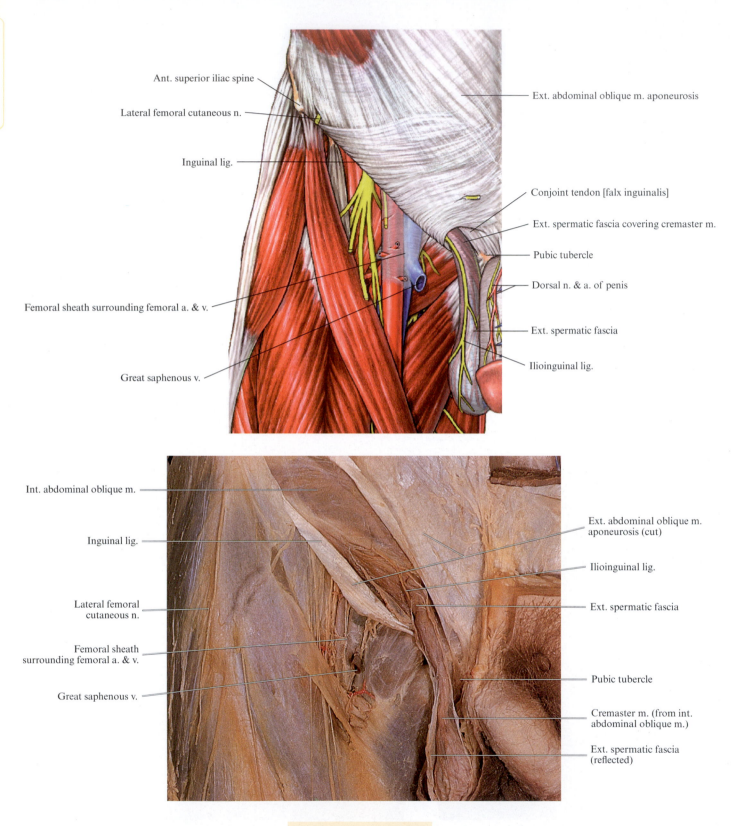

Ant. superior iliac spine

Lateral femoral cutaneous n.

Inguinal lig.

Femoral sheath surrounding femoral a. & v.

Great saphenous v.

Ext. abdominal oblique m. aponeurosis

Conjoint tendon [falx inguinalis]

Ext. spermatic fascia covering cremaster m.

Pubic tubercle

Dorsal n. & a. of penis

Ext. spermatic fascia

Ilioinguinal lig.

Int. abdominal oblique m.

Inguinal lig.

Lateral femoral cutaneous n.

Femoral sheath surrounding femoral a. & v.

Great saphenous v.

Ext. abdominal oblique m. aponeurosis (cut)

Ilioinguinal lig.

Ext. spermatic fascia

Pubic tubercle

Cremaster m. (from int. abdominal oblique m.)

Ext. spermatic fascia (reflected)

Anterior Views of Right Side

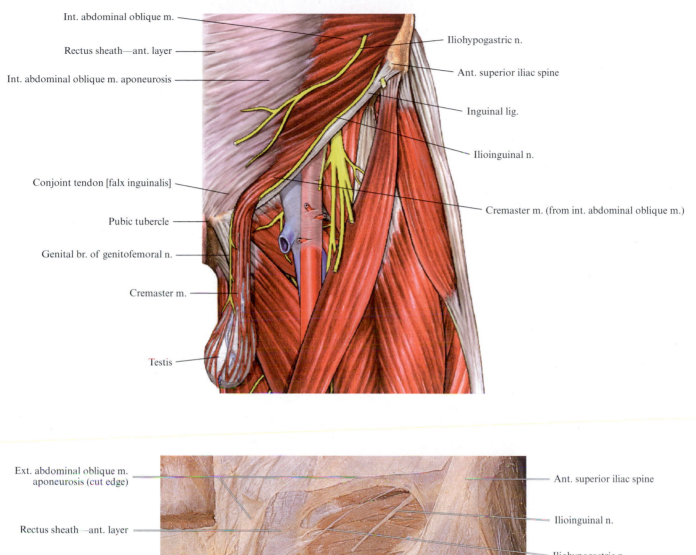

Int. abdominal oblique m.

Rectus sheath—ant. layer

Int. abdominal oblique m. aponeurosis

Conjoint tendon [falx inguinalis]

Pubic tubercle

Genital br. of genitofemoral n.

Cremaster m.

Testis

Iliohypogastric n.

Ant. superior iliac spine

Inguinal lig.

Ilioinguinal n.

Cremaster m. (from int. abdominal oblique m.)

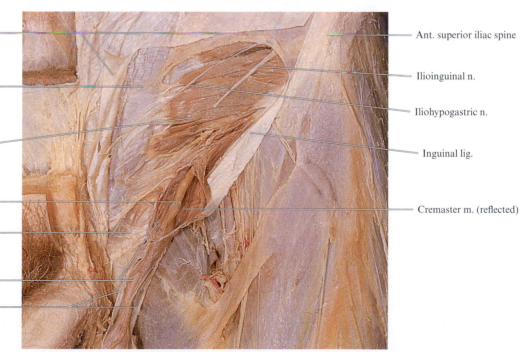

Ext. abdominal oblique m. aponeurosis (cut edge)

Rectus sheath —ant. layer

Int. abdominal oblique m.

Int. spermatic fascia

Conjoint tendon [falx inguinalis]

Cremaster m. (from int. abdominal oblique m.)

Ext. spermatic fascia (cut)

Ant. superior iliac spine

Ilioinguinal n.

Iliohypogastric n.

Inguinal lig.

Cremaster m. (reflected)

Anterior Views of Left Side

PLATE 1.51   INGUINAL REGION—INTERNAL SPERMATIC FASCIA

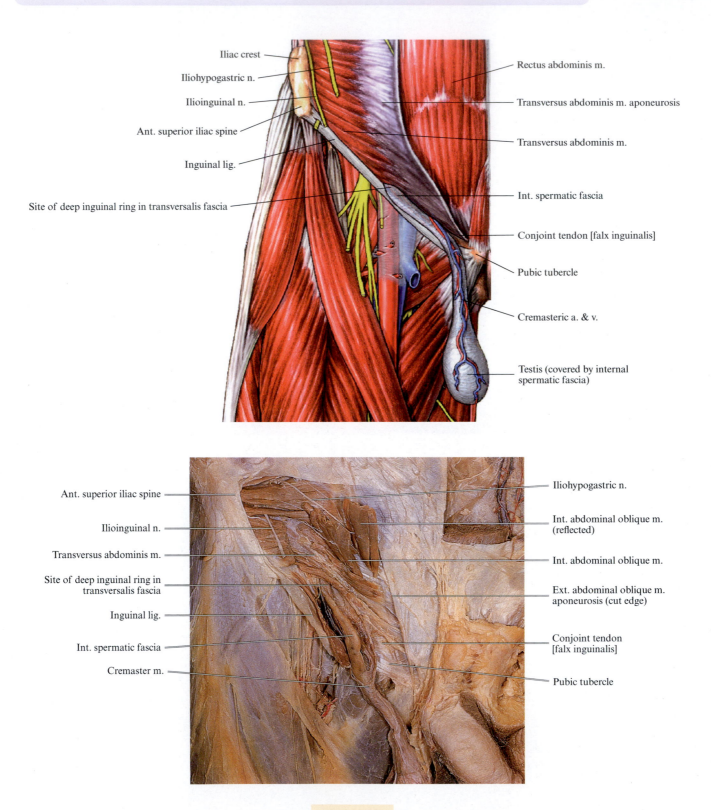

Iliac crest

Iliohypogastric n.

Ilioinguinal n.

Ant. superior iliac spine

Inguinal lig.

Site of deep inguinal ring in transversalis fascia

Rectus abdominis m.

Transversus abdominis m. aponeurosis

Transversus abdominis m.

Int. spermatic fascia

Conjoint tendon [falx inguinalis]

Pubic tubercle

Cremasteric a. & v.

Testis (covered by internal spermatic fascia)

Ant. superior iliac spine

Ilioinguinal n.

Transversus abdominis m.

Site of deep inguinal ring in transversalis fascia

Inguinal lig.

Int. spermatic fascia

Cremaster m.

Iliohypogastric n.

Int. abdominal oblique m. (reflected)

Int. abdominal oblique m.

Ext. abdominal oblique m. aponeurosis (cut edge)

Conjoint tendon [falx inguinalis]

Pubic tubercle

Anterior Views

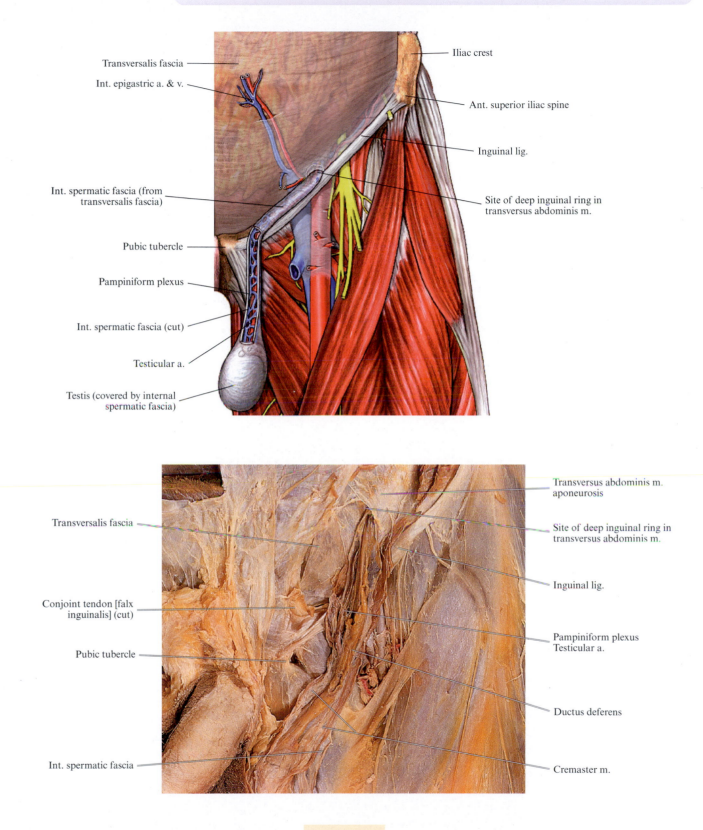

Transversalis fascia

Int. epigastric a. & v.

Int. spermatic fascia (from transversalis fascia)

Pubic tubercle

Pampiniform plexus

Int. spermatic fascia (cut)

Testicular a.

Testis (covered by internal spermatic fascia)

Iliac crest

Ant. superior iliac spine

Inguinal lig.

Site of deep inguinal ring in transversus abdominis m.

Transversalis fascia

Conjoint tendon [falx inguinalis] (cut)

Pubic tubercle

Int. spermatic fascia

Transversus abdominis m. aponeurosis

Site of deep inguinal ring in transversus abdominis m.

Inguinal lig.

Pampiniform plexus
Testicular a.

Ductus deferens

Cremaster m.

Anterior Views

PLATE 1.53   SUPERFICIAL BACK

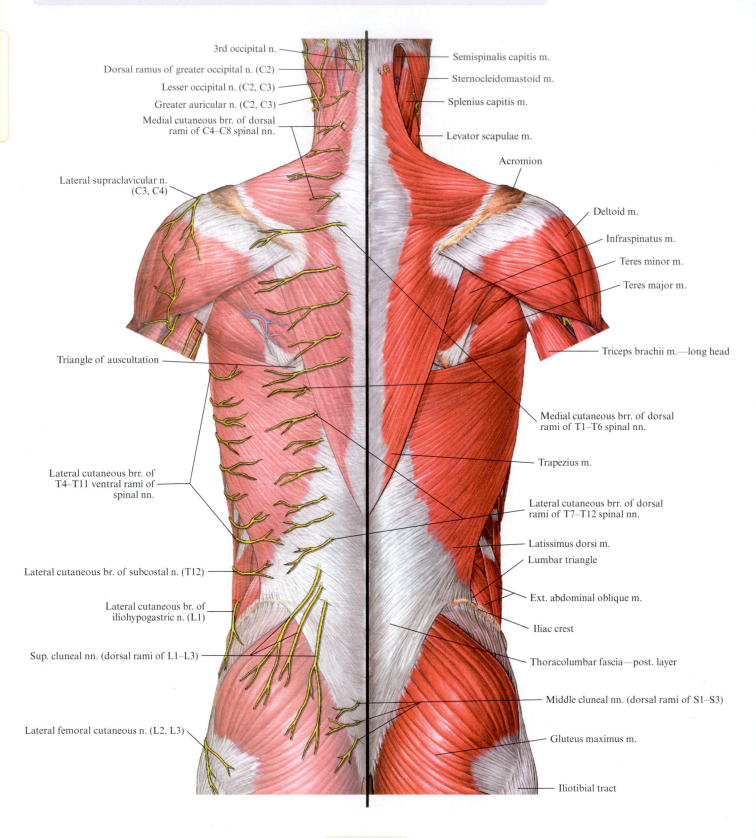

3rd occipital n.

Dorsal ramus of greater occipital n. (C2)

Lesser occipital n. (C2, C3)

Greater auricular n. (C2, C3)

Medial cutaneous brr. of dorsal
rami of C4–C8 spinal nn.

Lateral supraclavicular n.
(C3, C4)

Triangle of auscultation

Lateral cutaneous brr. of
T4–T11 ventral rami of
spinal nn.

Lateral cutaneous br. of subcostal n. (T12)

Lateral cutaneous br. of
iliohypogastric n. (L1)

Sup. cluneal nn. (dorsal rami of L1–L3)

Lateral femoral cutaneous n. (L2, L3)

Semispinalis capitis m.

Sternocleidomastoid m.

Splenius capitis m.

Levator scapulae m.

Acromion

Deltoid m.

Infraspinatus m.

Teres minor m.

Teres major m.

Triceps brachii m.—long head

Medial cutaneous brr. of dorsal
rami of T1–T6 spinal nn.

Trapezius m.

Lateral cutaneous brr. of dorsal
rami of T7–T12 spinal nn.

Latissimus dorsi m.

Lumbar triangle

Ext. abdominal oblique m.

Iliac crest

Thoracolumbar fascia—post. layer

Middle cluneal nn. (dorsal rami of S1–S3)

Gluteus maximus m.

Iliotibial tract

Posterior View

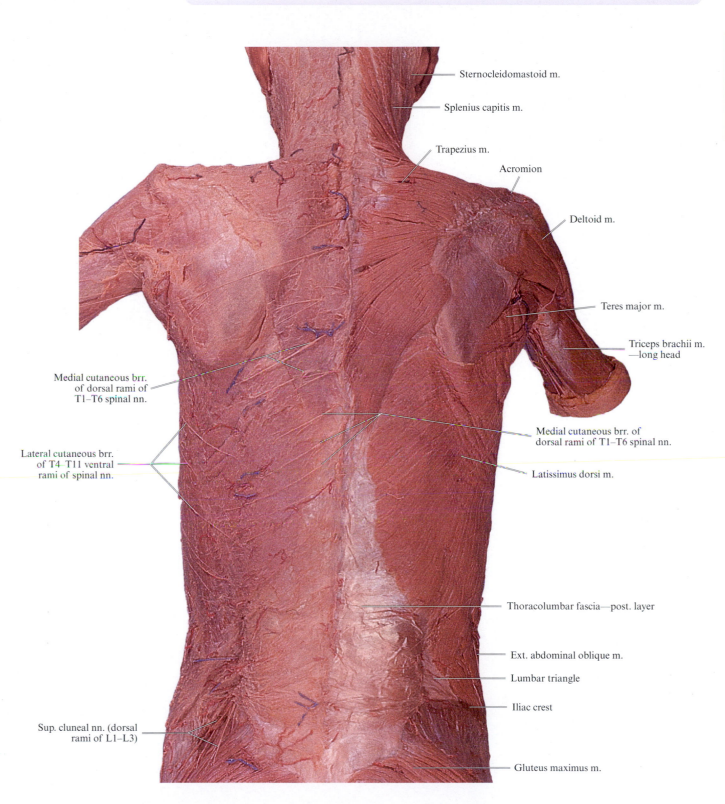

Sternocleidomastoid m.

Splenius capitis m.

Trapezius m.

Acromion

Deltoid m.

Teres major m.

Triceps brachii m.
—long head

Medial cutaneous brr.
of dorsal rami of
T1–T6 spinal nn.

Medial cutaneous brr. of
dorsal rami of T1–T6 spinal nn.

Lateral cutaneous brr.
of T4–T11 ventral
rami of spinal nn.

Latissimus dorsi m.

Thoracolumbar fascia—post. layer

Ext. abdominal oblique m.

Lumbar triangle

Iliac crest

Sup. cluneal nn. (dorsal
rami of L1–L3)

Gluteus maximus m.

Posterior View

PLATE 1.55   INTERMEDIATE BACK

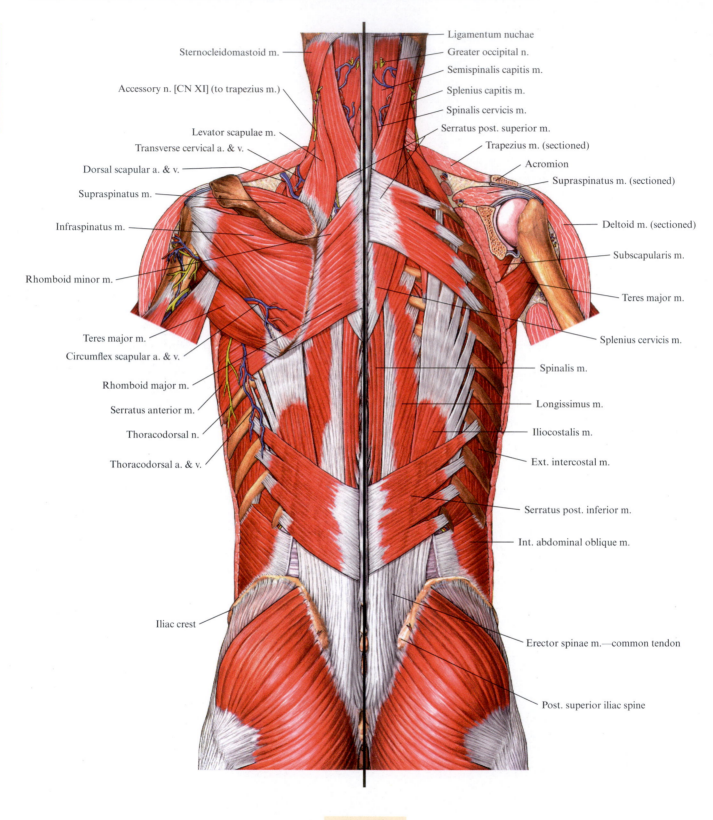

Sternocleidomastoid m.

Accessory n. [CN XI] (to trapezius m.)

Levator scapulae m.
Transverse cervical a. & v.
Dorsal scapular a. & v.
Supraspinatus m.
Infraspinatus m.

Rhomboid minor m.

Teres major m.
Circumflex scapular a. & v.
Rhomboid major m.
Serratus anterior m.
Thoracodorsal n.
Thoracodorsal a. & v.

Iliac crest

Ligamentum nuchae
Greater occipital n.
Semispinalis capitis m.
Splenius capitis m.
Spinalis cervicis m.
Serratus post. superior m.
Trapezius m. (sectioned)
Acromion
Supraspinatus m. (sectioned)

Deltoid m. (sectioned)

Subscapularis m.

Teres major m.

Splenius cervicis m.

Spinalis m.

Longissimus m.

Iliocostalis m.

Ext. intercostal m.

Serratus post. inferior m.

Int. abdominal oblique m.

Erector spinae m.—common tendon

Post. superior iliac spine

Posterior View

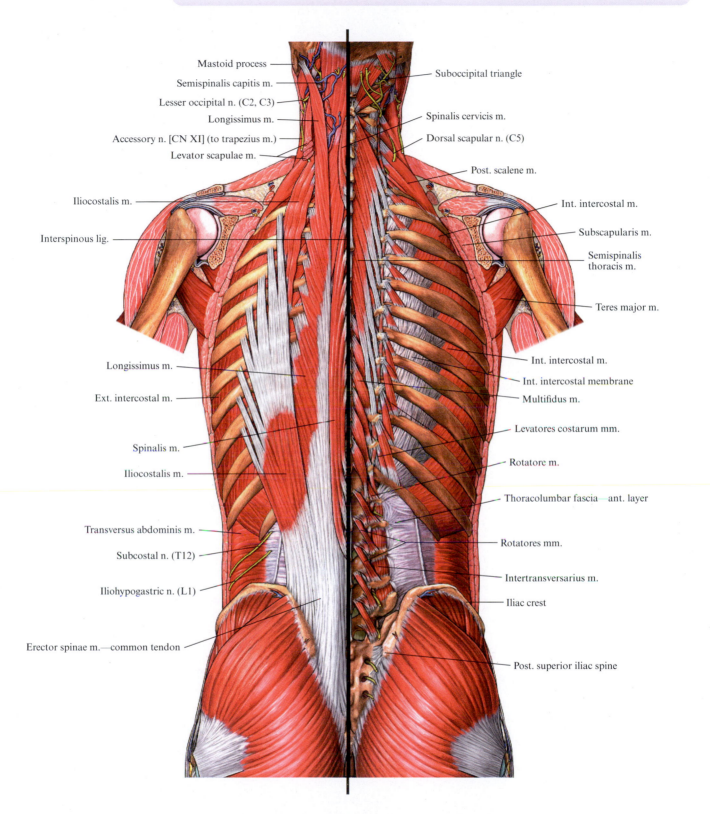

Mastoid process

Semispinalis capitis m.

Lesser occipital n. (C2, C3)

Longissimus m.

Accessory n. [CN XI] (to trapezius m.)

Levator scapulae m.

Iliocostalis m.

Interspinous lig.

Longissimus m.

Ext. intercostal m.

Spinalis m.

Iliocostalis m.

Transversus abdominis m.

Subcostal n. (T12)

Iliohypogastric n. (L1)

Erector spinae m.—common tendon

Suboccipital triangle

Spinalis cervicis m.

Dorsal scapular n. (C5)

Post. scalene m.

Int. intercostal m.

Subscapularis m.

Semispinalis thoracis m.

Teres major m.

Int. intercostal m.

Int. intercostal membrane

Multifidus m.

Levatores costarum mm.

Rotatore m.

Thoracolumbar fascia—ant. layer

Rotatores mm.

Intertransversarius m.

Iliac crest

Post. superior iliac spine

Posterior View

PLATE 1.57   SUBOCCIPITAL REGION

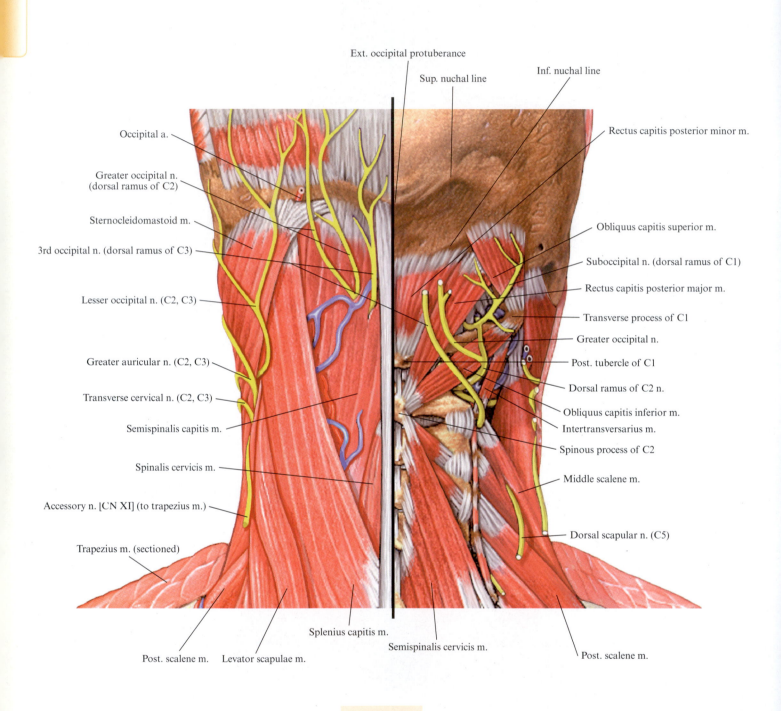

Ext. occipital protuberance

Sup. nuchal line

Inf. nuchal line

Occipital a.

Greater occipital n.
(dorsal ramus of C2)

Sternocleidomastoid m.

3rd occipital n. (dorsal ramus of C3)

Lesser occipital n. (C2, C3)

Greater auricular n. (C2, C3)

Transverse cervical n. (C2, C3)

Semispinalis capitis m.

Spinalis cervicis m.

Accessory n. [CN XI] (to trapezius m.)

Trapezius m. (sectioned)

Rectus capitis posterior minor m.

Obliquus capitis superior m.

Suboccipital n. (dorsal ramus of C1)

Rectus capitis posterior major m.

Transverse process of C1

Greater occipital n.

Post. tubercle of C1

Dorsal ramus of C2 n.

Obliquus capitis inferior m.

Intertransversarius m.

Spinous process of C2

Middle scalene m.

Dorsal scapular n. (C5)

Post. scalene m.   Levator scapulae m.

Splenius capitis m.

Semispinalis cervicis m.

Post. scalene m.

Posterior View

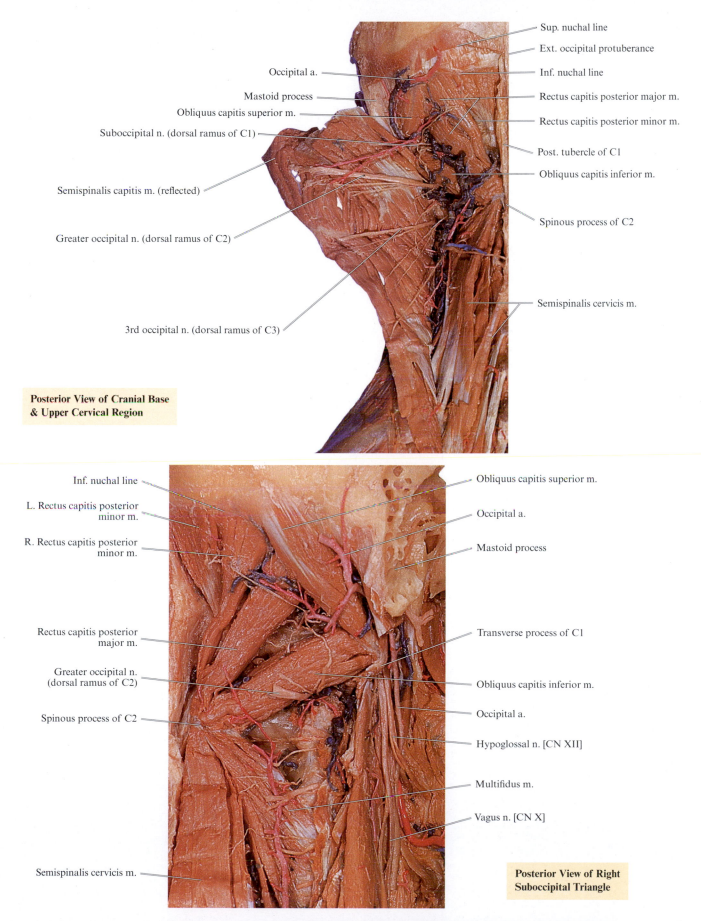

Posterior View of Cranial Base & Upper Cervical Region

Sup. nuchal line
Ext. occipital protuberance
Occipital a.
Inf. nuchal line
Mastoid process
Rectus capitis posterior major m.
Obliquus capitis superior m.
Rectus capitis posterior minor m.
Suboccipital n. (dorsal ramus of C1)
Post. tubercle of C1
Semispinalis capitis m. (reflected)
Obliquus capitis inferior m.
Greater occipital n. (dorsal ramus of C2)
Spinous process of C2
Semispinalis cervicis m.
3rd occipital n. (dorsal ramus of C3)

Posterior View of Right Suboccipital Triangle

Inf. nuchal line
Obliquus capitis superior m.
L. Rectus capitis posterior minor m.
Occipital a.
R. Rectus capitis posterior minor m.
Mastoid process
Rectus capitis posterior major m.
Transverse process of C1
Greater occipital n. (dorsal ramus of C2)
Obliquus capitis inferior m.
Spinous process of C2
Occipital a.
Hypoglossal n. [CN XII]
Multifidus m.
Semispinalis cervicis m.
Vagus n. [CN X]

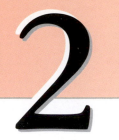

2 THORAX

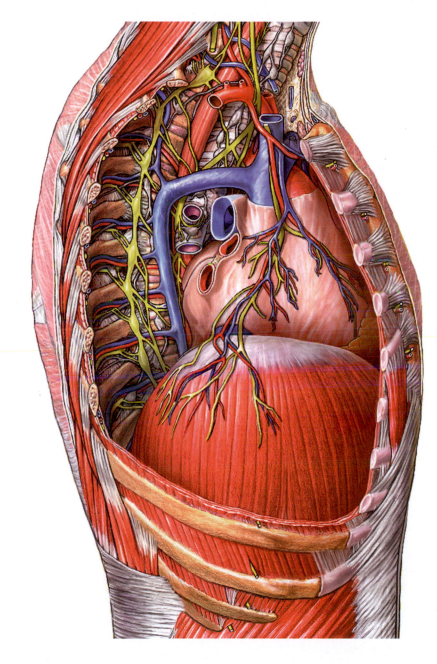

PLATE 2.1   SURFACE ANATOMY

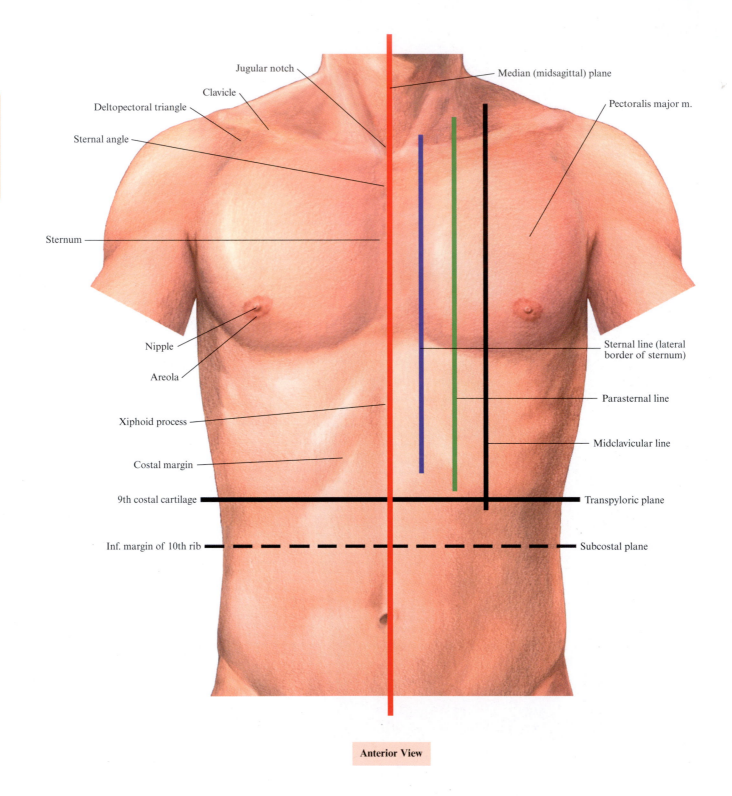

Jugular notch

Clavicle

Deltopectoral triangle

Sternal angle

Median (midsagittal) plane

Pectoralis major m.

Sternum

Nipple

Areola

Xiphoid process

Costal margin

9th costal cartilage

Inf. margin of 10th rib

Sternal line (lateral border of sternum)

Parasternal line

Midclavicular line

Transpyloric plane

Subcostal plane

Anterior View

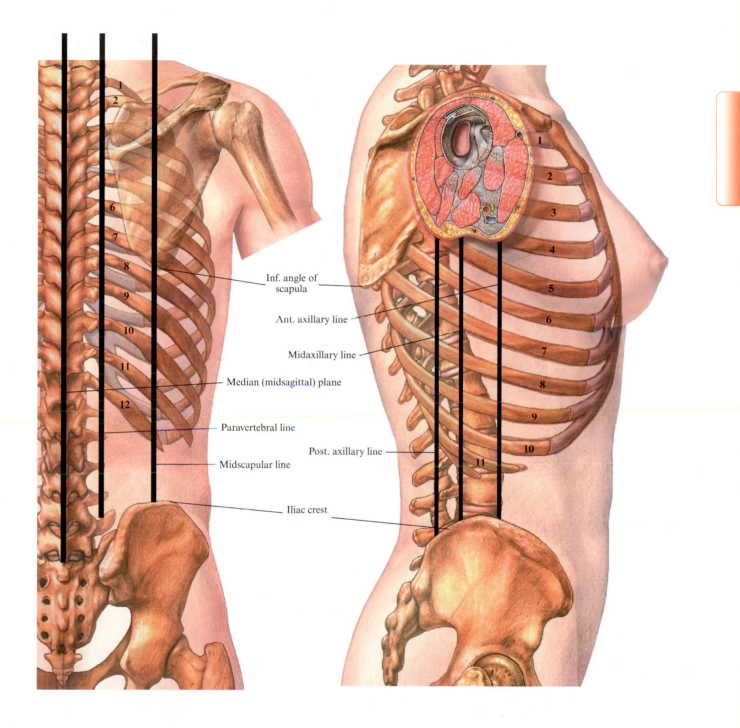

Inf. angle of
scapula

Ant. axillary line

Midaxillary line

Median (midsagittal) plane

Paravertebral line

Midscapular line

Post. axillary line

Iliac crest

Posterior View

Right Lateral View

PLATE 2.3   TOPOGRAPHY OF VISCERA

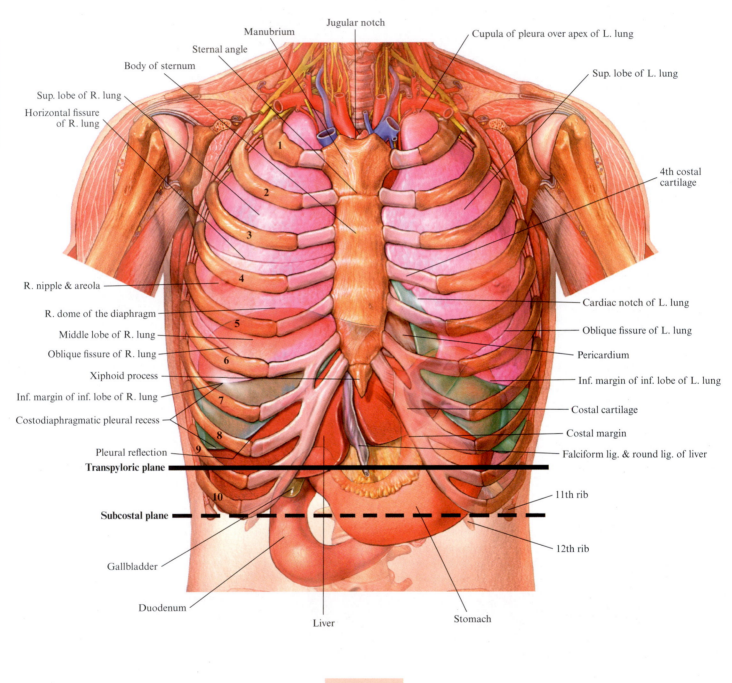

Jugular notch

Manubrium

Sternal angle

Body of sternum

Sup. lobe of R. lung

Horizontal fissure
of R. lung

Cupula of pleura over apex of L. lung

Sup. lobe of L. lung

4th costal
cartilage

R. nipple & areola

R. dome of the diaphragm

Middle lobe of R. lung

Oblique fissure of R. lung

Xiphoid process

Inf. margin of inf. lobe of R. lung

Costodiaphragmatic pleural recess

Pleural reflection

Transpyloric plane

Subcostal plane

Gallbladder

Duodenum

Liver

Cardiac notch of L. lung

Oblique fissure of L. lung

Pericardium

Inf. margin of inf. lobe of L. lung

Costal cartilage

Costal margin

Falciform lig. & round lig. of liver

11th rib

12th rib

Stomach

Anterior View

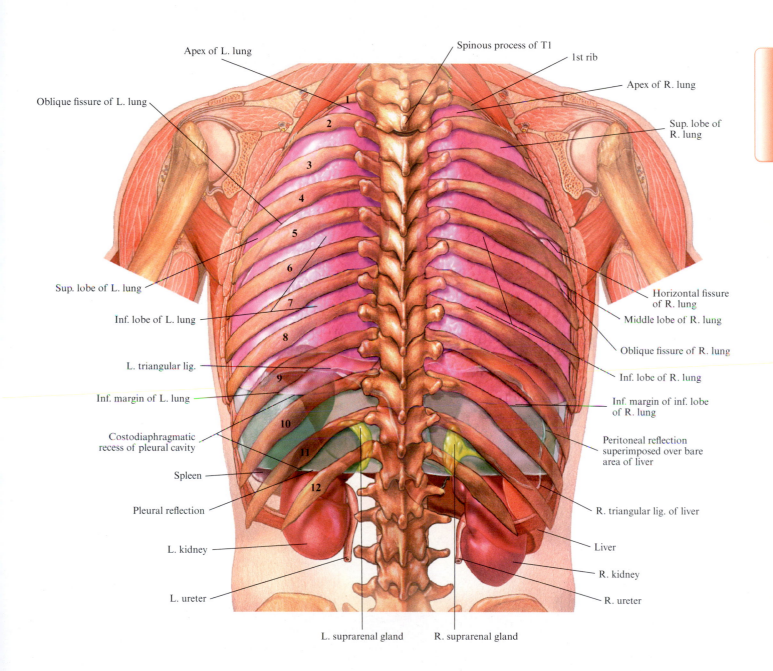

Apex of L. lung

Spinous process of T1

1st rib

Apex of R. lung

Oblique fissure of L. lung

Sup. lobe of
R. lung

Sup. lobe of L. lung

Horizontal fissure
of R. lung

Inf. lobe of L. lung

Middle lobe of R. lung

Oblique fissure of R. lung

L. triangular lig.

Inf. lobe of R. lung

Inf. margin of L. lung

Inf. margin of inf. lobe
of R. lung

Costodiaphragmatic
recess of pleural cavity

Peritoneal reflection
superimposed over bare
area of liver

Spleen

Pleural reflection

R. triangular lig. of liver

L. kidney

Liver

R. kidney

L. ureter

R. ureter

L. suprarenal gland

R. suprarenal gland

Posterior View

PLATE 2.5   TOPOGRAPHY OF VISCERA

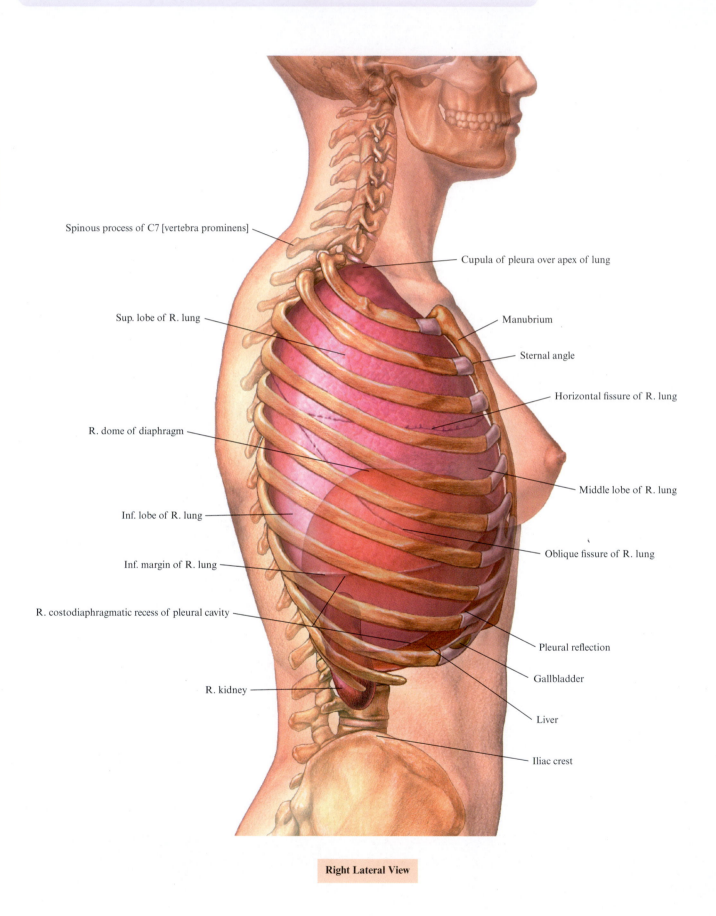

Spinous process of C7 [vertebra prominens]

Cupula of pleura over apex of lung

Sup. lobe of R. lung

Manubrium

Sternal angle

Horizontal fissure of R. lung

R. dome of diaphragm

Middle lobe of R. lung

Inf. lobe of R. lung

Oblique fissure of R. lung

Inf. margin of R. lung

R. costodiaphragmatic recess of pleural cavity

Pleural reflection

Gallbladder

R. kidney

Liver

Iliac crest

Right Lateral View

A.D.A.M. | Student Atlas of Anatomy

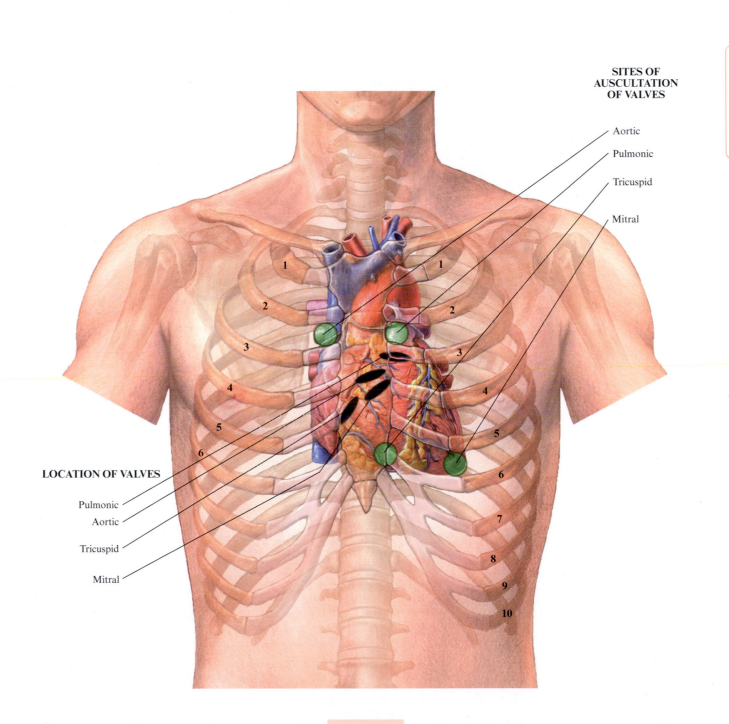

SITES OF
AUSCULTATION
OF VALVES

Aortic

Pulmonic

Tricuspid

Mitral

LOCATION OF VALVES

Pulmonic

Aortic

Tricuspid

Mitral

Anterior View

PLATE 2.7   THORACIC VISCERA IN SITU

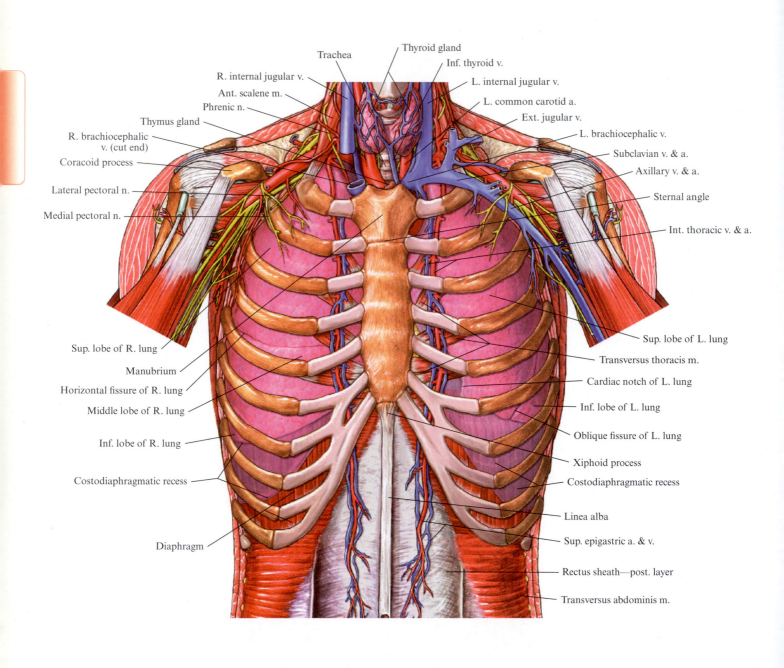

Trachea
Thyroid gland
Inf. thyroid v.
R. internal jugular v.
Ant. scalene m.
Phrenic n.
Thymus gland
R. brachiocephalic v. (cut end)
Coracoid process
Lateral pectoral n.
Medial pectoral n.
L. internal jugular v.
L. common carotid a.
Ext. jugular v.
L. brachiocephalic v.
Subclavian v. & a.
Axillary v. & a.
Sternal angle
Int. thoracic v. & a.
Sup. lobe of R. lung
Manubrium
Horizontal fissure of R. lung
Middle lobe of R. lung
Inf. lobe of R. lung
Costodiaphragmatic recess
Diaphragm
Sup. lobe of L. lung
Transversus thoracis m.
Cardiac notch of L. lung
Inf. lobe of L. lung
Oblique fissure of L. lung
Xiphoid process
Costodiaphragmatic recess
Linea alba
Sup. epigastric a. & v.
Rectus sheath—post. layer
Transversus abdominis m.

Anterior View

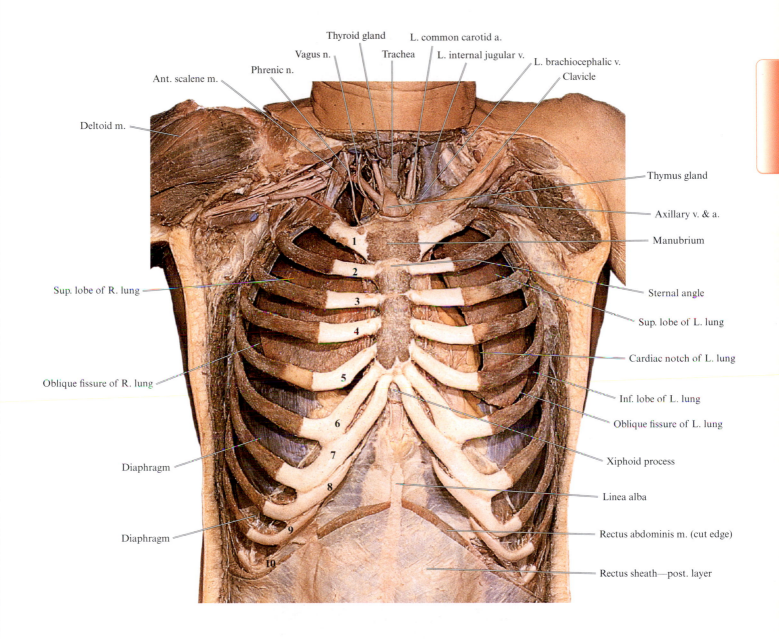

Thyroid gland

L. common carotid a.

Vagus n.

Trachea

L. internal jugular v.

L. brachiocephalic v.

Clavicle

Phrenic n.

Ant. scalene m.

Deltoid m.

Thymus gland

Axillary v. & a.

Manubrium

1

2

3

4

5

6

7

8

9

10

Sup. lobe of R. lung

Sternal angle

Sup. lobe of L. lung

Cardiac notch of L. lung

Oblique fissure of R. lung

Inf. lobe of L. lung

Oblique fissure of L. lung

Xiphoid process

Diaphragm

Linea alba

Diaphragm

Rectus abdominis m. (cut edge)

Rectus sheath—post. layer

Anterior View

PLATE 2.11   TRACHEA, BRONCHI & LUNGS

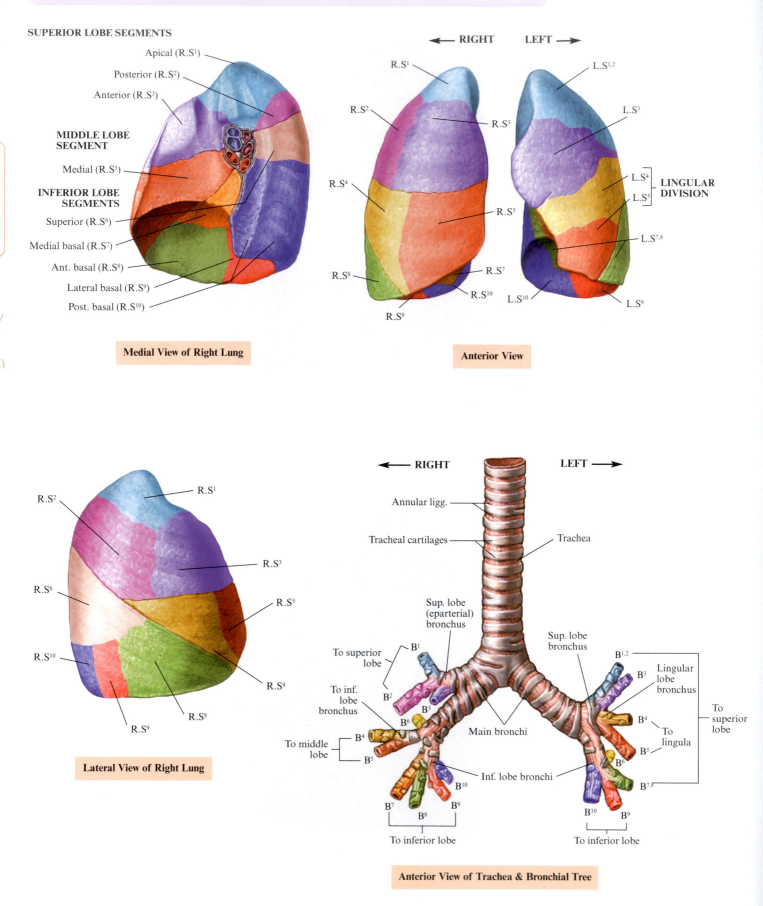

SUPERIOR LOBE SEGMENTS

Apical (R.S¹)
Posterior (R.S²)
Anterior (R.S³)

MIDDLE LOBE
SEGMENT

Medial (R.S⁵)

INFERIOR LOBE
SEGMENTS

Superior (R.S⁶)
Medial basal (R.S⁷)
Ant. basal (R.S⁸)
Lateral basal (R.S⁹)
Post. basal (R.S¹⁰)

Medial View of Right Lung

← RIGHT   LEFT →

R.S¹
R.S²   R.S³   L.S¹,²
R.S⁴   L.S³
R.S⁵   L.S⁴ LINGULAR
           L.S⁵ DIVISION
R.S⁸   R.S⁷ L.S⁷,⁸
R.S⁹   R.S¹⁰ L.S¹⁰ L.S⁹

Anterior View

R.S²   R.S¹
R.S⁶   R.S³
R.S¹⁰   R.S⁵
           R.S⁴
R.S⁹ R.S⁸

Lateral View of Right Lung

← RIGHT   LEFT →

Annular ligg.
Tracheal cartilages   Trachea

Sup. lobe
(eparterial)
bronchus   Sup. lobe
                            bronchus
To superior   B¹   B¹,²   Lingular
lobe   lobe
                     B²   B³   B³   bronchus
To inf.   B³   To
lobe   B⁶   B⁴   superior
bronchus   lobe
To middle   B⁴   Main bronchi   B⁵ To
lobe   B⁵   lingula
                                   B⁶
                     Inf. lobe bronchi B⁷,⁸
               B¹⁰
         B⁷   B⁹   B¹⁰   B⁹
              B⁸
To inferior lobe   To inferior lobe

Anterior View of Trachea & Bronchial Tree

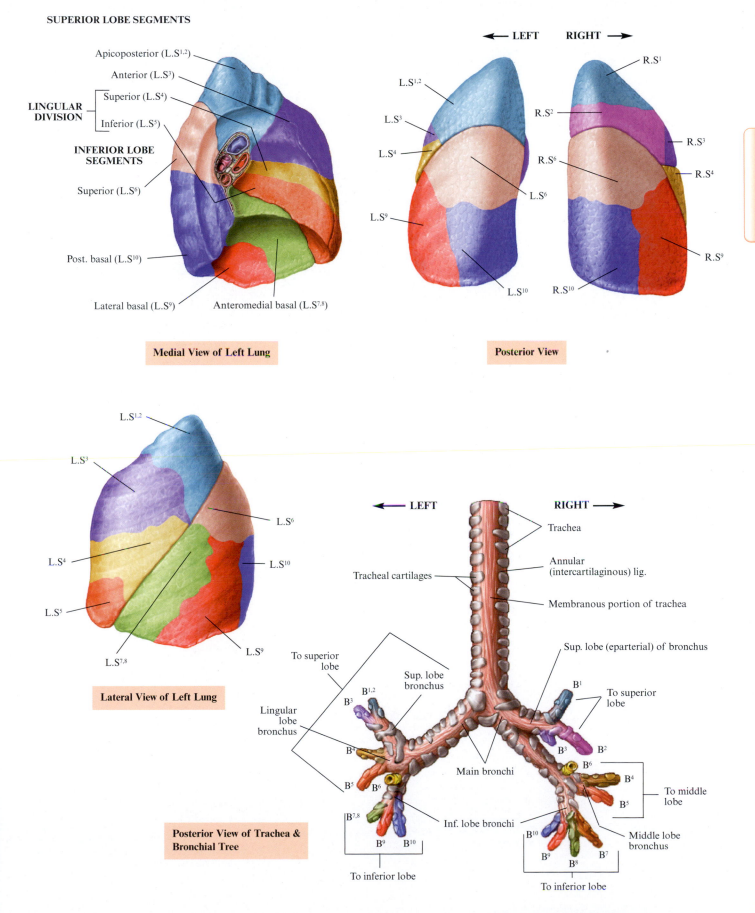

SUPERIOR LOBE SEGMENTS

Apicoposterior (L.S¹,²)

Anterior (L.S³)

LINGULAR DIVISION — Superior (L.S⁴)

Inferior (L.S⁵)

INFERIOR LOBE SEGMENTS

Superior (L.S⁶)

Post. basal (L.S¹⁰)

Lateral basal (L.S⁹)

Anteromedial basal (L.S⁷,⁸)

Medial View of Left Lung

← LEFT   RIGHT →

L.S¹,²   R.S¹
L.S³   R.S²
L.S⁴   R.S³
              R.S⁶
              R.S⁴
L.S⁶
L.S⁹
              R.S⁹
L.S¹⁰   R.S¹⁰

Posterior View

L.S¹,²
L.S³
L.S⁶
L.S⁴
L.S¹⁰
L.S⁵
L.S⁹
L.S⁷,⁸

Lateral View of Left Lung

← LEFT   RIGHT →

Trachea

Tracheal cartilages

Annular (intercartilaginous) lig.

Membranous portion of trachea

Sup. lobe (eparterial) of bronchus

To superior lobe

Sup. lobe bronchus

B¹,²
B³
B¹
To superior lobe

Lingular lobe bronchus

B⁴
B³   B²
B⁶
B⁴

B⁵
B⁶
B⁵
To middle lobe

Main bronchi

Middle lobe bronchus

B⁷,⁸
Inf. lobe bronchi

B¹⁰
B⁹   B¹⁰

B⁹   B⁸   B⁷

To inferior lobe

Posterior View of Trachea & Bronchial Tree

To inferior lobe

PLATE 2.13   TRACHEA, BRONCHI & LUNGS—LYMPHATICS

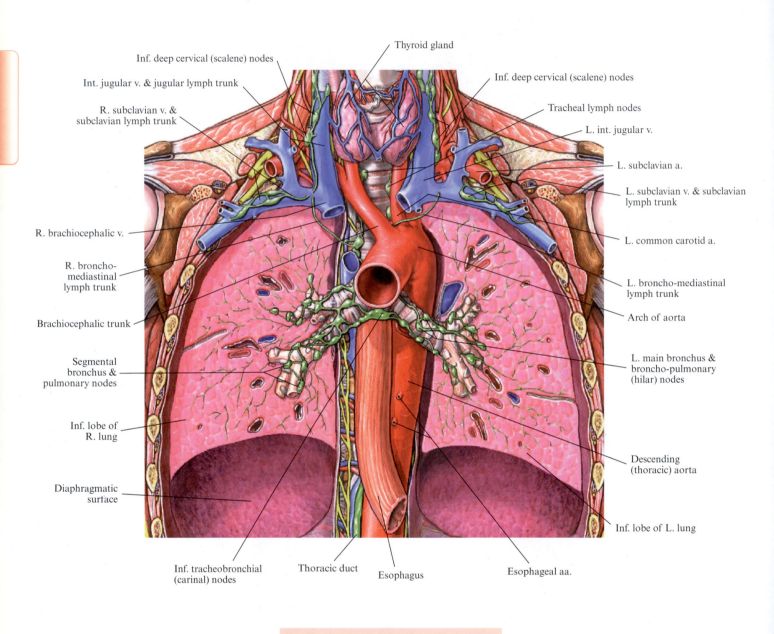

Thyroid gland

Inf. deep cervical (scalene) nodes

Int. jugular v. & jugular lymph trunk

R. subclavian v. &
subclavian lymph trunk

R. brachiocephalic v.

R. broncho-
mediastinal
lymph trunk

Brachiocephalic trunk

Segmental
bronchus &
pulmonary nodes

Inf. lobe of
R. lung

Diaphragmatic
surface

Inf. deep cervical (scalene) nodes

Tracheal lymph nodes

L. int. jugular v.

L. subclavian a.

L. subclavian v. & subclavian
lymph trunk

L. common carotid a.

L. broncho-mediastinal
lymph trunk

Arch of aorta

L. main bronchus &
broncho-pulmonary
(hilar) nodes

Descending
(thoracic) aorta

Inf. lobe of L. lung

Inf. tracheobronchial
(carinal) nodes

Thoracic duct

Esophagus

Esophageal aa.

Anterior View with Coronally Sectioned Lungs

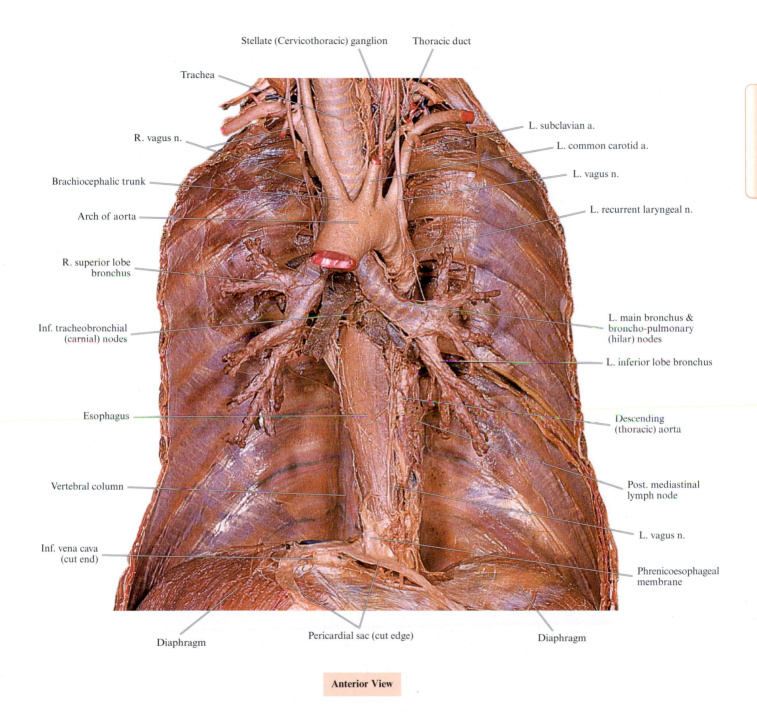

Stellate (Cervicothoracic) ganglion

Thoracic duct

Trachea

R. vagus n.

Brachiocephalic trunk

Arch of aorta

R. superior lobe bronchus

Inf. tracheobronchial (carnial) nodes

Esophagus

Vertebral column

Inf. vena cava (cut end)

Diaphragm

Pericardial sac (cut edge)

Diaphragm

L. subclavian a.

L. common carotid a.

L. vagus n.

L. recurrent laryngeal n.

L. main bronchus & broncho-pulmonary (hilar) nodes

L. inferior lobe bronchus

Descending (thoracic) aorta

Post. mediastinal lymph node

L. vagus n.

Phrenicoesophageal membrane

Anterior View

PLATE 2.15   LUNGS & HEART—CROSS SECTION

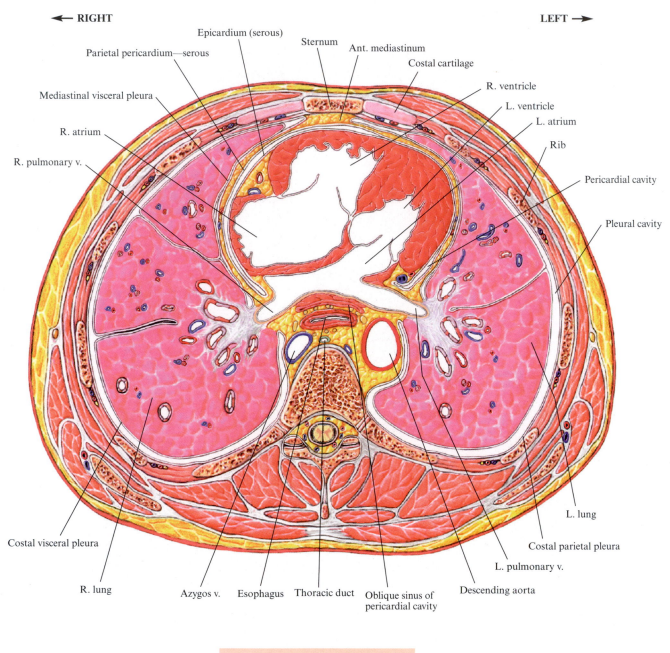

← RIGHT   LEFT →

Epicardium (serous)

Parietal pericardium—serous

Sternum   Ant. mediastinum

Costal cartilage

Mediastinal visceral pleura

R. ventricle

R. atrium

L. ventricle

R. pulmonary v.

L. atrium

Rib

Pericardial cavity

Pleural cavity

L. lung

Costal visceral pleura

Costal parietal pleura

R. lung   Azygos v.   Esophagus   Thoracic duct   Oblique sinus of
                                                          pericardial cavity

L. pulmonary v.

Descending aorta

Transverse Section at T8—Inferior View

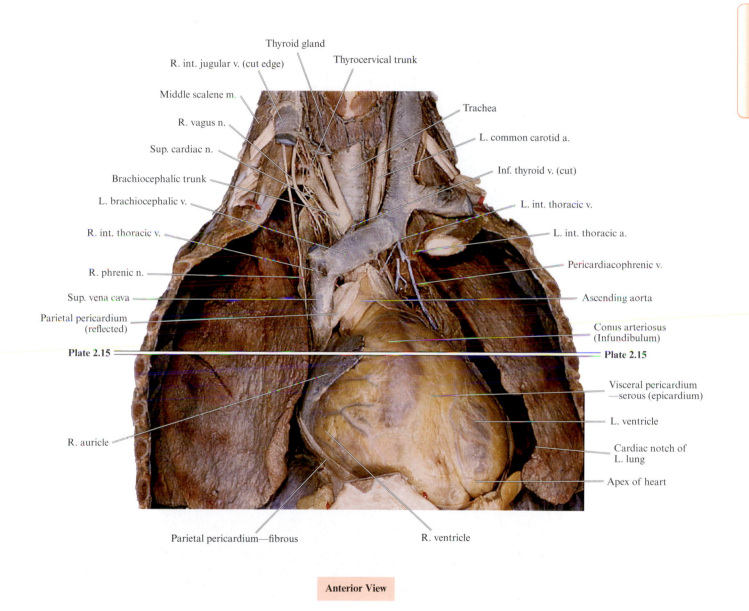

Thyroid gland

R. int. jugular v. (cut edge)

Thyrocervical trunk

Middle scalene m.

Trachea

R. vagus n.

L. common carotid a.

Sup. cardiac n.

Inf. thyroid v. (cut)

Brachiocephalic trunk

L. brachiocephalic v.

L. int. thoracic v.

R. int. thoracic v.

L. int. thoracic a.

R. phrenic n.

Pericardiacophrenic v.

Sup. vena cava

Ascending aorta

Parietal pericardium
(reflected)

Conus arteriosus
(Infundibulum)

Plate 2.15

Plate 2.15

Visceral pericardium
—serous (epicardium)

L. ventricle

R. auricle

Cardiac notch of
L. lung

Apex of heart

Parietal pericardium—fibrous

R. ventricle

Anterior View

PLATE 2.19   HEART IN SYSTOLE & DIASTOLE

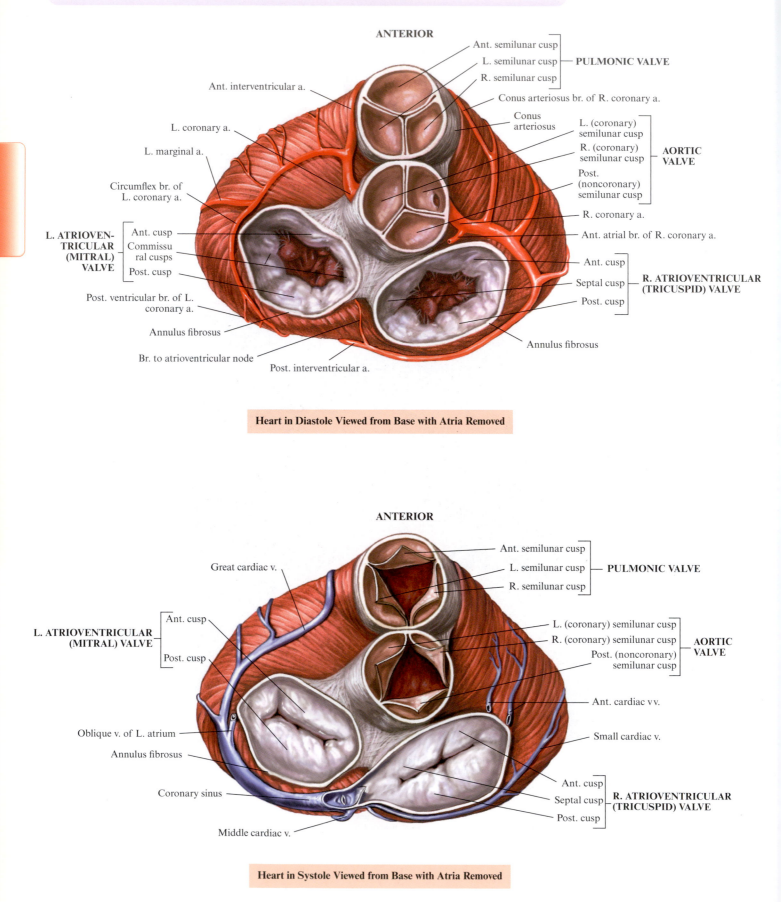

ANTERIOR

Ant. interventricular a.

L. coronary a.

L. marginal a.

Circumflex br. of
L. coronary a.

**L. ATRIOVEN-
TRICULAR
(MITRAL)
VALVE**
Ant. cusp
Commissu
ral cusps
Post. cusp

Post. ventricular br. of L.
coronary a.

Annulus fibrosus

Br. to atrioventricular node

Post. interventricular a.

Ant. semilunar cusp
L. semilunar cusp   **PULMONIC VALVE**
R. semilunar cusp

Conus arteriosus br. of R. coronary a.

Conus
arteriosus

L. (coronary)
semilunar cusp
R. (coronary)
semilunar cusp   **AORTIC
VALVE**
Post.
(noncoronary)
semilunar cusp

R. coronary a.

Ant. atrial br. of R. coronary a.

Ant. cusp
Septal cusp   **R. ATRIOVENTRICULAR
(TRICUSPID) VALVE**
Post. cusp

Annulus fibrosus

Heart in Diastole Viewed from Base with Atria Removed

ANTERIOR

Great cardiac v.

**L. ATRIOVENTRICULAR
(MITRAL) VALVE**
Ant. cusp

Post. cusp

Oblique v. of L. atrium

Annulus fibrosus

Coronary sinus

Middle cardiac v.

Ant. semilunar cusp
L. semilunar cusp   **PULMONIC VALVE**
R. semilunar cusp

L. (coronary) semilunar cusp
R. (coronary) semilunar cusp   **AORTIC
VALVE**
Post. (noncoronary)
semilunar cusp

Ant. cardiac vv.

Small cardiac v.

Ant. cusp
Septal cusp   **R. ATRIOVENTRICULAR
(TRICUSPID) VALVE**
Post. cusp

Heart in Systole Viewed from Base with Atria Removed

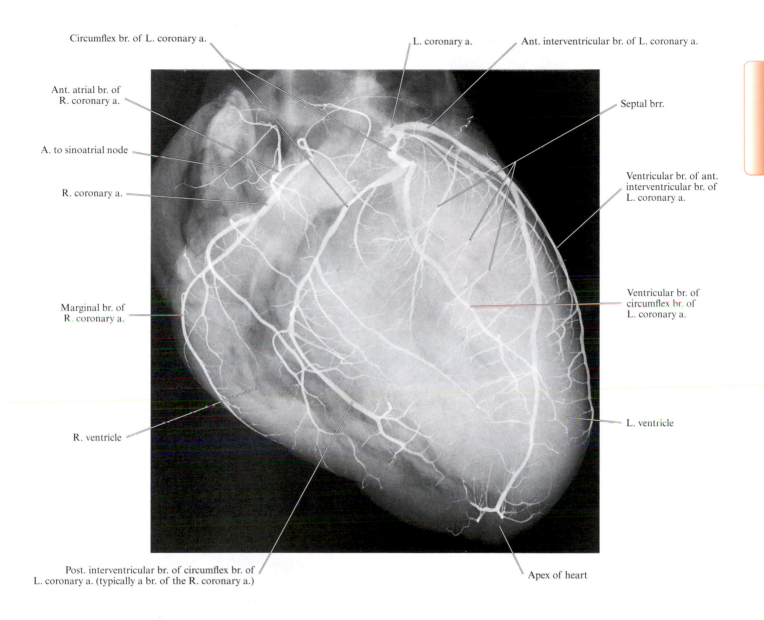

Circumflex br. of L. coronary a.

L. coronary a.

Ant. interventricular br. of L. coronary a.

Ant. atrial br. of
R. coronary a.

Septal brr.

A. to sinoatrial node

R. coronary a.

Ventricular br. of ant.
interventricular br. of
L. coronary a.

Marginal br. of
R. coronary a.

Ventricular br. of
circumflex br. of
L. coronary a.

R. ventricle

L. ventricle

Post. interventricular br. of circumflex br. of
L. coronary a. (typically a br. of the R. coronary a.)

Apex of heart

Anteroposterior View

PLATE 2.23 RIGHT ATRIUM

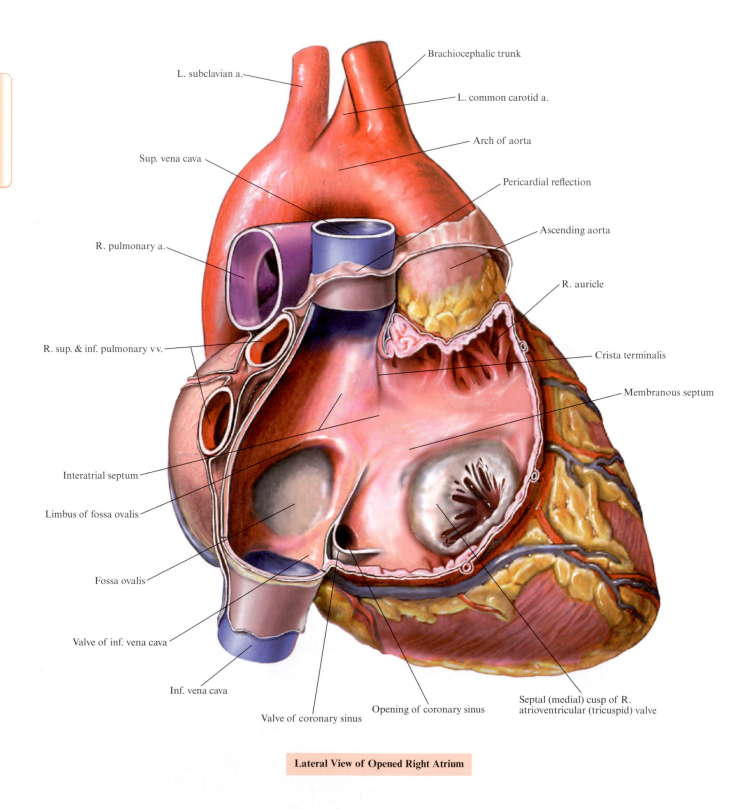

L. subclavian a.

Brachiocephalic trunk

L. common carotid a.

Arch of aorta

Sup. vena cava

Pericardial reflection

Ascending aorta

R. pulmonary a.

R. auricle

R. sup. & inf. pulmonary v v.

Crista terminalis

Membranous septum

Interatrial septum

Limbus of fossa ovalis

Fossa ovalis

Valve of inf. vena cava

Inf. vena cava

Septal (medial) cusp of R.
atrioventricular (tricuspid) valve

Valve of coronary sinus

Opening of coronary sinus

Lateral View of Opened Right Atrium

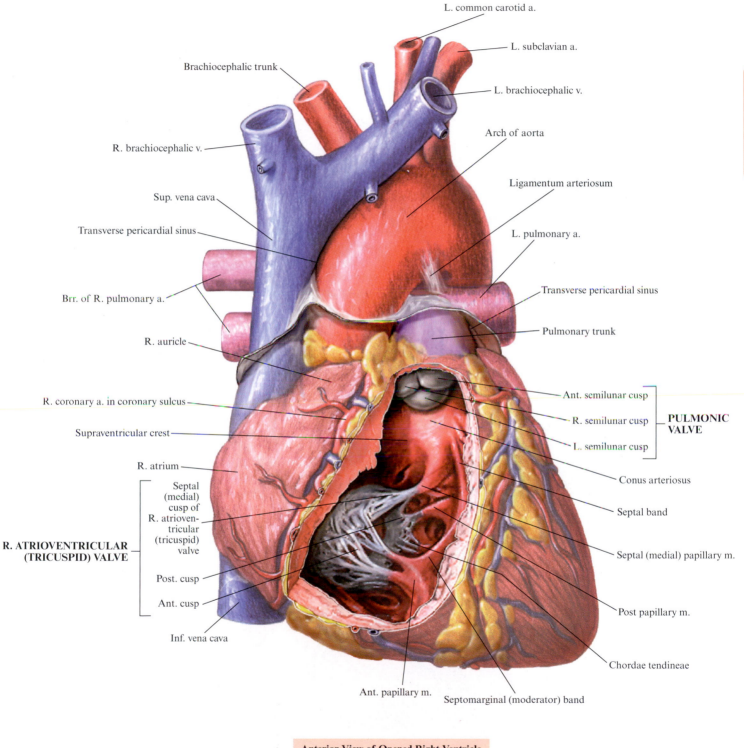

L. common carotid a.

L. subclavian a.

Brachiocephalic trunk

L. brachiocephalic v.

Arch of aorta

R. brachiocephalic v.

Ligamentum arteriosum

Sup. vena cava

L. pulmonary a.

Transverse pericardial sinus

Transverse pericardial sinus

Brr. of R. pulmonary a.

Pulmonary trunk

R. auricle

Ant. semilunar cusp

R. coronary a. in coronary sulcus

R. semilunar cusp

PULMONIC VALVE

Supraventricular crest

L. semilunar cusp

R. atrium

Conus arteriosus

Septal (medial) cusp of R. atrioventricular (tricuspid) valve

Septal band

R. ATRIOVENTRICULAR (TRICUSPID) VALVE

Septal (medial) papillary m.

Post. cusp

Ant. cusp

Post papillary m.

Inf. vena cava

Chordae tendineae

Ant. papillary m.

Septomarginal (moderator) band

Anterior View of Opened Right Ventricle

PLATE 2.27   PERICARDIAL CAVITY

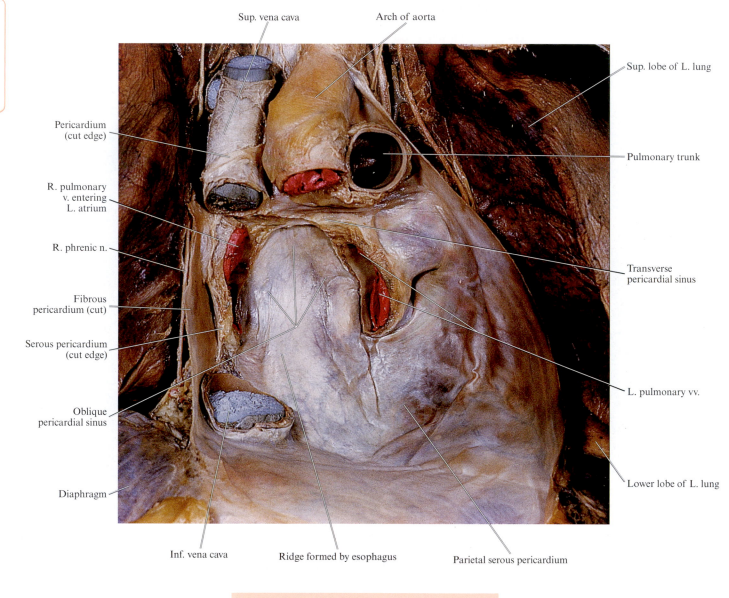

Sup. vena cava

Arch of aorta

Sup. lobe of L. lung

Pericardium (cut edge)

Pulmonary trunk

R. pulmonary v. entering L. atrium

R. phrenic n.

Transverse pericardial sinus

Fibrous pericardium (cut)

Serous pericardium (cut edge)

L. pulmonary vv.

Oblique pericardial sinus

Diaphragm

Lower lobe of L. lung

Inf. vena cava

Ridge formed by esophagus

Parietal serous pericardium

Anterior View of Pericardial Cavity with Heart Removed

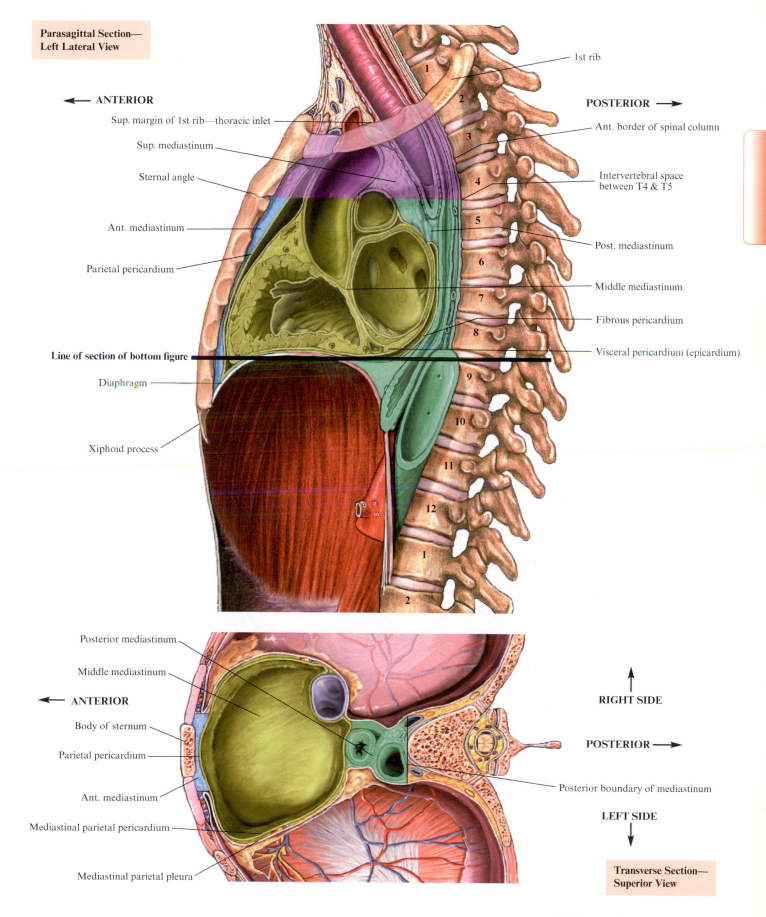

Parasagittal Section—Left Lateral View

← ANTERIOR

POSTERIOR →

1st rib

Sup. margin of 1st rib—thoracic inlet

Sup. mediastinum

Sternal angle

Ant. border of spinal column

Intervertebral space between T4 & T5

Ant. mediastinum

Parietal pericardium

Post. mediastinum

Middle mediastinum

Fibrous pericardium

Line of section of bottom figure

Visceral pericardium (epicardium)

Diaphragm

Xiphoid process

Posterior mediastinum

Middle mediastinum

← ANTERIOR

RIGHT SIDE

Body of sternum

POSTERIOR →

Parietal pericardium

Ant. mediastinum

Posterior boundary of mediastinum

Mediastinal parietal pericardium

LEFT SIDE

Mediastinal parietal pleura

Transverse Section—Superior View

PLATE 2.35 ESOPHAGUS

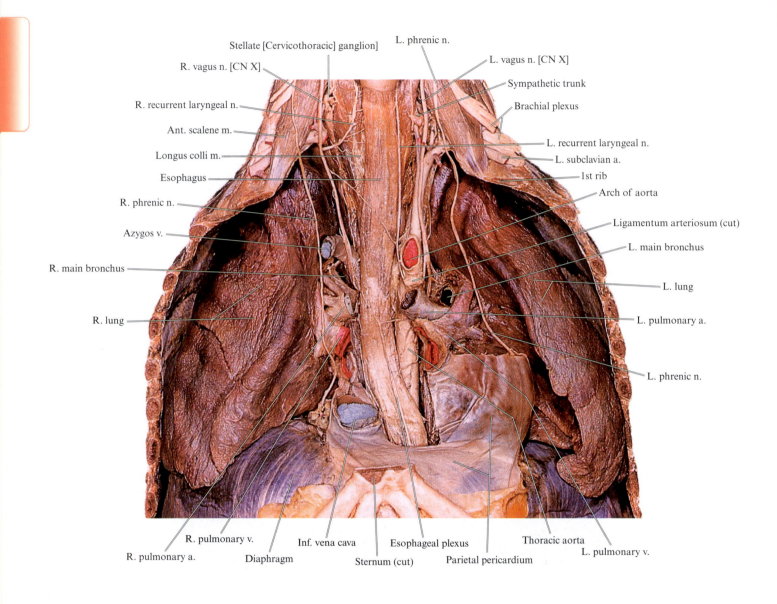

Stellate [Cervicothoracic] ganglion]

L. phrenic n.

R. vagus n. [CN X]

L. vagus n. [CN X]

Sympathetic trunk

R. recurrent laryngeal n.

Brachial plexus

Ant. scalene m.

L. recurrent laryngeal n.

Longus colli m.

L. subclavian a.

Esophagus

1st rib

R. phrenic n.

Arch of aorta

Azygos v.

Ligamentum arteriosum (cut)

L. main bronchus

R. main bronchus

L. lung

R. lung

L. pulmonary a.

L. phrenic n.

R. pulmonary v.

Esophageal plexus

Thoracic aorta

R. pulmonary a.

Diaphragm

Inf. vena cava

Sternum (cut)

Parietal pericardium

L. pulmonary v.

Anterior View of Posterior Mediastinal Structures

A.D.A.M. | Student Atlas of Anatomy

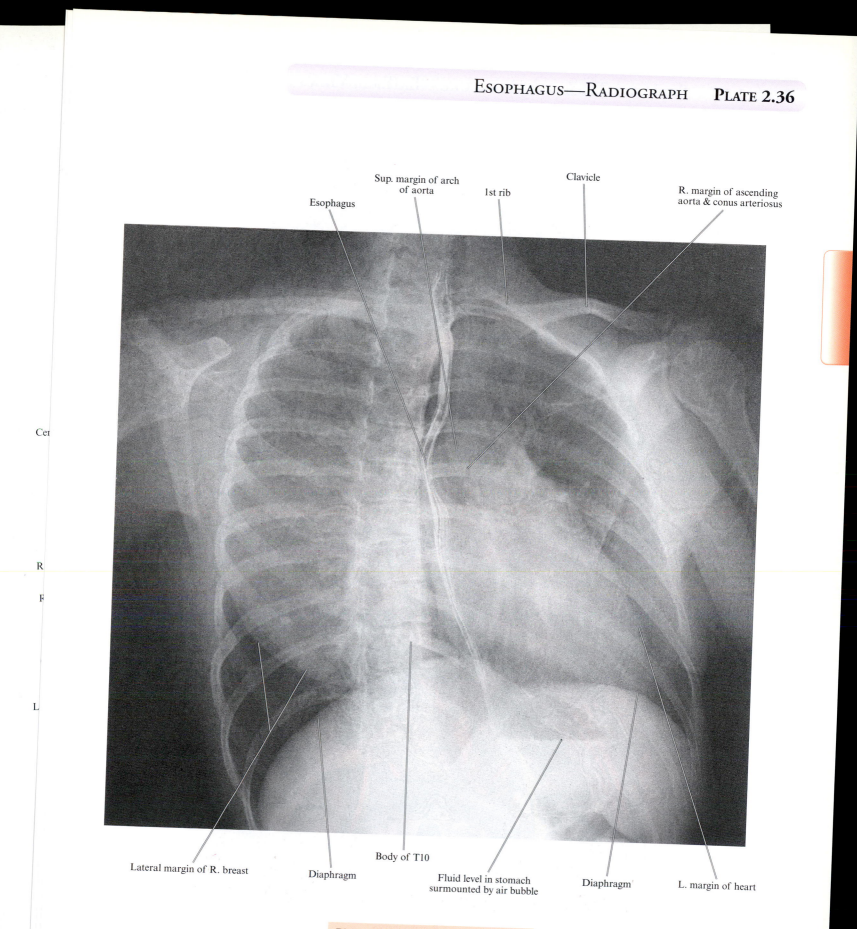

Sup. margin of arch of aorta

Esophagus

1st rib

Clavicle

R. margin of ascending aorta & conus arteriosus

Lateral margin of R. breast

Diaphragm

Body of T10

Fluid level in stomach surmounted by air bubble

Diaphragm

L. margin of heart

Right Anterior Oblique View of Esophagus

G

Le

ABDOMEN

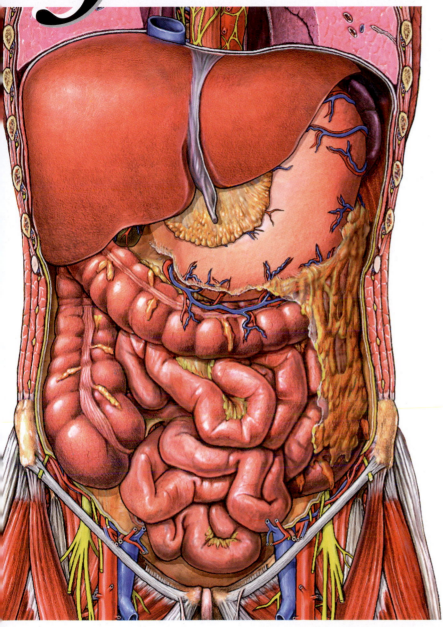

TOPOGRAPHY

PERITONEAL CAVITY

STOMACH

PANCREAS

GALLBLADDER &
DUCTS

LIVER

SMALL INTESTINES

LARGE INTESTINES

POSTERIOR ABDOMINAL
WALL

KIDNEYS &
SUPRARENAL GLANDS

PLATE 3.1 TOPOGRAPHY—ABDOMINAL PLANES & LINES

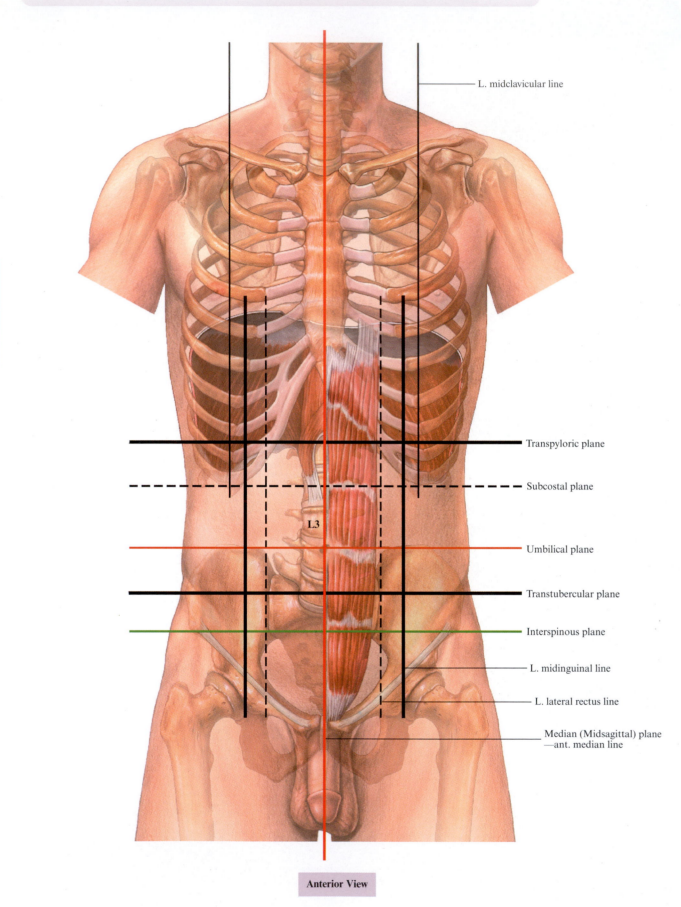

L. midclavicular line

Transpyloric plane

Subcostal plane

L3

Umbilical plane

Transtubercular plane

Interspinous plane

L. midinguinal line

L. lateral rectus line

Median (Midsagittal) plane
—ant. median line

Anterior View

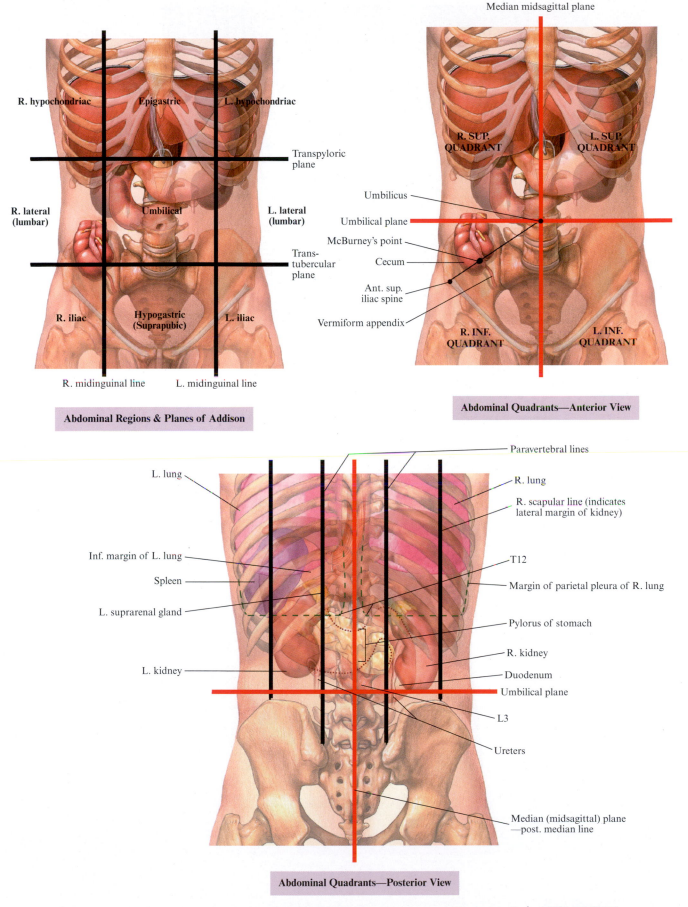

Median midsagittal plane

R. hypochondriac   Epigastric   L. hypochondriac

Transpyloric plane

R. lateral (lumbar)   Umbilical   L. lateral (lumbar)

Trans-tubercular plane

R. iliac   Hypogastric (Suprapubic)   L. iliac

R. midinguinal line   L. midinguinal line

Abdominal Regions & Planes of Addison

R. SUP. QUADRANT   L. SUP. QUADRANT

Umbilicus
Umbilical plane
McBurney's point
Cecum
Ant. sup. iliac spine
Vermiform appendix

R. INF. QUADRANT   L. INF. QUADRANT

Abdominal Quadrants—Anterior View

Paravertebral lines
L. lung
R. lung
R. scapular line (indicates lateral margin of kidney)
Inf. margin of L. lung
Spleen
T12
Margin of parietal pleura of R. lung
L. suprarenal gland
Pylorus of stomach
R. kidney
L. kidney
Duodenum
Umbilical plane
L3
Ureters
Median (midsagittal) plane —post. median line

Abdominal Quadrants—Posterior View

PLATE 3.3   PERITONEAL CAVITY

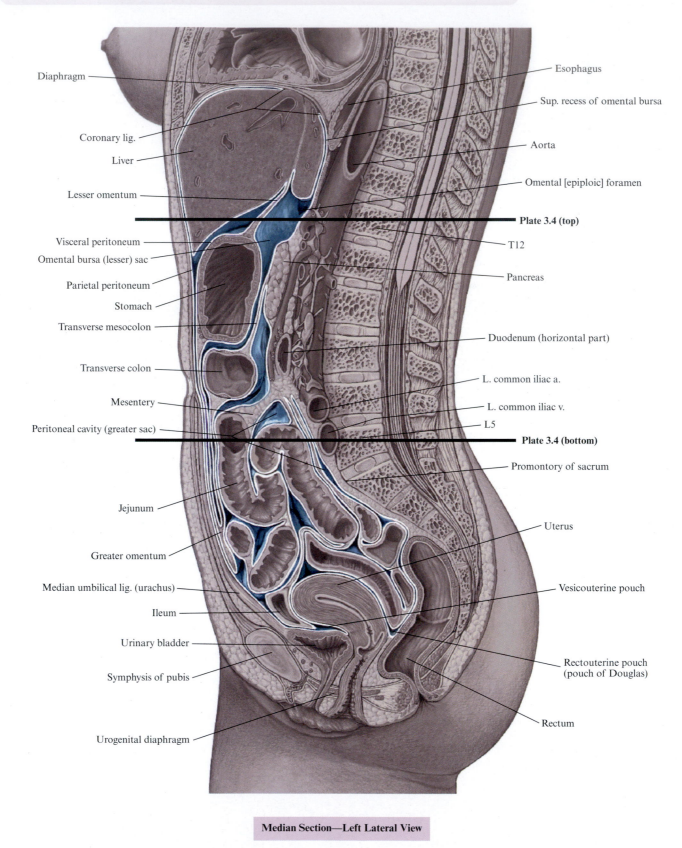

Diaphragm

Coronary lig.

Liver

Lesser omentum

Visceral peritoneum

Omental bursa (lesser) sac

Parietal peritoneum

Stomach

Transverse mesocolon

Transverse colon

Mesentery

Peritoneal cavity (greater sac)

Jejunum

Greater omentum

Median umbilical lig. (urachus)

Ileum

Urinary bladder

Symphysis of pubis

Urogenital diaphragm

Esophagus

Sup. recess of omental bursa

Aorta

Omental [epiploic] foramen

Plate 3.4 (top)

T12

Pancreas

Duodenum (horizontal part)

L. common iliac a.

L. common iliac v.

L5

Plate 3.4 (bottom)

Promontory of sacrum

Uterus

Vesicouterine pouch

Rectouterine pouch
(pouch of Douglas)

Rectum

Median Section—Left Lateral View

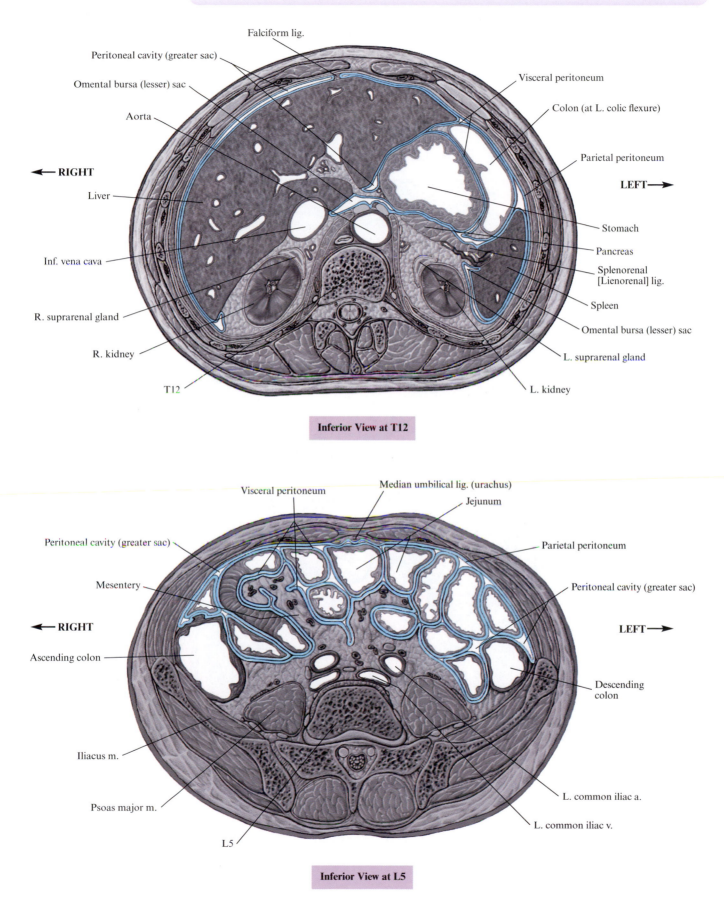

Falciform lig.

Peritoneal cavity (greater sac)

Omental bursa (lesser) sac

Aorta

Visceral peritoneum

Colon (at L. colic flexure)

Parietal peritoneum

← **RIGHT**

LEFT →

Liver

Inf. vena cava

Stomach

Pancreas

Splenorenal [Lienorenal] lig.

Spleen

Omental bursa (lesser) sac

R. suprarenal gland

R. kidney

L. suprarenal gland

T12

L. kidney

Inferior View at T12

Visceral peritoneum

Median umbilical lig. (urachus)

Jejunum

Peritoneal cavity (greater sac)

Parietal peritoneum

Mesentery

Peritoneal cavity (greater sac)

← **RIGHT**

LEFT →

Ascending colon

Descending colon

Iliacus m.

Psoas major m.

L. common iliac a.

L. common iliac v.

L5

Inferior View at L5

PLATE 3.7   PERITONEAL CAVITY—CONTENTS

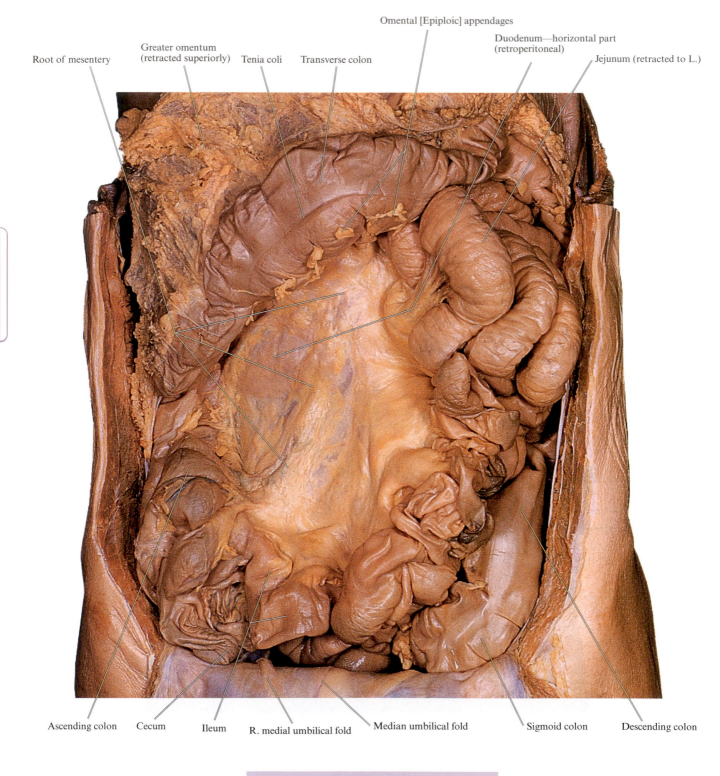

Omental [Epiploic] appendages

Duodenum—horizontal part
(retroperitoneal)

Root of mesentery   Greater omentum   Tenia coli   Transverse colon   Jejunum (retracted to L.)
(retracted superiorly)

Ascending colon   Cecum   Ileum   R. medial umbilical fold   Median umbilical fold   Sigmoid colon   Descending colon

Anterior View with Small Intestines Retracted to Left

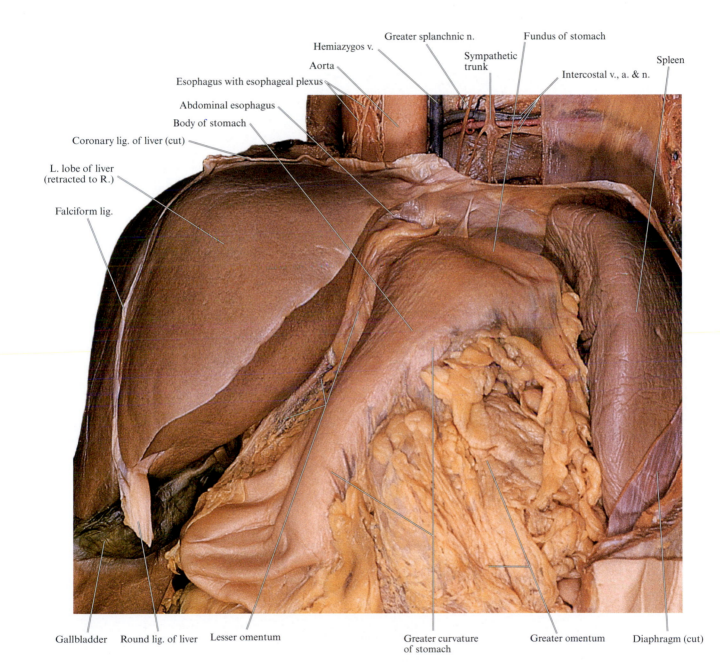

Greater splanchnic n.

Fundus of stomach

Hemiazygos v.

Sympathetic trunk

Spleen

Aorta

Intercostal v., a. & n.

Esophagus with esophageal plexus

Abdominal esophagus

Body of stomach

Coronary lig. of liver (cut)

L. lobe of liver (retracted to R.)

Falciform lig.

Gallbladder   Round lig. of liver   Lesser omentum

Greater curvature of stomach

Greater omentum

Diaphragm (cut)

Left Anterolateral View

PLATE 3.9   STOMACH

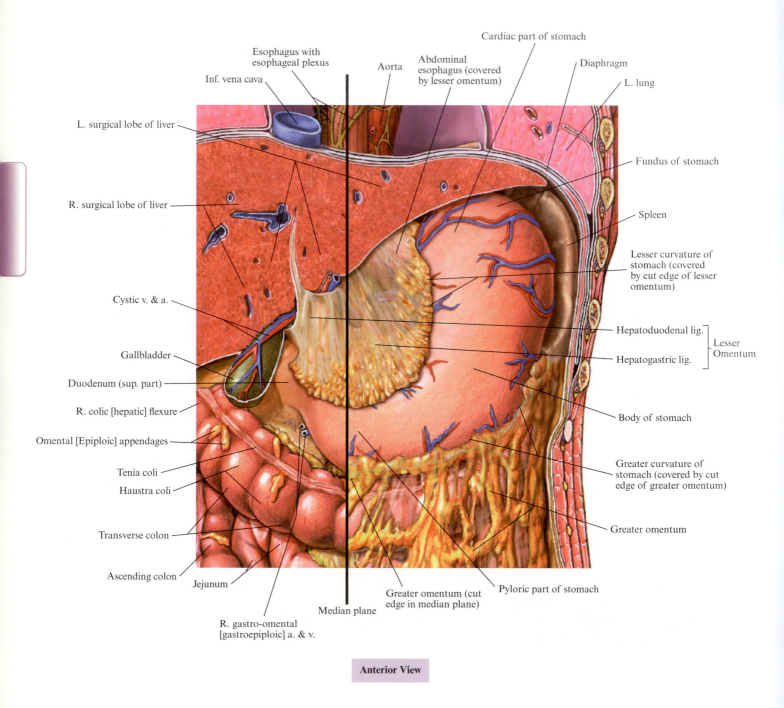

Esophagus with esophageal plexus

Inf. vena cava

Aorta

Abdominal esophagus (covered by lesser omentum)

Cardiac part of stomach

Diaphragm

L. lung

L. surgical lobe of liver

R. surgical lobe of liver

Fundus of stomach

Spleen

Lesser curvature of stomach (covered by cut edge of lesser omentum)

Cystic v. & a.

Gallbladder

Duodenum (sup. part)

R. colic [hepatic] flexure

Omental [Epiploic] appendages

Tenia coli

Haustra coli

Transverse colon

Ascending colon

Jejunum

Hepatoduodenal lig.
Hepatogastric lig.
} Lesser Omentum

Body of stomach

Greater curvature of stomach (covered by cut edge of greater omentum)

Greater omentum

Median plane

R. gastro-omental [gastroepiploic] a. & v.

Greater omentum (cut edge in median plane)

Pyloric part of stomach

Anterior View

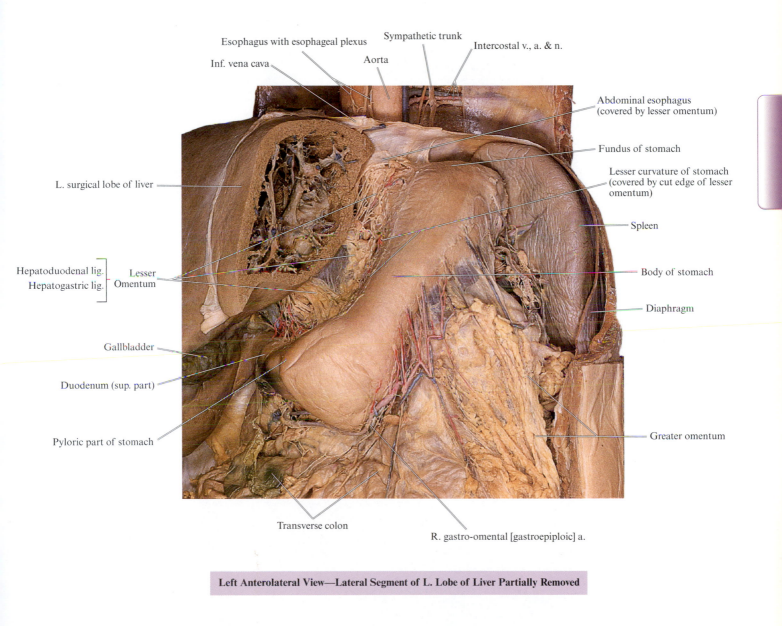

Esophagus with esophageal plexus

Sympathetic trunk

Intercostal v., a. & n.

Inf. vena cava

Aorta

Abdominal esophagus
(covered by lesser omentum)

L. surgical lobe of liver

Fundus of stomach

Lesser curvature of stomach
(covered by cut edge of lesser
omentum)

Spleen

Hepatoduodenal lig.

Hepatogastric lig.

Lesser
Omentum

Body of stomach

Diaphragm

Gallbladder

Duodenum (sup. part)

Pyloric part of stomach

Greater omentum

Transverse colon

R. gastro-omental [gastroepiploic] a.

Left Anterolateral View—Lateral Segment of L. Lobe of Liver Partially Removed

PLATE 3.11   STOMACH

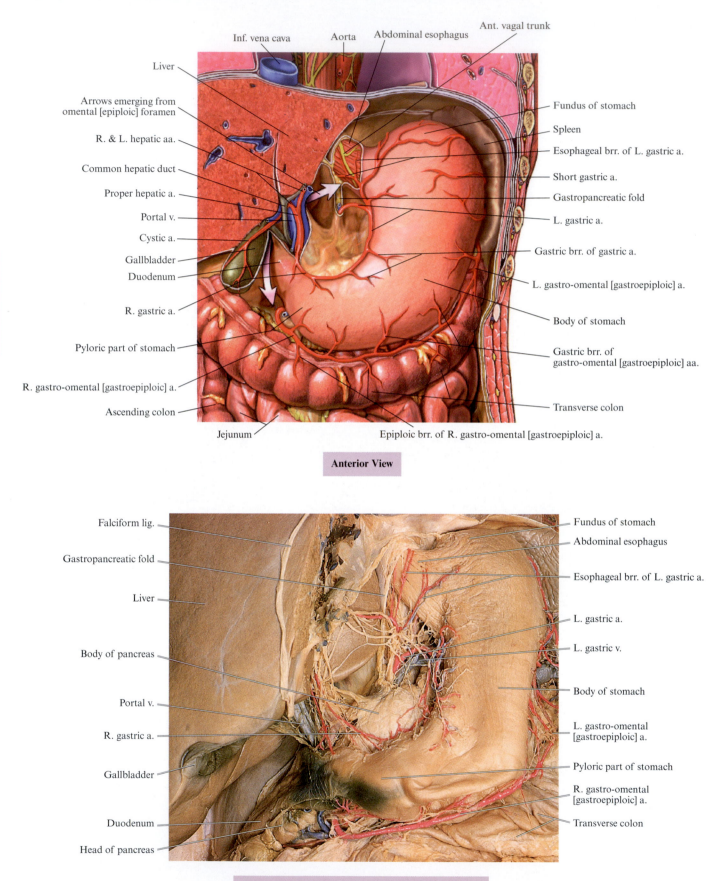

Inf. vena cava

Aorta

Abdominal esophagus

Ant. vagal trunk

Liver

Arrows emerging from omental [epiploic] foramen

R. & L. hepatic aa.

Common hepatic duct

Proper hepatic a.

Portal v.

Cystic a.

Gallbladder

Duodenum

R. gastric a.

Pyloric part of stomach

R. gastro-omental [gastroepiploic] a.

Ascending colon

Jejunum

Fundus of stomach

Spleen

Esophageal brr. of L. gastric a.

Short gastric a.

Gastropancreatic fold

L. gastric a.

Gastric brr. of gastric a.

L. gastro-omental [gastroepiploic] a.

Body of stomach

Gastric brr. of gastro-omental [gastroepiploic] aa.

Transverse colon

Epiploic brr. of R. gastro-omental [gastroepiploic] a.

Anterior View

Falciform lig.

Gastropancreatic fold

Liver

Body of pancreas

Portal v.

R. gastric a.

Gallbladder

Duodenum

Head of pancreas

Fundus of stomach

Abdominal esophagus

Esophageal brr. of L. gastric a.

L. gastric a.

L. gastric v.

Body of stomach

L. gastro-omental [gastroepiploic] a.

Pyloric part of stomach

R. gastro-omental [gastroepiploic] a.

Transverse colon

Anterior View—Liver Left of Falciform Lig. Removed

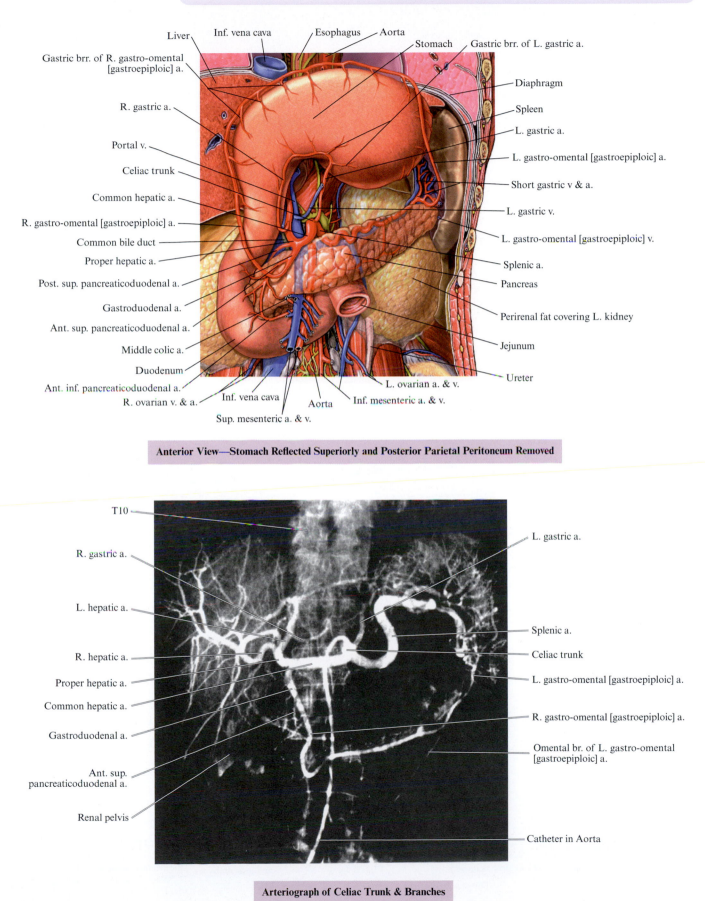

Liver — Inf. vena cava — Esophagus — Aorta

Stomach — Gastric brr. of L. gastric a.

Gastric brr. of R. gastro-omental [gastroepiploic] a.

Diaphragm

R. gastric a.

Spleen

L. gastric a.

Portal v.

L. gastro-omental [gastroepiploic] a.

Celiac trunk

Short gastric v & a.

Common hepatic a.

L. gastric v.

R. gastro-omental [gastroepiploic] a.

L. gastro-omental [gastroepiploic] v.

Common bile duct

Splenic a.

Proper hepatic a.

Pancreas

Post. sup. pancreaticoduodenal a.

Perirenal fat covering L. kidney

Gastroduodenal a.

Ant. sup. pancreaticoduodenal a.

Jejunum

Middle colic a.

Duodenum

Ureter

Ant. inf. pancreaticoduodenal a.

L. ovarian a. & v.

R. ovarian v. & a. — Inf. vena cava — Aorta — Inf. mesenteric a. & v.

Sup. mesenteric a. & v.

Anterior View—Stomach Reflected Superiorly and Posterior Parietal Peritoneum Removed

T10

L. gastric a.

R. gastric a.

L. hepatic a.

Splenic a.

R. hepatic a.

Celiac trunk

Proper hepatic a.

L. gastro-omental [gastroepiploic] a.

Common hepatic a.

R. gastro-omental [gastroepiploic] a.

Gastroduodenal a.

Omental br. of L. gastro-omental [gastroepiploic] a.

Ant. sup. pancreaticoduodenal a.

Renal pelvis

Catheter in Aorta

Arteriograph of Celiac Trunk & Branches

PLATE 3.13   PANCREAS

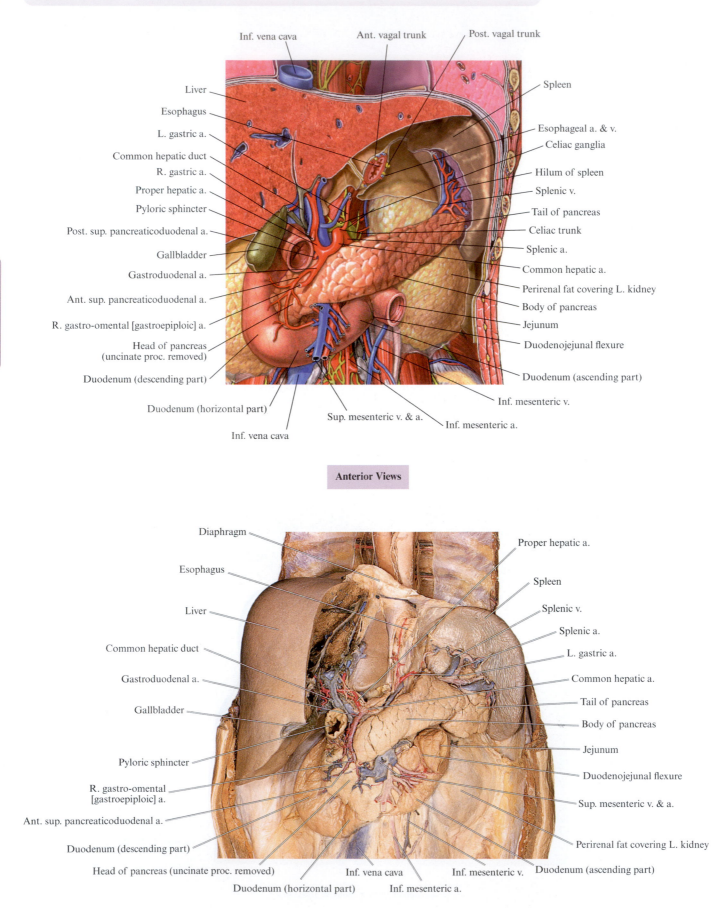

Inf. vena cava

Ant. vagal trunk

Post. vagal trunk

Liver

Esophagus

L. gastric a.

Common hepatic duct

R. gastric a.

Proper hepatic a.

Pyloric sphincter

Post. sup. pancreaticoduodenal a.

Gallbladder

Gastroduodenal a.

Ant. sup. pancreaticoduodenal a.

R. gastro-omental [gastroepiploic] a.

Head of pancreas
(uncinate proc. removed)

Duodenum (descending part)

Duodenum (horizontal part)

Sup. mesenteric v. & a.

Inf. vena cava

Spleen

Esophageal a. & v.

Celiac ganglia

Hilum of spleen

Splenic v.

Tail of pancreas

Celiac trunk

Splenic a.

Common hepatic a.

Perirenal fat covering L. kidney

Body of pancreas

Jejunum

Duodenojejunal flexure

Duodenum (ascending part)

Inf. mesenteric v.

Inf. mesenteric a.

Anterior Views

Diaphragm

Esophagus

Liver

Common hepatic duct

Gastroduodenal a.

Gallbladder

Pyloric sphincter

R. gastro-omental
[gastroepiploic] a.

Ant. sup. pancreaticoduodenal a.

Duodenum (descending part)

Head of pancreas (uncinate proc. removed)

Duodenum (horizontal part)

Inf. vena cava

Inf. mesenteric a.

Proper hepatic a.

Spleen

Splenic v.

Splenic a.

L. gastric a.

Common hepatic a.

Tail of pancreas

Body of pancreas

Jejunum

Duodenojejunal flexure

Sup. mesenteric v. & a.

Perirenal fat covering L. kidney

Duodenum (ascending part)

Inf. mesenteric v.

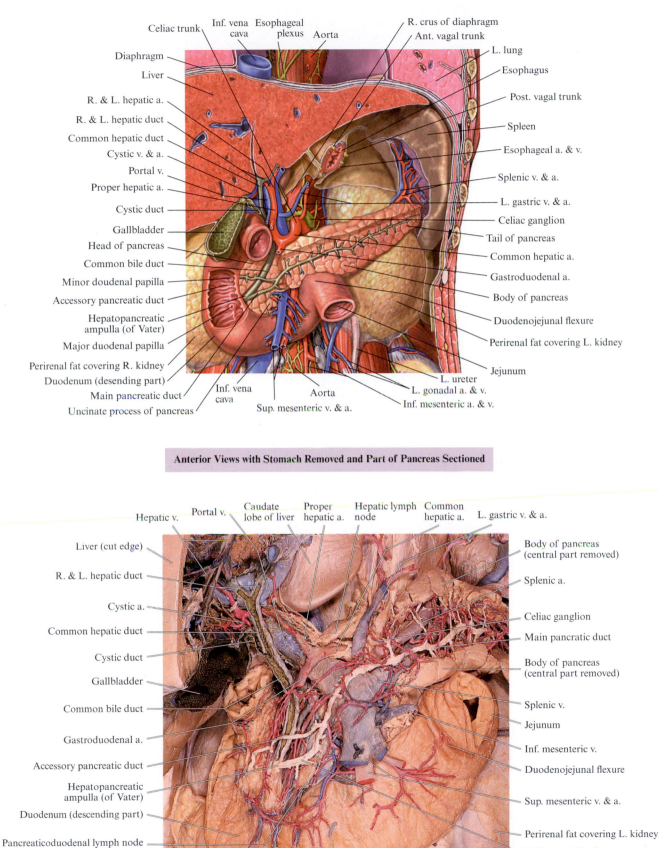

Celiac trunk
Inf. vena cava
Esophageal plexus
Aorta
R. crus of diaphragm
Ant. vagal trunk
L. lung
Diaphragm
Esophagus
Liver
Post. vagal trunk
R. & L. hepatic a.
R. & L. hepatic duct
Spleen
Common hepatic duct
Esophageal a. & v.
Cystic v. & a.
Splenic v. & a.
Portal v.
Proper hepatic a.
L. gastric v. & a.
Cystic duct
Celiac ganglion
Gallbladder
Tail of pancreas
Head of pancreas
Common hepatic a.
Common bile duct
Gastroduodenal a.
Minor doudenal papilla
Body of pancreas
Accessory pancreatic duct
Hepatopancreatic ampulla (of Vater)
Duodenojejunal flexure
Major duodenal papilla
Perirenal fat covering L. kidney
Perirenal fat covering R. kidney
Jejunum
Duodenum (desending part)
L. ureter
Inf. vena cava
Aorta
L. gonadal a. & v.
Main pancreatic duct
Inf. mesenteric a. & v.
Uncinate process of pancreas
Sup. mesenteric v. & a.

Anterior Views with Stomach Removed and Part of Pancreas Sectioned

Hepatic v.
Portal v.
Caudate lobe of liver
Proper hepatic a.
Hepatic lymph node
Common hepatic a.
L. gastric v. & a.
Liver (cut edge)
Body of pancreas (central part removed)
R. & L. hepatic duct
Splenic a.
Cystic a.
Celiac ganglion
Common hepatic duct
Main pancratic duct
Cystic duct
Body of pancreas (central part removed)
Gallbladder
Splenic v.
Common bile duct
Jejunum
Gastroduodenal a.
Inf. mesenteric v.
Accessory pancreatic duct
Duodenojejunal flexure
Hepatopancreatic ampulla (of Vater)
Sup. mesenteric v. & a.
Duodenum (descending part)
Perirenal fat covering L. kidney
Pancreaticoduodenal lymph node
Main pancratic duct

PLATE 3.15   PORTAL VEIN

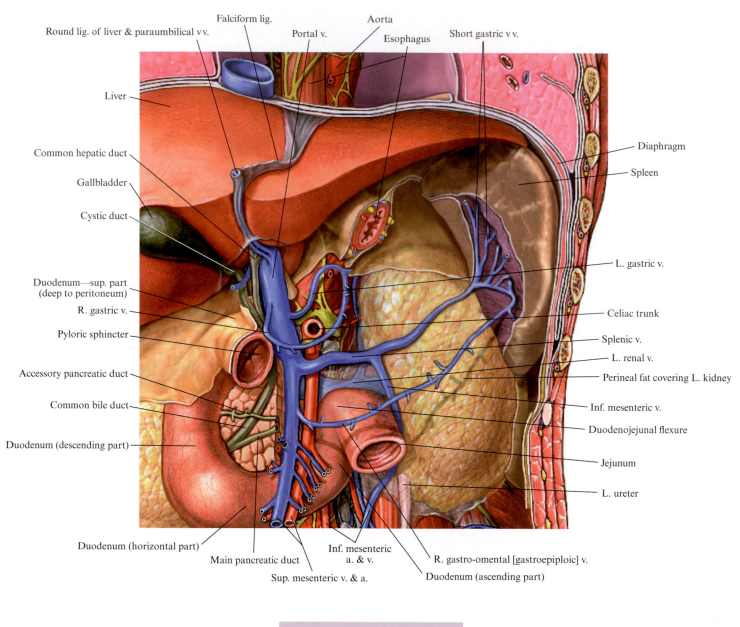

Round lig. of liver & paraumbilical v v.

Falciform lig.

Aorta

Portal v.

Esophagus

Short gastric v v.

Liver

Common hepatic duct

Gallbladder

Cystic duct

Duodenum—sup. part
(deep to peritoneum)

R. gastric v.

Pyloric sphincter

Accessory pancreatic duct

Common bile duct

Duodenum (descending part)

Diaphragm

Spleen

L. gastric v.

Celiac trunk

Splenic v.

L. renal v.

Perineal fat covering L. kidney

Inf. mesenteric v.

Duodenojejunal flexure

Jejunum

L. ureter

Duodenum (horizontal part)

Main pancreatic duct

Inf. mesenteric
a. & v.

Sup. mesenteric v. & a.

R. gastro-omental [gastroepiploic] v.

Duodenum (ascending part)

Anterior View with Stomach Removed

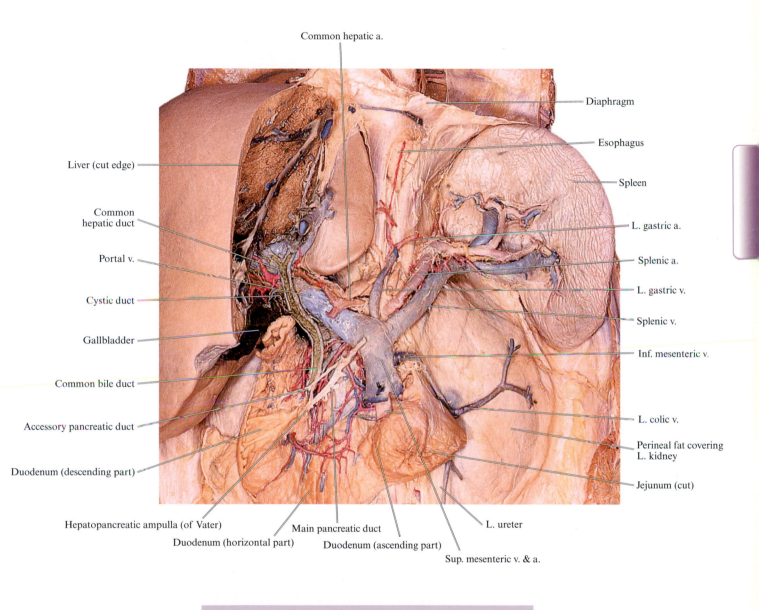

Common hepatic a.

Diaphragm

Esophagus

Liver (cut edge)

Spleen

Common
hepatic duct

L. gastric a.

Portal v.

Splenic a.

Cystic duct

L. gastric v.

Splenic v.

Gallbladder

Inf. mesenteric v.

Common bile duct

Accessory pancreatic duct

L. colic v.

Perineal fat covering
L. kidney

Duodenum (descending part)

Jejunum (cut)

Hepatopancreatic ampulla (of Vater)

Main pancreatic duct

L. ureter

Duodenum (horizontal part)

Duodenum (ascending part)

Sup. mesenteric v. & a.

Anterior View with Stomach, Left Half of Liver, and Pancreas Removed

PLATE 3.17 LIVER

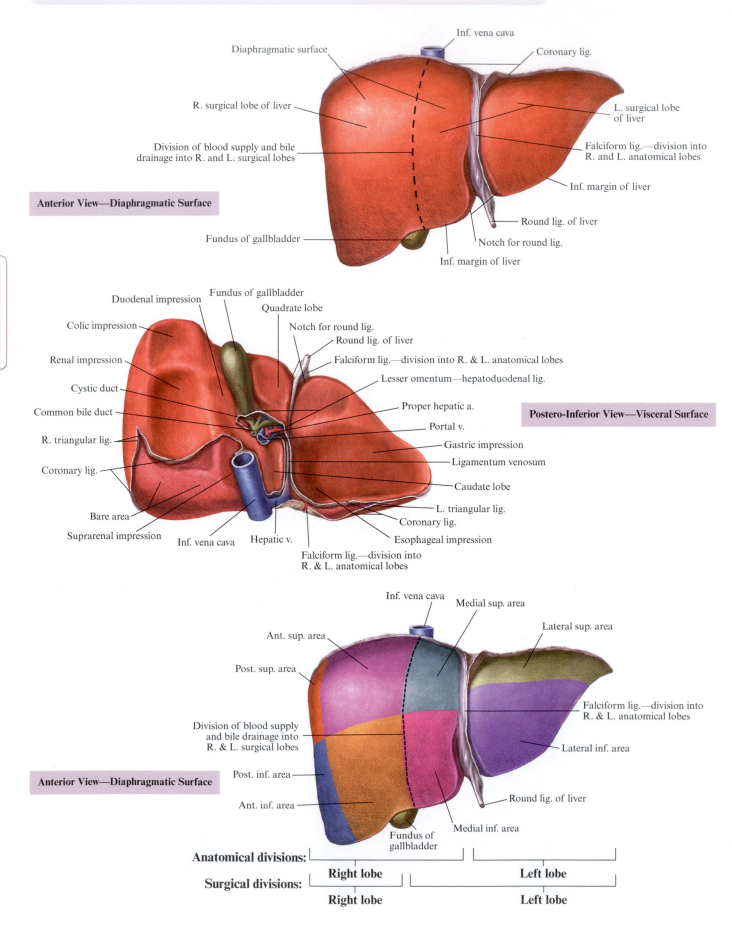

Inf. vena cava

Diaphragmatic surface

Coronary lig.

R. surgical lobe of liver

L. surgical lobe
of liver

Division of blood supply and bile
drainage into R. and L. surgical lobes

Falciform lig.—division into
R. and L. anatomical lobes

Inf. margin of liver

Anterior View—Diaphragmatic Surface

Round lig. of liver

Fundus of gallbladder

Notch for round lig.

Inf. margin of liver

Duodenal impression

Fundus of gallbladder

Colic impression

Quadrate lobe

Notch for round lig.

Renal impression

Round lig. of liver

Cystic duct

Falciform lig.—division into R. & L. anatomical lobes

Common bile duct

Lesser omentum—hepatoduodenal lig.

R. triangular lig.

Proper hepatic a.

Postero-Inferior View—Visceral Surface

Portal v.

Coronary lig.

Gastric impression

Ligamentum venosum

Caudate lobe

Bare area

L. triangular lig.

Coronary lig.

Suprarenal impression

Inf. vena cava

Hepatic v.

Esophageal impression

Falciform lig.—division into
R. & L. anatomical lobes

Inf. vena cava

Medial sup. area

Ant. sup. area

Lateral sup. area

Post. sup. area

Falciform lig.—division into
R. & L. anatomical lobes

Division of blood supply
and bile drainage into
R. & L. surgical lobes

Lateral inf. area

Anterior View—Diaphragmatic Surface

Post. inf. area

Ant. inf. area

Round lig. of liver

Medial inf. area

Fundus of
gallbladder

Anatomical divisions:	**Right lobe**	**Left lobe**
Surgical divisions:	**Right lobe**	**Left lobe**

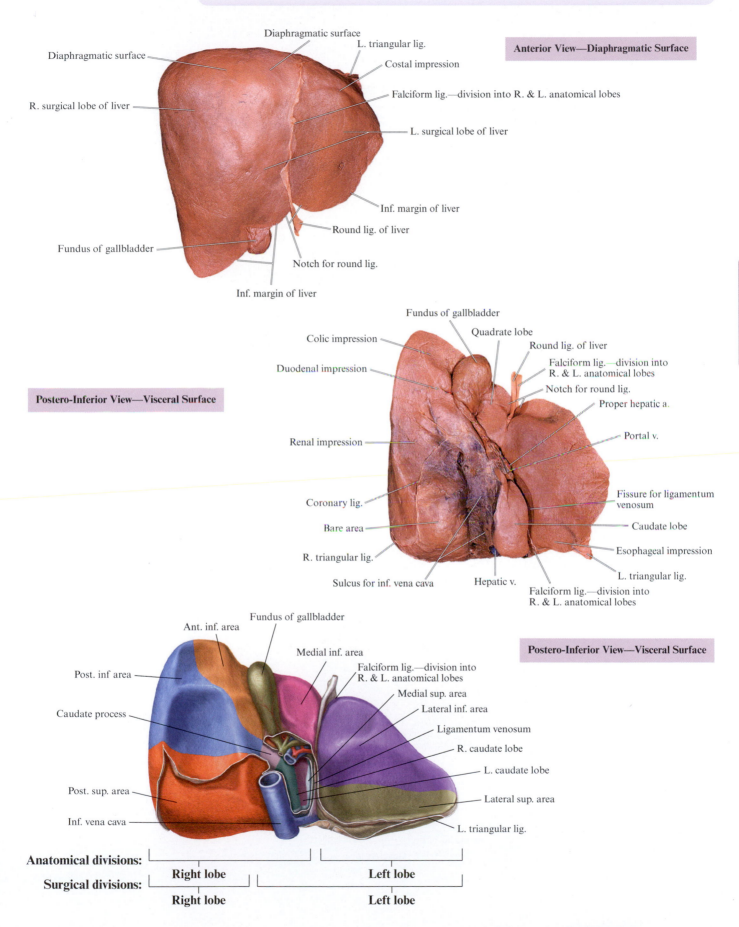

Diaphragmatic surface

Diaphragmatic surface

L. triangular lig.

Costal impression

Falciform lig.—division into R. & L. anatomical lobes

R. surgical lobe of liver

L. surgical lobe of liver

Inf. margin of liver

Round lig. of liver

Fundus of gallbladder

Notch for round lig.

Inf. margin of liver

Fundus of gallbladder

Colic impression

Quadrate lobe

Round lig. of liver

Falciform lig.—division into R. & L. anatomical lobes

Duodenal impression

Notch for round lig.

Proper hepatic a.

Postero-Inferior View—Visceral Surface

Renal impression

Portal v.

Coronary lig.

Fissure for ligamentum venosum

Caudate lobe

Bare area

Esophageal impression

R. triangular lig.

L. triangular lig.

Sulcus for inf. vena cava

Hepatic v.

Falciform lig.—division into R. & L. anatomical lobes

Ant. inf. area

Fundus of gallbladder

Postero-Inferior View—Visceral Surface

Post. inf area

Medial inf. area

Falciform lig.—division into R. & L. anatomical lobes

Medial sup. area

Caudate process

Lateral inf. area

Ligamentum venosum

R. caudate lobe

Post. sup. area

L. caudate lobe

Inf. vena cava

Lateral sup. area

L. triangular lig.

Anatomical divisions:

Surgical divisions:

Right lobe

Left lobe

Right lobe

Left lobe

PLATE 3.19   LIVER—PERITONEAL LIGAMENTS

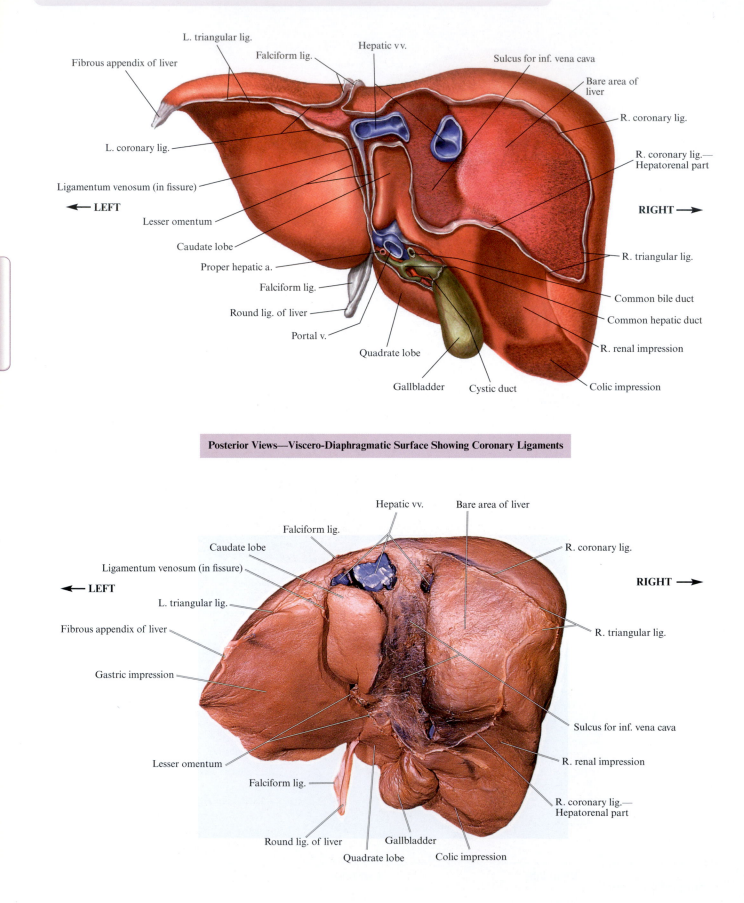

L. triangular lig.

Fibrous appendix of liver

Falciform lig.

Hepatic vv.

Sulcus for inf. vena cava

Bare area of liver

L. coronary lig.

R. coronary lig.

R. coronary lig.—Hepatorenal part

Ligamentum venosum (in fissure)

← LEFT

RIGHT →

Lesser omentum

Caudate lobe

R. triangular lig.

Proper hepatic a.

Falciform lig.

Common bile duct

Round lig. of liver

Common hepatic duct

Portal v.

R. renal impression

Quadrate lobe

Gallbladder   Cystic duct   Colic impression

Posterior Views—Viscero-Diaphragmatic Surface Showing Coronary Ligaments

Hepatic vv.   Bare area of liver

Falciform lig.

Caudate lobe

R. coronary lig.

Ligamentum venosum (in fissure)

← LEFT

RIGHT →

L. triangular lig.

Fibrous appendix of liver

R. triangular lig.

Gastric impression

Sulcus for inf. vena cava

Lesser omentum

R. renal impression

Falciform lig.

R. coronary lig.—Hepatorenal part

Round lig. of liver   Gallbladder

Quadrate lobe   Colic impression

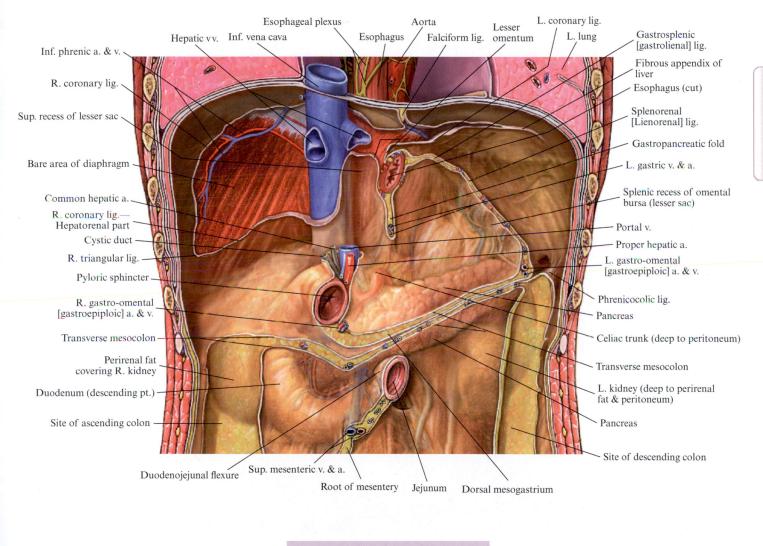

Esophageal plexus

Aorta

L. coronary lig.

Hepatic v v.   Inf. vena cava

Esophagus   Falciform lig.   Lesser omentum   L. lung

Gastrosplenic [gastrolienal] lig.

Inf. phrenic a. & v.

Fibrous appendix of liver

R. coronary lig.

Esophagus (cut)

Sup. recess of lesser sac

Splenorenal [Lienorenal] lig.

Gastropancreatic fold

Bare area of diaphragm

L. gastric v. & a.

Common hepatic a.

Splenic recess of omental bursa (lesser sac)

R. coronary lig.—
Hepatorenal part

Portal v.

Cystic duct

Proper hepatic a.

R. triangular lig.

L. gastro-omental [gastroepiploic] a. & v.

Pyloric sphincter

Phrenicocolic lig.

R. gastro-omental [gastroepiploic] a. & v.

Pancreas

Transverse mesocolon

Celiac trunk (deep to peritoneum)

Perirenal fat covering R. kidney

Transverse mesocolon

L. kidney (deep to perirenal fat & peritoneum)

Duodenum (descending pt.)

Site of ascending colon

Pancreas

Site of descending colon

Duodenojejunal flexure   Sup. mesenteric v. & a.

Root of mesentery   Jejunum   Dorsal mesogastrium

Anterior View—Posterior Abdominal Wall

PLATE 3.21   STOMACH & SMALL INTESTINES

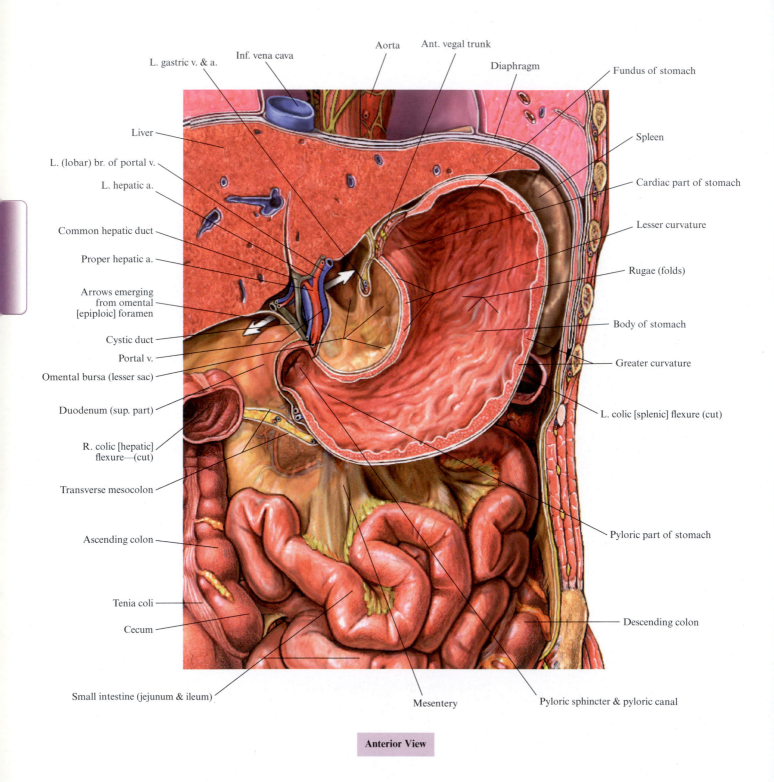

Aorta

Ant. vegal trunk

Inf. vena cava

L. gastric v. & a.

Diaphragm

Fundus of stomach

Liver

Spleen

L. (lobar) br. of portal v.

Cardiac part of stomach

L. hepatic a.

Lesser curvature

Common hepatic duct

Rugae (folds)

Proper hepatic a.

Arrows emerging from omental [epiploic] foramen

Body of stomach

Cystic duct

Portal v.

Greater curvature

Omental bursa (lesser sac)

Duodenum (sup. part)

L. colic [splenic] flexure (cut)

R. colic [hepatic] flexure—(cut)

Transverse mesocolon

Ascending colon

Pyloric part of stomach

Tenia coli

Cecum

Descending colon

Small intestine (jejunum & ileum)

Mesentery

Pyloric sphincter & pyloric canal

Anterior View

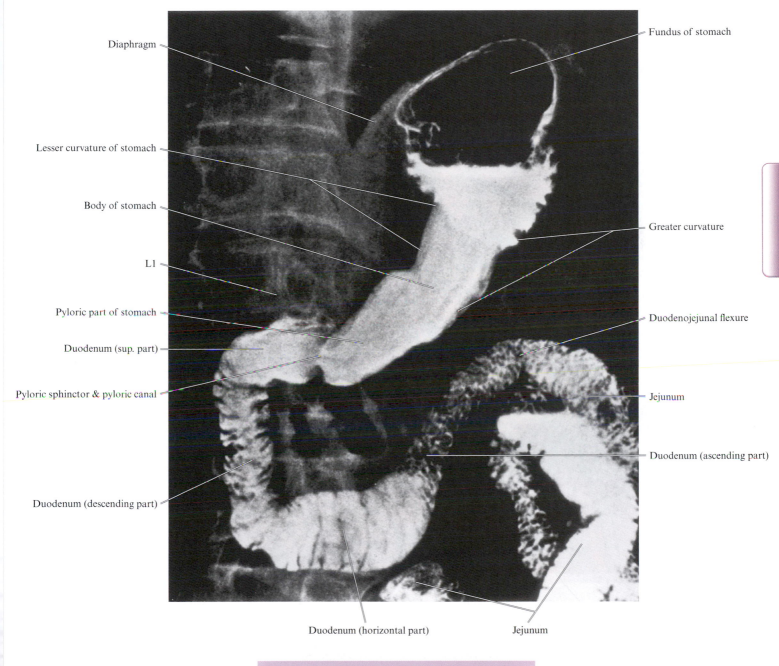

Diaphragm

Lesser curvature of stomach

Body of stomach

L1

Pyloric part of stomach

Duodenum (sup. part)

Pyloric sphincter & pyloric canal

Duodenum (descending part)

Fundus of stomach

Greater curvature

Duodenojejunal flexure

Jejunum

Duodenum (ascending part)

Duodenum (horizontal part)

Jejunum

Radiograph of Upper G.I. Tract Following Barium Swallow

PLATE 3.25   LARGE INTESTINES—VASCULATURE

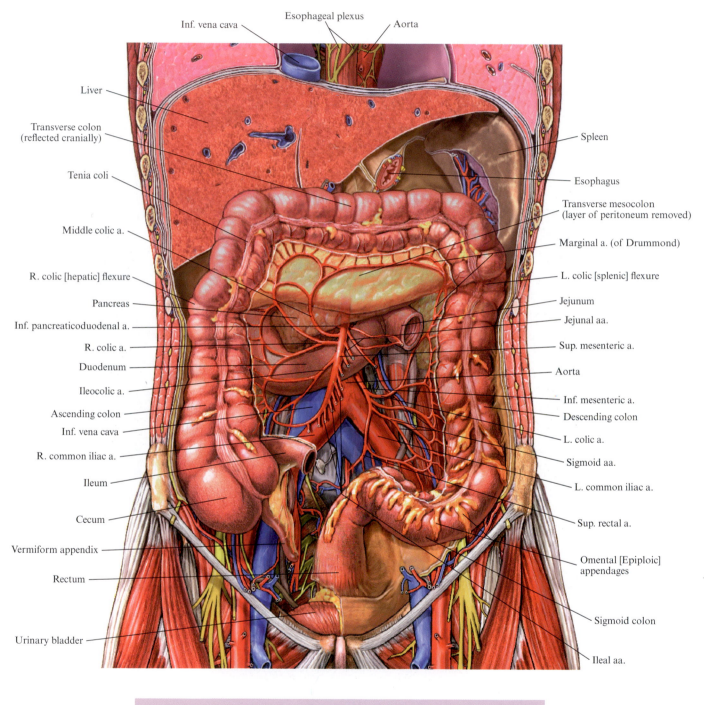

Inf. vena cava

Esophageal plexus

Aorta

Liver

Transverse colon
(reflected cranially)

Tenia coli

Middle colic a.

R. colic [hepatic] flexure

Pancreas

Inf. pancreaticoduodenal a.

R. colic a.

Duodenum

Ileocolic a.

Ascending colon

Inf. vena cava

R. common iliac a.

Ileum

Cecum

Vermiform appendix

Rectum

Urinary bladder

Spleen

Esophagus

Transverse mesocolon
(layer of peritoneum removed)

Marginal a. (of Drummond)

L. colic [splenic] flexure

Jejunum

Jejunal aa.

Sup. mesenteric a.

Aorta

Inf. mesenteric a.

Descending colon

L. colic a.

Sigmoid aa.

L. common iliac a.

Sup. rectal a.

Omental [Epiploic]
appendages

Sigmoid colon

Ileal aa.

Anterior View—Transverse Colon Reflected Superiorly & the Mesentery Proper Removed

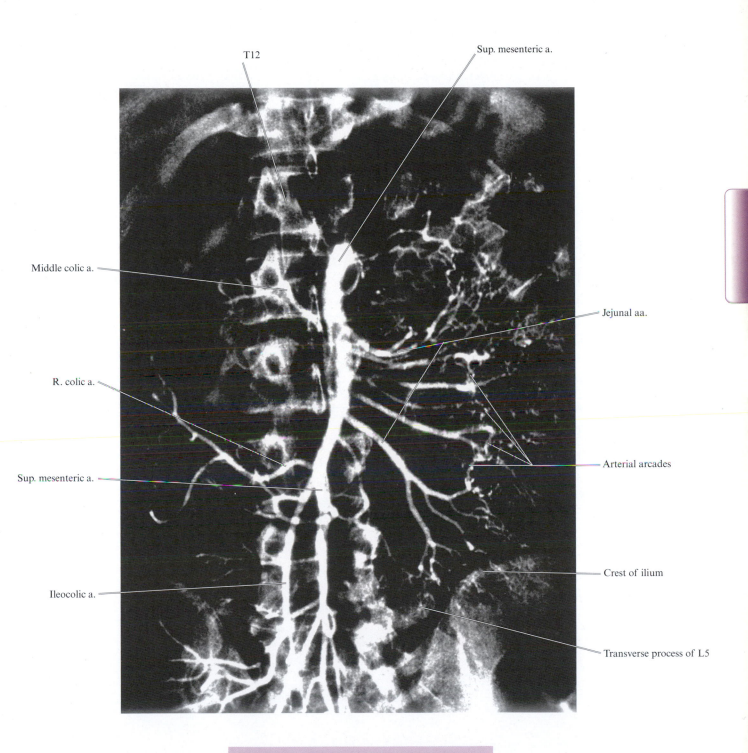

T12

Sup. mesenteric a.

Middle colic a.

Jejunal aa.

R. colic a.

Arterial arcades

Sup. mesenteric a.

Crest of ilium

Ileocolic a.

Transverse process of L5

Arteriograph of Superior Mesenteric Artery & Branches

PLATE 3.27   LARGE INTESTINES

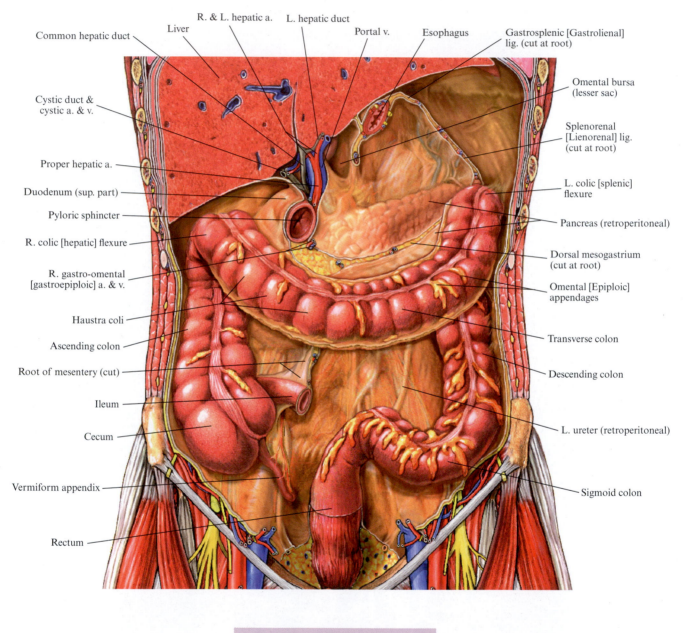

Common hepatic duct

Liver

R. & L. hepatic a.

L. hepatic duct

Portal v.

Esophagus

Gastrosplenic [Gastrolienal] lig. (cut at root)

Cystic duct & cystic a. & v.

Omental bursa (lesser sac)

Proper hepatic a.

Splenorenal [Lienorenal] lig. (cut at root)

Duodenum (sup. part)

L. colic [splenic] flexure

Pyloric sphincter

Pancreas (retroperitoneal)

R. colic [hepatic] flexure

Dorsal mesogastrium (cut at root)

R. gastro-omental [gastroepiploic] a. & v.

Omental [Epiploic] appendages

Haustra coli

Ascending colon

Transverse colon

Root of mesentery (cut)

Descending colon

Ileum

Cecum

L. ureter (retroperitoneal)

Vermiform appendix

Sigmoid colon

Rectum

Anterior View—Small Intestines Removed

R. colic [hepatic] flexure   Haustra coli   L. colic [splenic] flexure

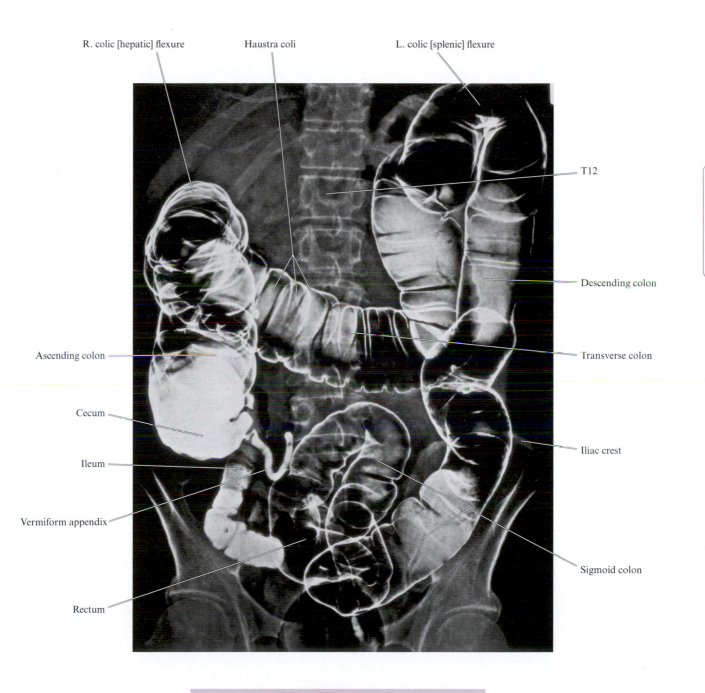

T12

Descending colon

Ascending colon

Transverse colon

Cecum

Ileum

Iliac crest

Vermiform appendix

Sigmoid colon

Rectum

Double Contrast (Air & Barium) Radiograph of Large Intestine

PLATE 3.29   LARGE INTESTINES—PORTAL VASCULATURE

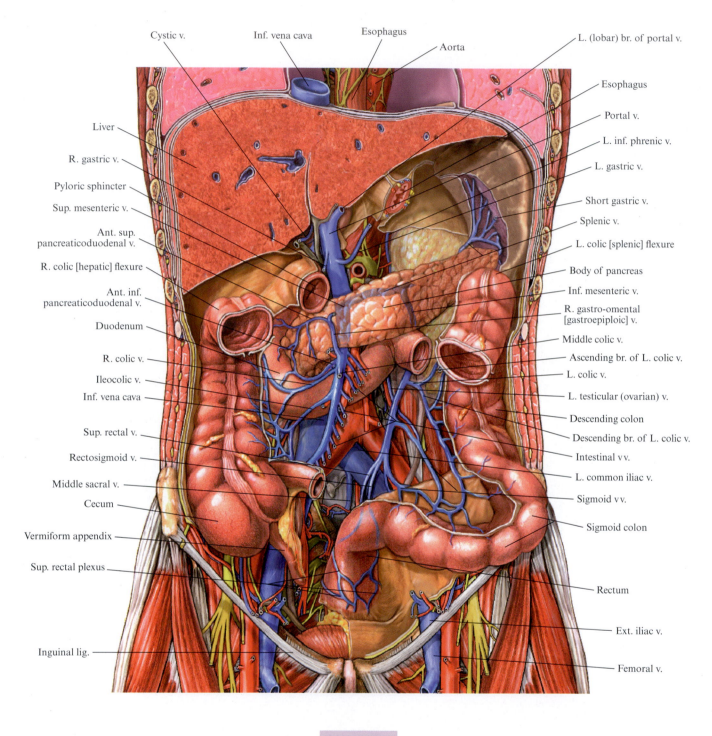

Cystic v.

Inf. vena cava

Esophagus

Aorta

L. (lobar) br. of portal v.

Esophagus

Liver

Portal v.

R. gastric v.

L. inf. phrenic v.

Pyloric sphincter

L. gastric v.

Sup. mesenteric v.

Short gastric v.

Ant. sup.
pancreaticoduodenal v.

Splenic v.

R. colic [hepatic] flexure

L. colic [splenic] flexure

Ant. inf.
pancreaticoduodenal v.

Body of pancreas

Duodenum

Inf. mesenteric v.

R. gastro-omental
[gastroepiploic] v.

R. colic v.

Middle colic v.

Ileocolic v.

Ascending br. of L. colic v.

Inf. vena cava

L. colic v.

Sup. rectal v.

L. testicular (ovarian) v.

Rectosigmoid v.

Descending colon

Middle sacral v.

Descending br. of L. colic v.

Cecum

Intestinal vv.

Vermiform appendix

L. common iliac v.

Sup. rectal plexus

Sigmoid vv.

Sigmoid colon

Rectum

Inguinal lig.

Ext. iliac v.

Femoral v.

Anterior View

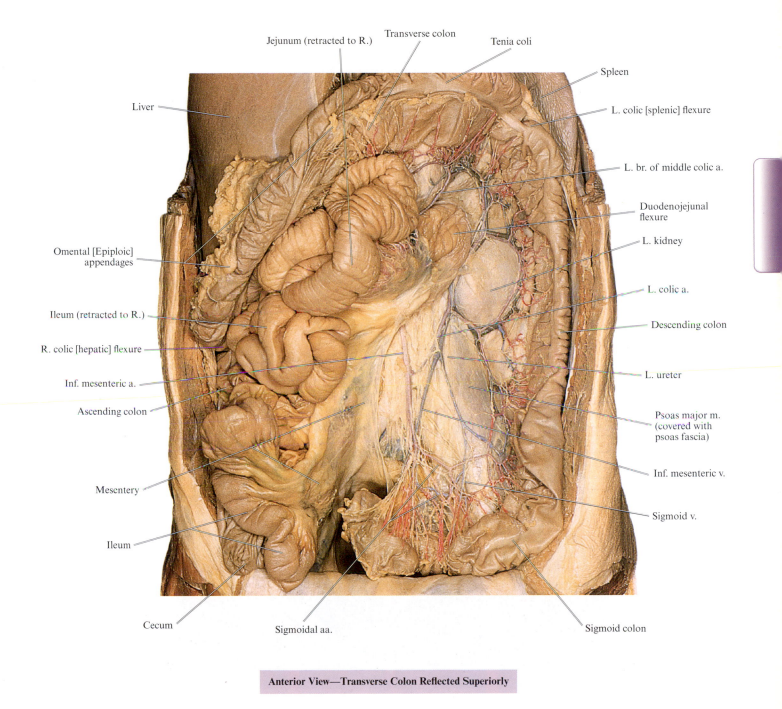

Jejunum (retracted to R.)

Transverse colon

Tenia coli

Spleen

Liver

L. colic [splenic] flexure

L. br. of middle colic a.

Duodenojejunal flexure

L. kidney

Omental [Epiploic] appendages

L. colic a.

Ileum (retracted to R.)

Descending colon

R. colic [hepatic] flexure

L. ureter

Inf. mesenteric a.

Psoas major m. (covered with psoas fascia)

Ascending colon

Inf. mesenteric v.

Mesentery

Sigmoid v.

Ileum

Cecum

Sigmoidal aa.

Sigmoid colon

Anterior View—Transverse Colon Reflected Superiorly

PLATE 3.33 POSTERIOR ABDOMINAL WALL

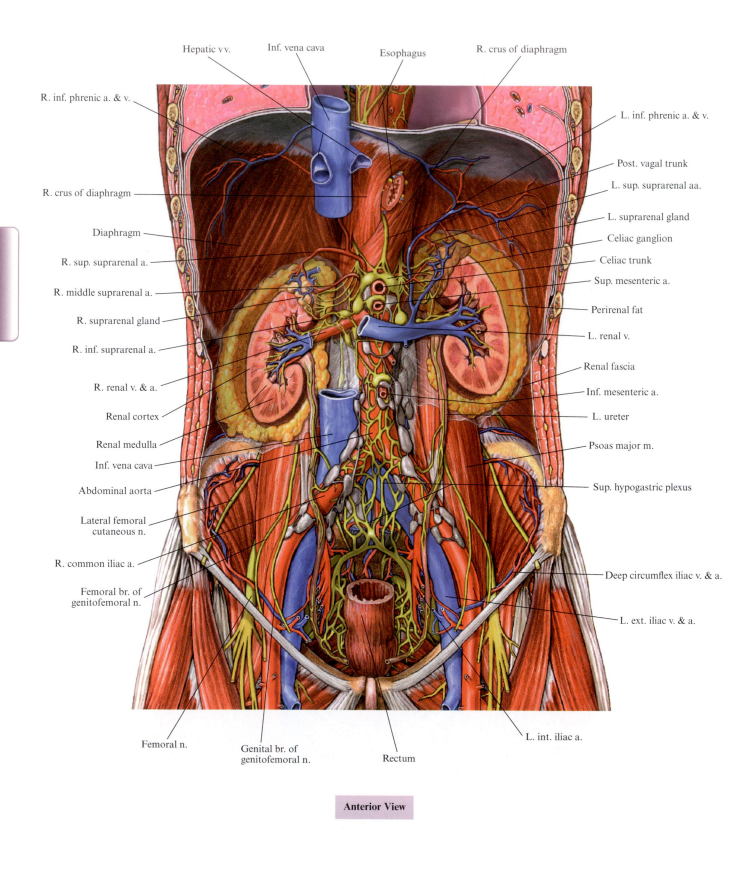

Hepatic v v.

Inf. vena cava

Esophagus

R. crus of diaphragm

R. inf. phrenic a. & v.

L. inf. phrenic a. & v.

Post. vagal trunk

R. crus of diaphragm

L. sup. suprarenal aa.

Diaphragm

L. suprarenal gland

R. sup. suprarenal a.

Celiac ganglion

Celiac trunk

R. middle suprarenal a.

Sup. mesenteric a.

R. suprarenal gland

Perirenal fat

R. inf. suprarenal a.

L. renal v.

R. renal v. & a.

Renal fascia

Renal cortex

Inf. mesenteric a.

Renal medulla

L. ureter

Inf. vena cava

Psoas major m.

Abdominal aorta

Sup. hypogastric plexus

Lateral femoral
cutaneous n.

R. common iliac a.

Deep circumflex iliac v. & a.

Femoral br. of
genitofemoral n.

L. ext. iliac v. & a.

Femoral n.

Genital br. of
genitofemoral n.

Rectum

L. int. iliac a.

Anterior View

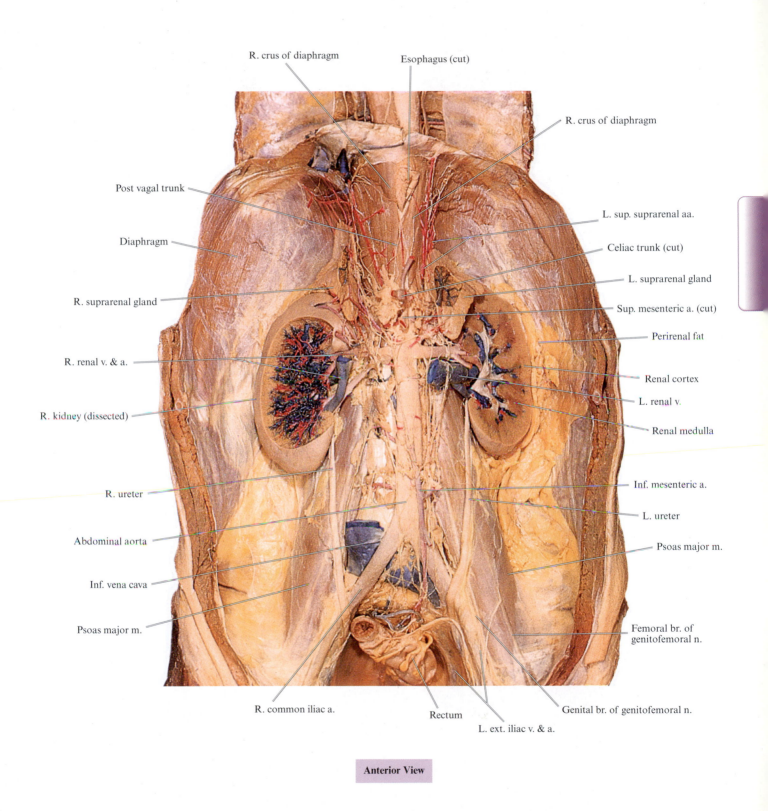

R. crus of diaphragm

Esophagus (cut)

R. crus of diaphragm

Post vagal trunk

L. sup. suprarenal aa.

Diaphragm

Celiac trunk (cut)

L. suprarenal gland

R. suprarenal gland

Sup. mesenteric a. (cut)

Perirenal fat

R. renal v. & a.

Renal cortex

L. renal v.

R. kidney (dissected)

Renal medulla

R. ureter

Inf. mesenteric a.

L. ureter

Abdominal aorta

Psoas major m.

Inf. vena cava

Psoas major m.

Femoral br. of genitofemoral n.

R. common iliac a.

Rectum

Genital br. of genitofemoral n.

L. ext. iliac v. & a.

Anterior View

PLATE 3.35   KIDNEYS

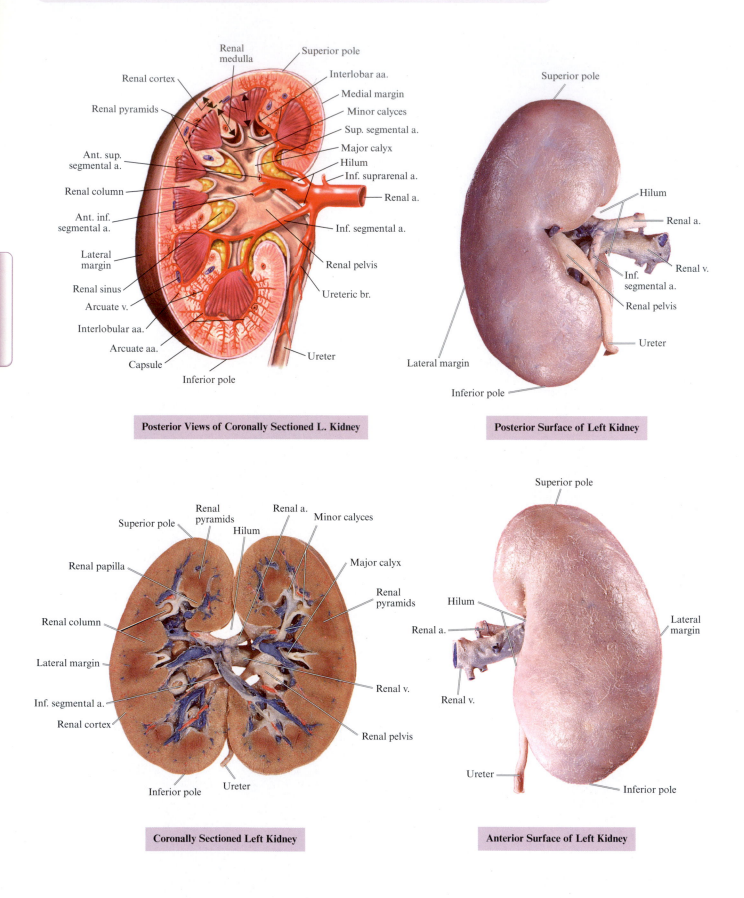

Posterior Views of Coronally Sectioned L. Kidney

Posterior Surface of Left Kidney

Coronally Sectioned Left Kidney

Anterior Surface of Left Kidney

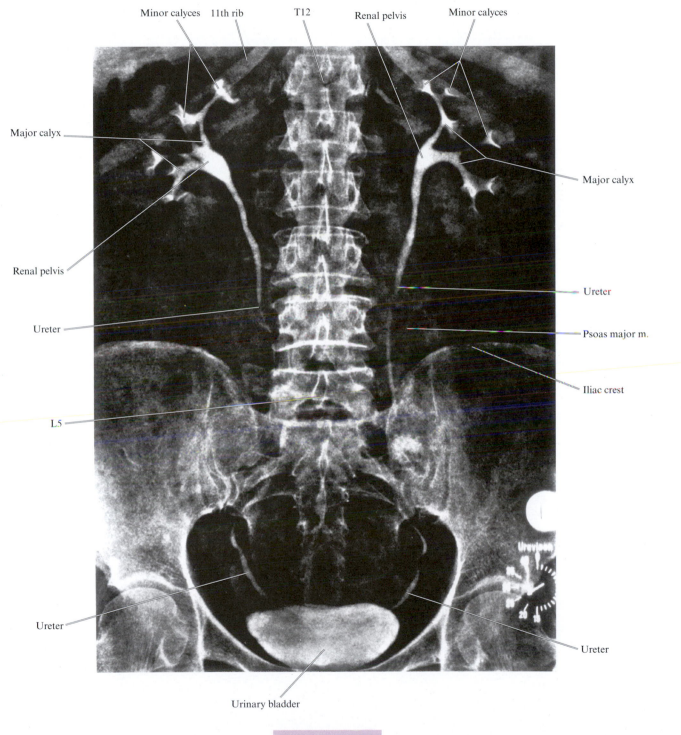

Minor calyces   11th rib   T12   Renal pelvis   Minor calyces

Major calyx

Renal pelvis

Ureter

L5

Ureter

Major calyx

Ureter

Psoas major m.

Iliac crest

Ureter

Urinary bladder

Intravenous Urogram

PLATE 3.37   SUPRARENAL GLANDS

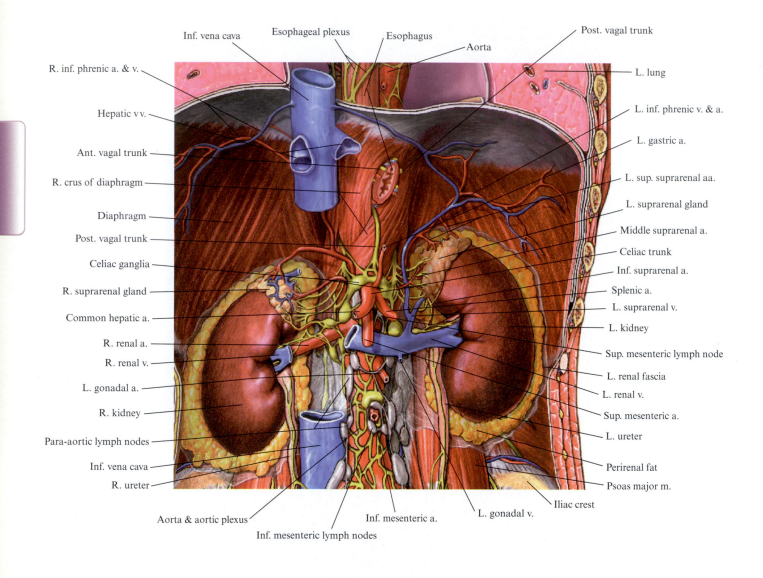

Inf. vena cava   Esophageal plexus   Esophagus   Aorta   Post. vagal trunk

R. inf. phrenic a. & v.   L. lung

Hepatic vv.   L. inf. phrenic v. & a.

Ant. vagal trunk   L. gastric a.

R. crus of diaphragm   L. sup. suprarenal aa.

Diaphragm   L. suprarenal gland

Post. vagal trunk   Middle suprarenal a.

Celiac ganglia   Celiac trunk

R. suprarenal gland   Inf. suprarenal a.

Common hepatic a.   Splenic a.

R. renal a.   L. suprarenal v.

R. renal v.   L. kidney

L. gonadal a.   Sup. mesenteric lymph node

R. kidney   L. renal fascia

Para-aortic lymph nodes   L. renal v.

Inf. vena cava   Sup. mesenteric a.

R. ureter   L. ureter

Aorta & aortic plexus   Perirenal fat

Inf. mesenteric lymph nodes   Psoas major m.

Inf. mesenteric a.   Iliac crest

L. gonadal v.

Anterior View

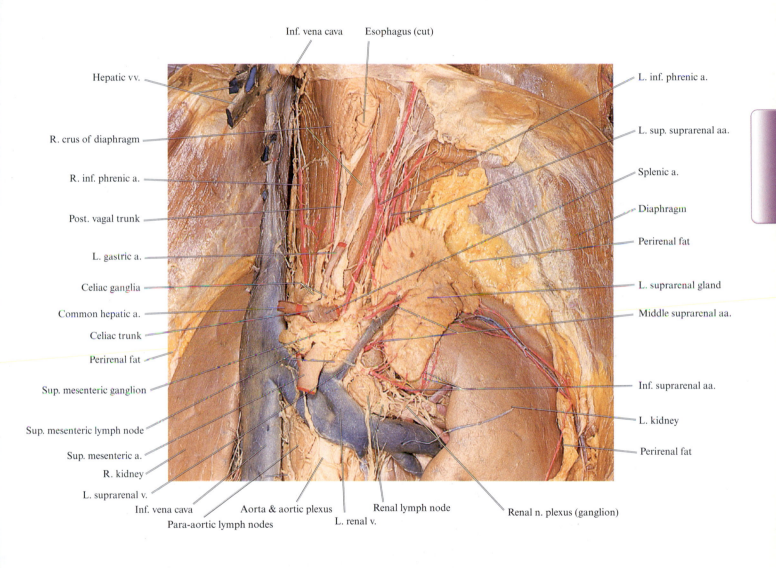

Inf. vena cava

Esophagus (cut)

Hepatic vv.

R. crus of diaphragm

R. inf. phrenic a.

Post. vagal trunk

L. gastric a.

Celiac ganglia

Common hepatic a.

Celiac trunk

Perirenal fat

Sup. mesenteric ganglion

Sup. mesenteric lymph node

Sup. mesenteric a.

R. kidney

L. suprarenal v.

Inf. vena cava

Para-aortic lymph nodes

Aorta & aortic plexus

L. renal v.

Renal lymph node

Renal n. plexus (ganglion)

L. inf. phrenic a.

L. sup. suprarenal aa.

Splenic a.

Diaphragm

Perirenal fat

L. suprarenal gland

Middle suprarenal aa.

Inf. suprarenal aa.

L. kidney

Perirenal fat

Anterior View of Superior Pole of L. Kidney

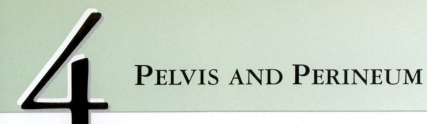

4 PELVIS AND PERINEUM

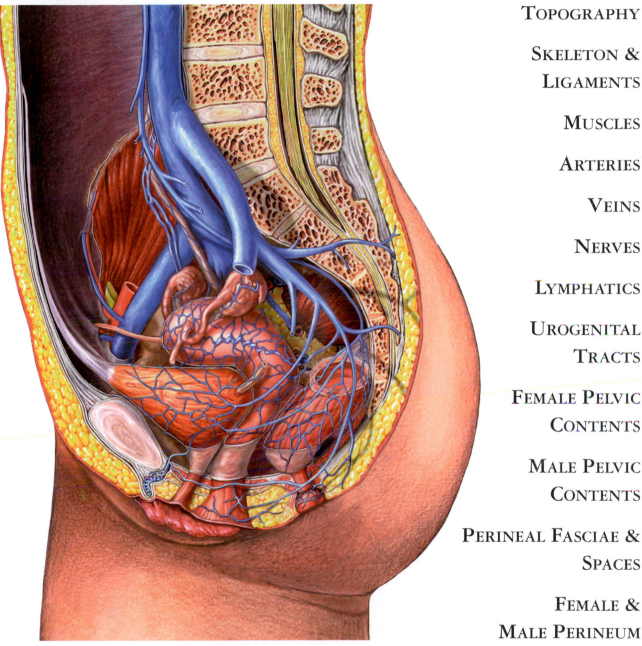

PLATE 4.1   TOPOGRAPHY—MALE

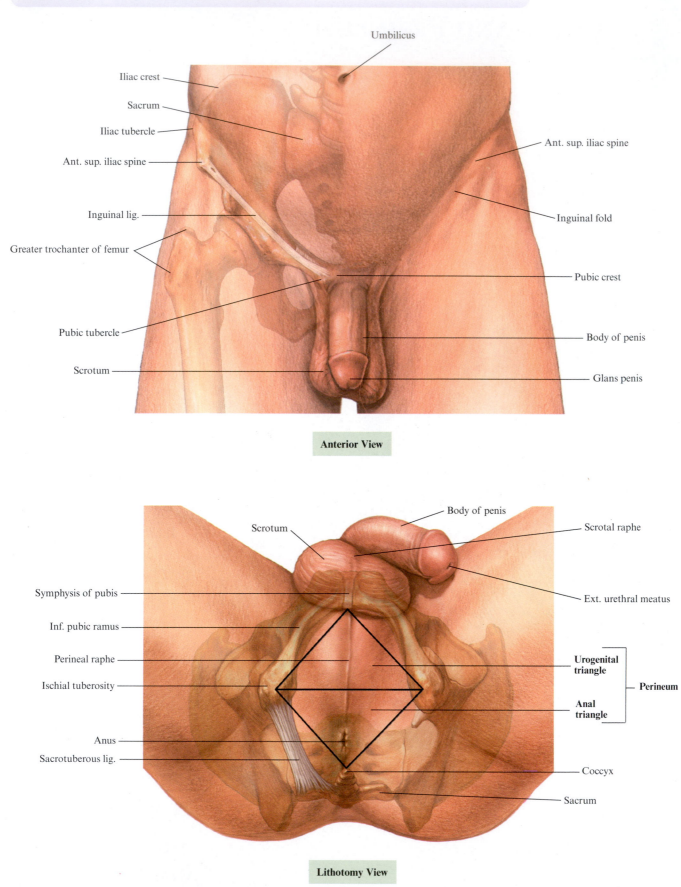

Umbilicus

Iliac crest

Sacrum

Iliac tubercle

Ant. sup. iliac spine

Ant. sup. iliac spine

Inguinal lig.

Inguinal fold

Greater trochanter of femur

Pubic crest

Pubic tubercle

Body of penis

Scrotum

Glans penis

Anterior View

Body of penis

Scrotum

Scrotal raphe

Symphysis of pubis

Ext. urethral meatus

Inf. pubic ramus

Perineal raphe

Urogenital
triangle

Ischial tuberosity

Perineum

Anal
triangle

Anus

Sacrotuberous lig.

Coccyx

Sacrum

Lithotomy View

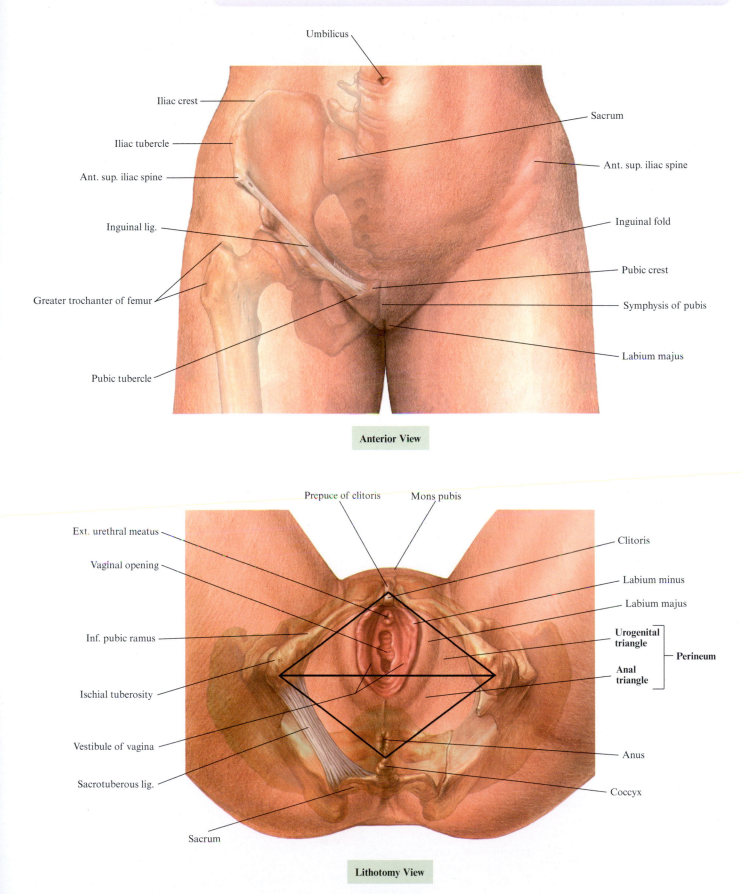

Umbilicus

Iliac crest

Iliac tubercle

Ant. sup. iliac spine

Inguinal lig.

Greater trochanter of femur

Pubic tubercle

Sacrum

Ant. sup. iliac spine

Inguinal fold

Pubic crest

Symphysis of pubis

Labium majus

Anterior View

Prepuce of clitoris   Mons pubis

Ext. urethral meatus

Vaginal opening

Inf. pubic ramus

Ischial tuberosity

Vestibule of vagina

Sacrotuberous lig.

Sacrum

Clitoris

Labium minus

Labium majus

Urogenital triangle

Anal triangle

Perineum

Anus

Coccyx

Lithotomy View

PLATE 4.3   SKELETON & LIGAMENTS

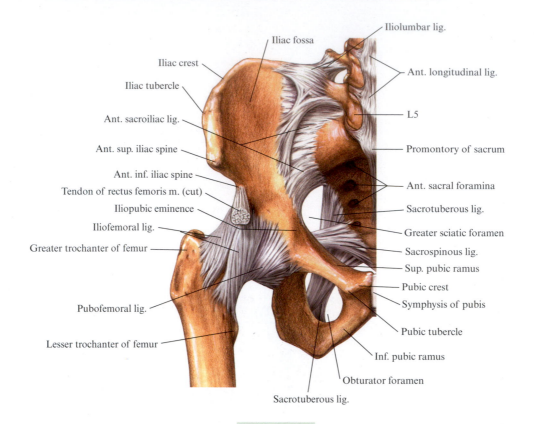

Iliac fossa

Iliolumbar lig.

Iliac crest

Ant. longitudinal lig.

Iliac tubercle

Ant. sacroiliac lig.

L5

Ant. sup. iliac spine

Promontory of sacrum

Ant. inf. iliac spine

Ant. sacral foramina

Tendon of rectus femoris m. (cut)

Iliopubic eminence

Sacrotuberous lig.

Iliofemoral lig.

Greater sciatic foramen

Greater trochanter of femur

Sacrospinous lig.

Sup. pubic ramus

Pubic crest

Symphysis of pubis

Pubofemoral lig.

Pubic tubercle

Lesser trochanter of femur

Inf. pubic ramus

Obturator foramen

Sacrotuberous lig.

Anterior View

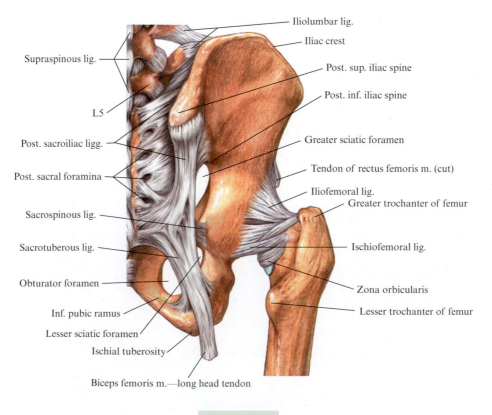

Iliolumbar lig.

Iliac crest

Supraspinous lig.

Post. sup. iliac spine

Post. inf. iliac spine

L5

Greater sciatic foramen

Post. sacroiliac ligg.

Tendon of rectus femoris m. (cut)

Post. sacral foramina

Iliofemoral lig.

Greater trochanter of femur

Sacrospinous lig.

Sacrotuberous lig.

Ischiofemoral lig.

Obturator foramen

Zona orbicularis

Inf. pubic ramus

Lesser trochanter of femur

Lesser sciatic foramen

Ischial tuberosity

Biceps femoris m.—long head tendon

Posterior View

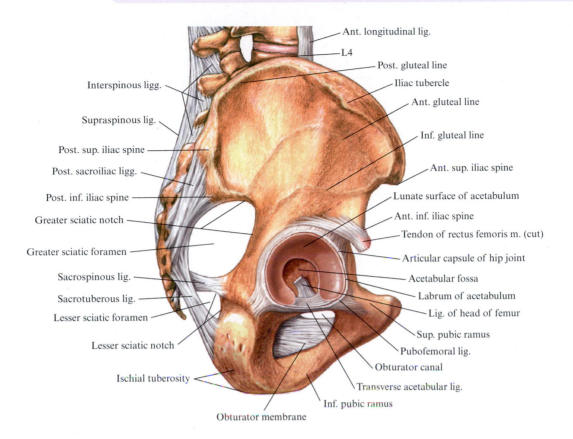

Ant. longitudinal lig.

L4

Post. gluteal line

Iliac tubercle

Ant. gluteal line

Inf. gluteal line

Interspinous ligg.

Supraspinous lig.

Post. sup. iliac spine

Post. sacroiliac ligg.

Post. inf. iliac spine

Greater sciatic notch

Greater sciatic foramen

Sacrospinous lig.

Sacrotuberous lig.

Lesser sciatic foramen

Lesser sciatic notch

Ischial tuberosity

Obturator membrane

Ant. sup. iliac spine

Lunate surface of acetabulum

Ant. inf. iliac spine

Tendon of rectus femoris m. (cut)

Articular capsule of hip joint

Acetabular fossa

Labrum of acetabulum

Lig. of head of femur

Sup. pubic ramus

Pubofemoral lig.

Obturator canal

Transverse acetabular lig.

Inf. pubic ramus

Right Lateral View

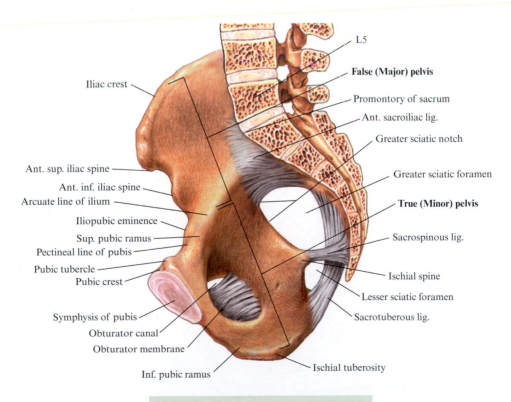

L5

Iliac crest

False (Major) pelvis

Promontory of sacrum

Ant. sacroiliac lig.

Greater sciatic notch

Greater sciatic foramen

Ant. sup. iliac spine

Ant. inf. iliac spine

Arcuate line of ilium

Iliopubic eminence

Sup. pubic ramus

Pectineal line of pubis

Pubic tubercle

Pubic crest

True (Minor) pelvis

Sacrospinous lig.

Ischial spine

Lesser sciatic foramen

Sacrotuberous lig.

Symphysis of pubis

Obturator canal

Obturator membrane

Inf. pubic ramus

Ischial tuberosity

Right Side of Hemisected Pelvis—Medial View

PLATE 4.5   BONY PELVIS—MALE

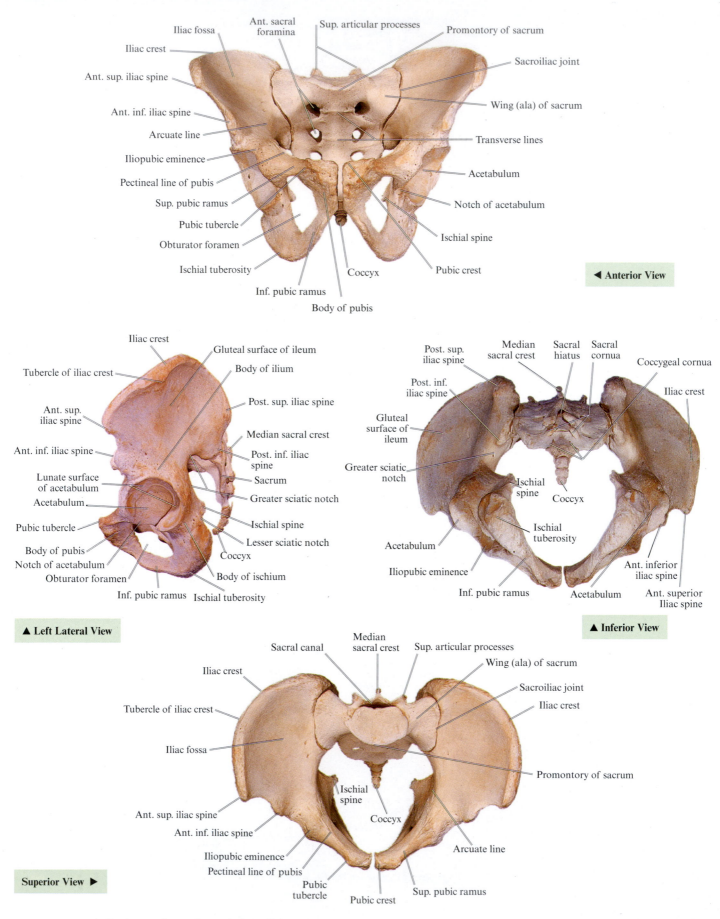

Anterior View

Iliac fossa
Ant. sacral foramina
Sup. articular processes
Promontory of sacrum
Iliac crest
Sacroiliac joint
Ant. sup. iliac spine
Wing (ala) of sacrum
Ant. inf. iliac spine
Transverse lines
Arcuate line
Iliopubic eminence
Acetabulum
Pectineal line of pubis
Notch of acetabulum
Sup. pubic ramus
Pubic tubercle
Ischial spine
Obturator foramen
Ischial tuberosity
Pubic crest
Coccyx
Inf. pubic ramus
Body of pubis

Left Lateral View

Iliac crest
Gluteal surface of ileum
Tubercle of iliac crest
Body of ilium
Post. sup. iliac spine
Ant. sup. iliac spine
Median sacral crest
Ant. inf. iliac spine
Post. inf. iliac spine
Lunate surface of acetabulum
Sacrum
Acetabulum
Greater sciatic notch
Pubic tubercle
Ischial spine
Body of pubis
Lesser sciatic notch
Notch of acetabulum
Coccyx
Obturator foramen
Body of ischium
Inf. pubic ramus
Ischial tuberosity

Inferior View

Post. sup. iliac spine
Median sacral crest
Sacral hiatus
Sacral cornua
Coccygeal cornua
Post. inf. iliac spine
Iliac crest
Gluteal surface of ileum
Greater sciatic notch
Ischial spine
Coccyx
Acetabulum
Ischial tuberosity
Iliopubic eminence
Ant. inferior iliac spine
Inf. pubic ramus
Acetabulum
Ant. superior Iliac spine

Superior View

Sacral canal
Median sacral crest
Sup. articular processes
Iliac crest
Wing (ala) of sacrum
Sacroiliac joint
Tubercle of iliac crest
Iliac crest
Iliac fossa
Promontory of sacrum
Ischial spine
Ant. sup. iliac spine
Coccyx
Ant. inf. iliac spine
Arcuate line
Iliopubic eminence
Pectineal line of pubis
Pubic tubercle
Sup. pubic ramus
Pubic crest

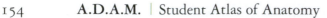

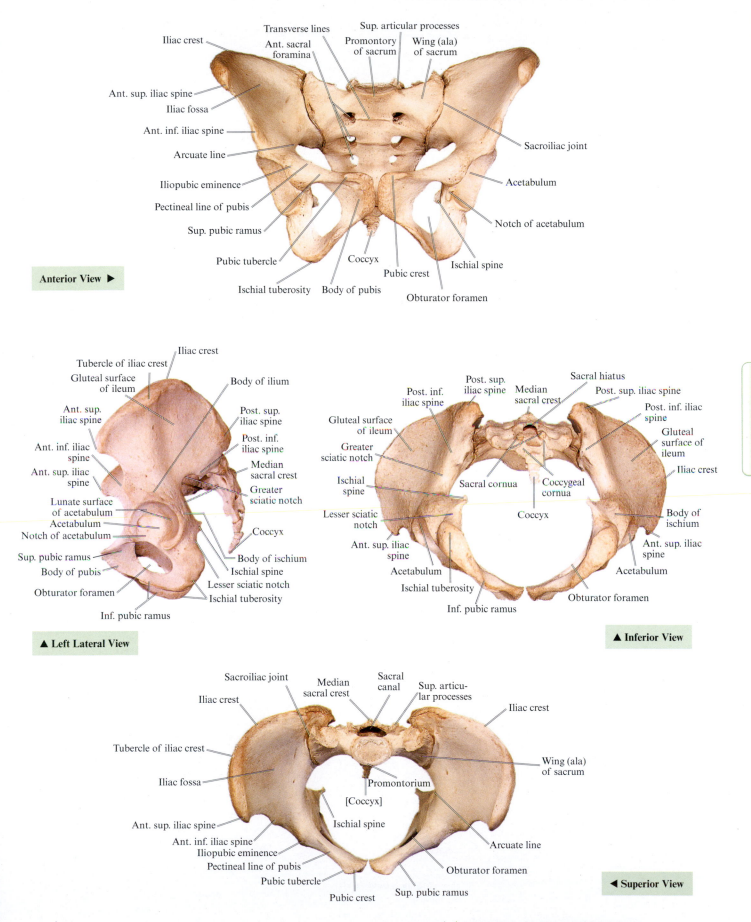

Anterior View ▶

Transverse lines
Ant. sacral foramina
Promontory of sacrum
Sup. articular processes
Wing (ala) of sacrum
Iliac crest
Ant. sup. iliac spine
Iliac fossa
Ant. inf. iliac spine
Arcuate line
Iliopubic eminence
Pectineal line of pubis
Sup. pubic ramus
Pubic tubercle
Ischial tuberosity
Body of pubis
Coccyx
Pubic crest
Ischial spine
Obturator foramen
Sacroiliac joint
Acetabulum
Notch of acetabulum

▲ Left Lateral View

Iliac crest
Tubercle of iliac crest
Gluteal surface of ileum
Ant. sup. iliac spine
Ant. inf. iliac spine
Ant. sup. iliac spine
Lunate surface of acetabulum
Acetabulum
Notch of acetabulum
Sup. pubic ramus
Body of pubis
Obturator foramen
Inf. pubic ramus
Body of ilium
Post. sup. iliac spine
Post. inf. iliac spine
Median sacral crest
Greater sciatic notch
Coccyx
Body of ischium
Ischial spine
Lesser sciatic notch
Ischial tuberosity

▲ Inferior View

Post. inf. iliac spine
Post. sup. iliac spine
Median sacral crest
Sacral hiatus
Post. sup. iliac spine
Post. inf. iliac spine
Gluteal surface of ileum
Greater sciatic notch
Ischial spine
Lesser sciatic notch
Ant. sup. iliac spine
Acetabulum
Ischial tuberosity
Inf. pubic ramus
Sacral cornua
Coccygeal cornua
Coccyx
Gluteal surface of ileum
Iliac crest
Body of ischium
Ant. sup. iliac spine
Acetabulum
Obturator foramen

◀ Superior View

Sacroiliac joint
Median sacral crest
Sacral canal
Sup. articular processes
Iliac crest
Tubercle of iliac crest
Iliac fossa
Ant. sup. iliac spine
Ant. inf. iliac spine
Iliopubic eminence
Pectineal line of pubis
Pubic tubercle
Pubic crest
Promontorium
[Coccyx]
Ischial spine
Sup. pubic ramus
Iliac crest
Wing (ala) of sacrum
Arcuate line
Obturator foramen

PLATE 4.7   PELVIC MUSCLES—SUPERFICIAL PERINEAL

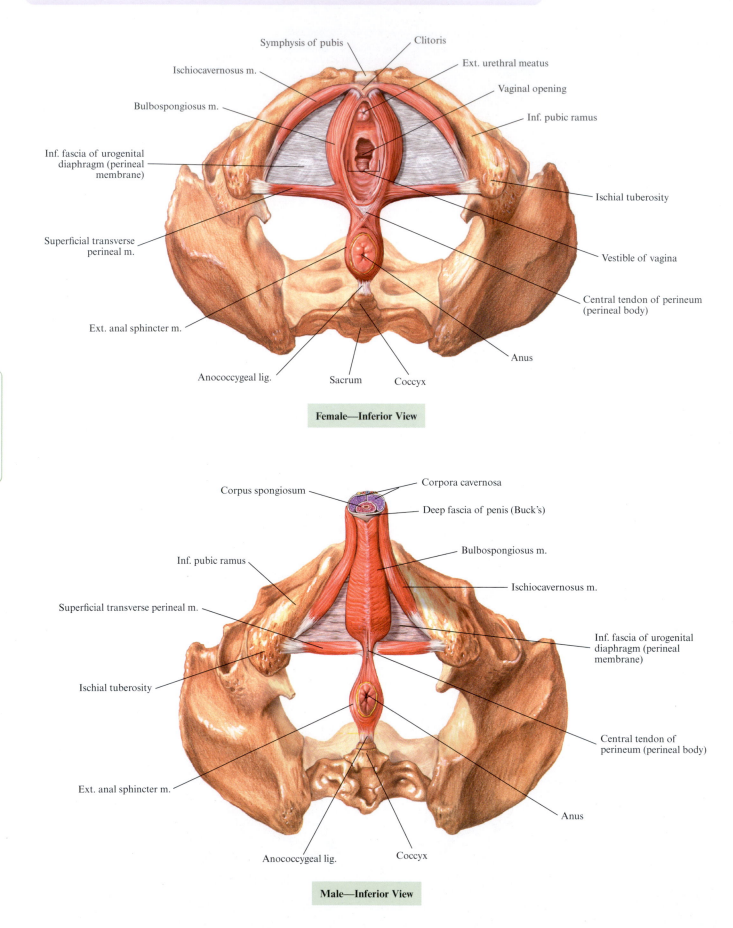

Symphysis of pubis

Clitoris

Ischiocavernosus m.

Ext. urethral meatus

Bulbospongiosus m.

Vaginal opening

Inf. pubic ramus

Inf. fascia of urogenital diaphragm (perineal membrane)

Ischial tuberosity

Superficial transverse perineal m.

Vestible of vagina

Central tendon of perineum (perineal body)

Ext. anal sphincter m.

Anus

Anococcygeal lig.   Sacrum   Coccyx

Female—Inferior View

Corpus spongiosum

Corpora cavernosa

Deep fascia of penis (Buck's)

Inf. pubic ramus

Bulbospongiosus m.

Ischiocavernosus m.

Superficial transverse perineal m.

Inf. fascia of urogenital diaphragm (perineal membrane)

Ischial tuberosity

Central tendon of perineum (perineal body)

Ext. anal sphincter m.

Anus

Anococcygeal lig.   Coccyx

Male—Inferior View

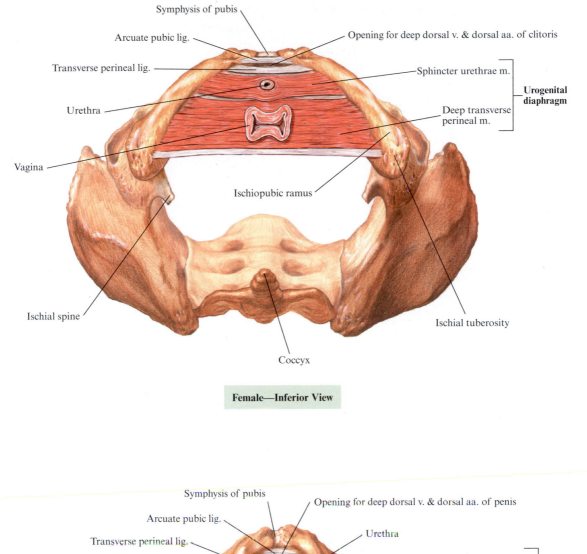

Symphysis of pubis

Arcuate pubic lig.

Transverse perineal lig.

Opening for deep dorsal v. & dorsal aa. of clitoris

Sphincter urethrae m.

Urethra

Deep transverse perineal m.

Urogenital diaphragm

Vagina

Ischiopubic ramus

Ischial spine

Ischial tuberosity

Coccyx

Female—Inferior View

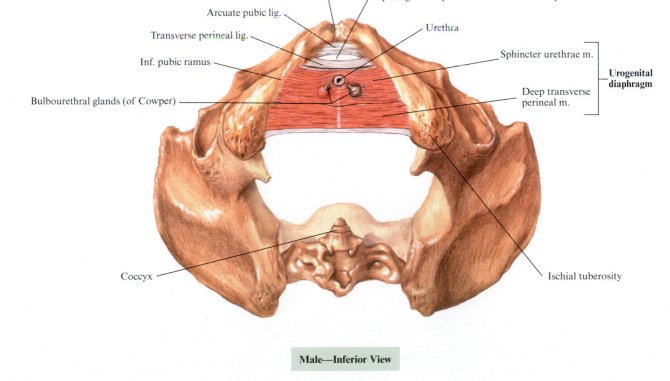

Symphysis of pubis

Arcuate pubic lig.

Transverse perineal lig.

Inf. pubic ramus

Opening for deep dorsal v. & dorsal aa. of penis

Urethra

Sphincter urethrae m.

Deep transverse perineal m.

Urogenital diaphragm

Bulbourethral glands (of Cowper)

Coccyx

Ischial tuberosity

Male—Inferior View

PLATE 4.9   PELVIC MUSCLES—PELVIC DIAPHRAGM

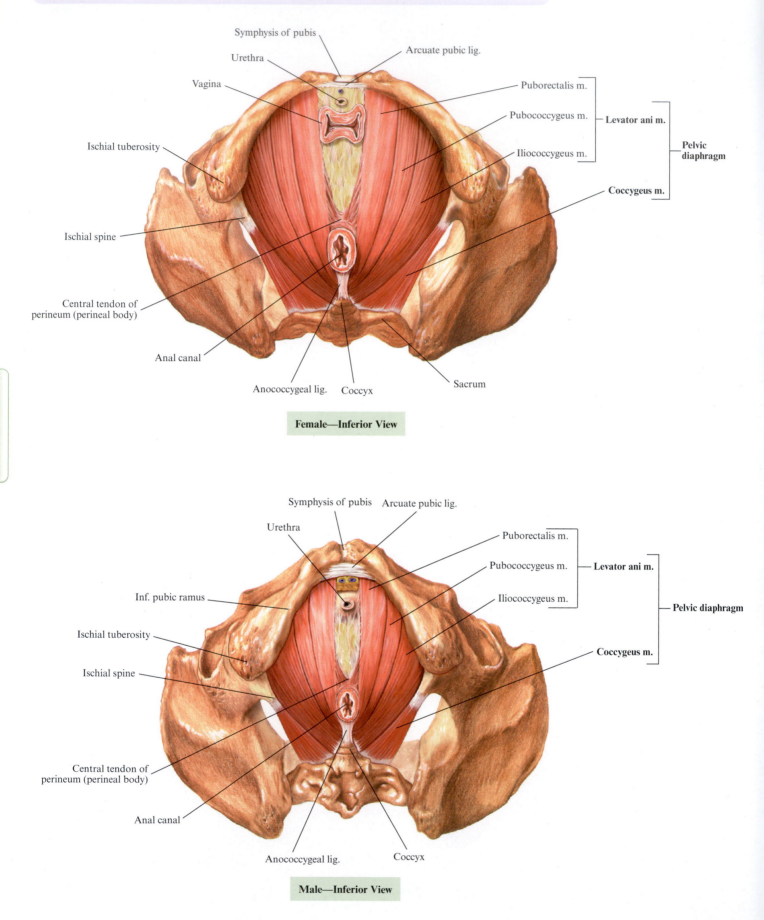

Female—Inferior View

Male—Inferior View

Muscle	Superior or Lateral Attachment	Inferior or Medial Attachment	Innervation	Action(s)
Ischiocavernosus	Int. surface of ischial ramus & tuberosity laterally	Sides & ventrum of crus of penis in ♂ or clitoris medially in ♀	Perineal brr. of pudendal n. (S2–4)	Maintains erection of penis or clitoris
Bulbospongiosus	Dorsum of clitoris in ♀; inf. fascia of urogenital diaphragm, sides & dorsum of penile bulb in ♂	Perineal body, inf. fascia of urogenital diaphragm & median raphe of penile bulb in ♂		Compresses vaginal orifice & erection of clitoris in ♀; compresses urethra, assist in erection & ejaculation in ♂
Superficial transverse perineal	Int. surface of ischial tuberosity laterally	Perineal body (central perineal tendon) medially		Supports pelvic viscera
Ext. anal sphincter	Anococcygeal lig. to coccyx & int. anal sphincter m. superiorly	Perineal body anteriorly & skin superficially	Inf. rectal n. (S2–3) and perineal br. of S4 spinal n.	Compresses anus
Sphincter urethrae	Inf. pubic ramus laterally	Perineal body posteriorly & fibers from opposite side medially	Perineal brr. of pudendal n. (S2–4)	Compresses urethra in ♂ & ♀ & vagina in ♀
Deep transverse perineal	Ischial ramus laterally	Perineal body medially		Supports pelvic viscera

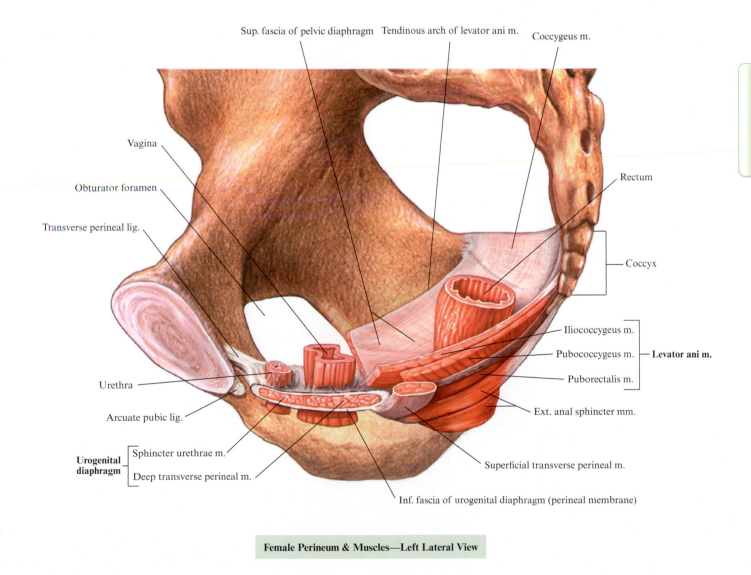

Female Perineum & Muscles—Left Lateral View

PLATE 4.10   PELVIC MUSCLES—MALE

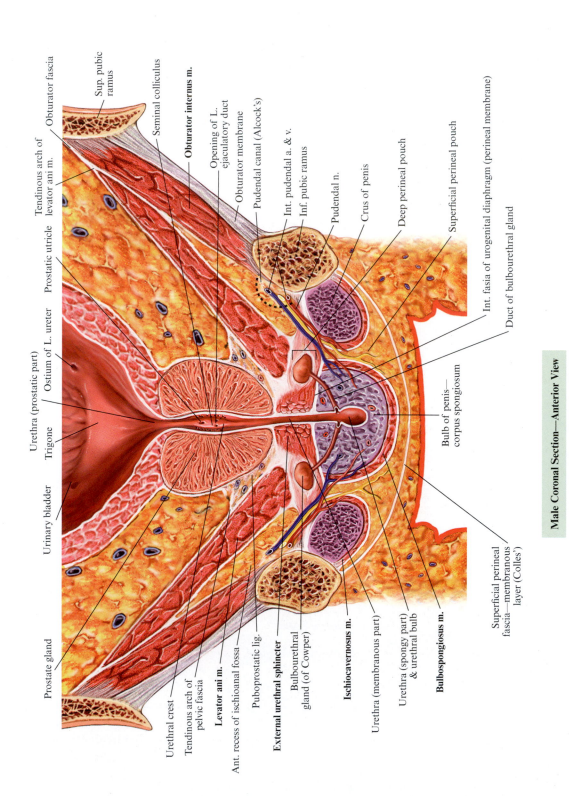

Obturator fascia
Sup. pubic ramus
Tendinous arch of levator ani m.
Obturator internus m.
Seminal colliculus
Opening of L. ejaculatory duct
Obturator membrane
Pudendal canal (Alcock's)
Int. pudendal a. & v.
Inf. pubic ramus
Pudendal n.
Crus of penis
Deep perineal pouch
Superficial perineal pouch
Int. fasia of urogenital diaphragm (perineal membrane)
Duct of bulbourethral gland
Bulb of penis— corpus spongiosum

Prostatic utricle
Urethra (prostatic part)
Ostium of L. ureter
Trigone
Urinary bladder
Prostate gland
Urethral crest
Tendinous arch of pelvic fascia
Levator ani m.
Ant. recess of ischioanal fossa
Puboprostatic lig.
External urethral sphincter
Bulbourethral gland (of Cowper)
Ischiocavernosus m.
Urethra (membranous part)
Urethra (spongy part) & urethral bulb
Bulbospongiosus m.
Superficial perineal fascia—membranous layer (Colles')

Male Coronal Section—Anterior View

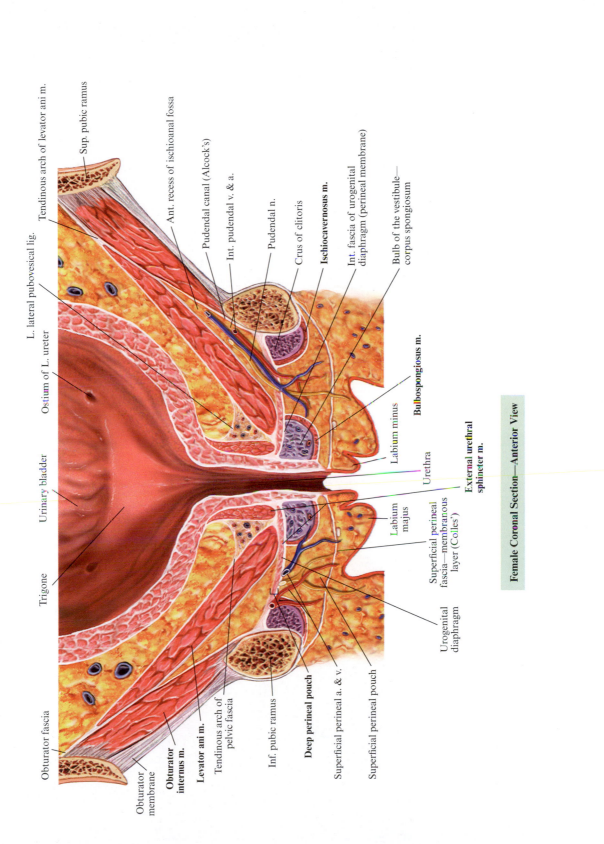

Tendinous arch of levator ani m.

Sup. pubic ramus

Ant. recess of ischioanal fossa

Pudendal canal (Alcock's)

Int. pudendal v. & a.

Pudendal n.

Crus of clitoris

Ischiocavernosus m.

Int. fascia of urogenital diaphragm (perineal membrane)

Bulb of the vestibule—corpus spongiosum

L. lateral pubovesical lig.

Ostium of L. ureter

Bulbospongiosus m.

Labium minus

Urinary bladder

Urethra

External urethral sphincter m.

Labium majus

Trigone

Superficial perineal fascia—membranous layer (Colles')

Urogenital diaphragm

Obturator fascia

Obturator membrane

Obturator internus m.

Levator ani m.

Tendinous arch of pelvic fascia

Inf. pubic ramus

Deep perineal pouch

Superficial perineal a. & v.

Superficial perineal pouch

Female Coronal Section—Anterior View

PLATE 4.12   FEMOROPELVIC MUSCLES

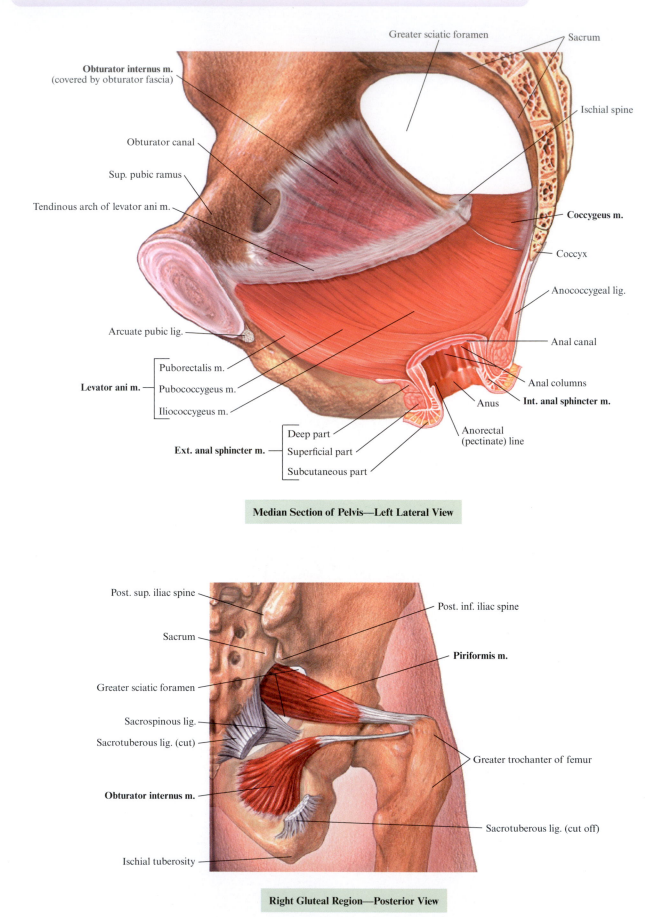

Greater sciatic foramen

Sacrum

Obturator internus m.
(covered by obturator fascia)

Ischial spine

Obturator canal

Sup. pubic ramus

Tendinous arch of levator ani m.

Coccygeus m.

Coccyx

Anococcygeal lig.

Arcuate pubic lig.

Anal canal

Puborectalis m.

Levator ani m.   Pubococcygeus m.

Iliococcygeus m.

Anal columns

Int. anal sphincter m.

Anus

Anorectal
(pectinate) line

Deep part

Ext. anal sphincter m.   Superficial part

Subcutaneous part

Median Section of Pelvis—Left Lateral View

Post. sup. iliac spine

Post. inf. iliac spine

Sacrum

Piriformis m.

Greater sciatic foramen

Sacrospinous lig.

Sacrotuberous lig. (cut)

Greater trochanter of femur

Obturator internus m.

Sacrotuberous lig. (cut off)

Ischial tuberosity

Right Gluteal Region—Posterior View

Muscles of the Pelvic Diaphragm

Muscle	Superior or Lateral Attachment	Inferior or Medial Attachment	Innervation	Action(s)
Puborectalis	Body of pubis anteriorly	Fibers of opposite side post. to rectum	Inf. rectal n. (S2, 3) & perineal brr. of S3, 4 spinal n.	Maintains anorectal flexure by drawing anal canal anteriorly
Pubococcygeus	Body of pubis and obturator fascia anteriorly	Coccyx & anococcygeal lig. posteriorly		Supports pelvic viscera
Iliococcygeus	Ischial spine & tendinous arch of pelvic fascia laterally	Coccyx & anococcygeal lig. posteriorly		Supports pelvic viscera
Coccygeus	Ischial spine & sacrospinous lig. laterally	Coccyx & S5 vertebra medially	Brr. of S3–5 spinal nn.	Supports pelvic viscera

Muscles of the Pelvic Walls

Muscle	Superior or Medial Attachment	Inferior or Lateral Attachment	Innervation	Action(s)
Obturator internus	Pelvic surfaces of ilium & ischium; obturator membrane	Greater trochanter of femur	N. to obturator internus (L5–S2)	Rotates thigh laterally
Piriformis	Pelvic surface of 2nd–4th sacral segments; sup. margin of greater sciatic notch, & sacrotuberous lig.		Ventral rami of S1 & S2	Rotates thigh laterally

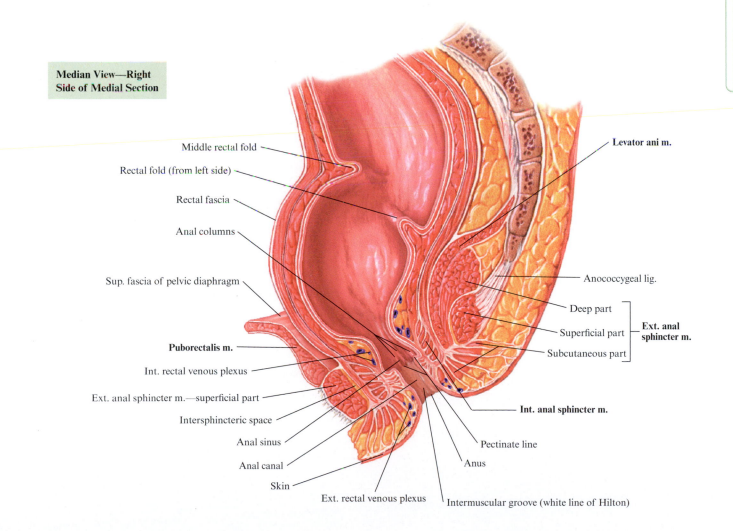

Median View—Right Side of Medial Section

Middle rectal fold

Rectal fold (from left side)

Rectal fascia

Anal columns

Sup. fascia of pelvic diaphragm

Puborectalis m.

Int. rectal venous plexus

Ext. anal sphincter m.—superficial part

Intersphincteric space

Anal sinus

Anal canal

Skin

Ext. rectal venous plexus

Levator ani m.

Anococcygeal lig.

Deep part

Superficial part } Ext. anal sphincter m.

Subcutaneous part

Int. anal sphincter m.

Pectinate line

Anus

Intermuscular groove (white line of Hilton)

PLATE 4.13   ARTERIES OF THE PELVIS—MALE

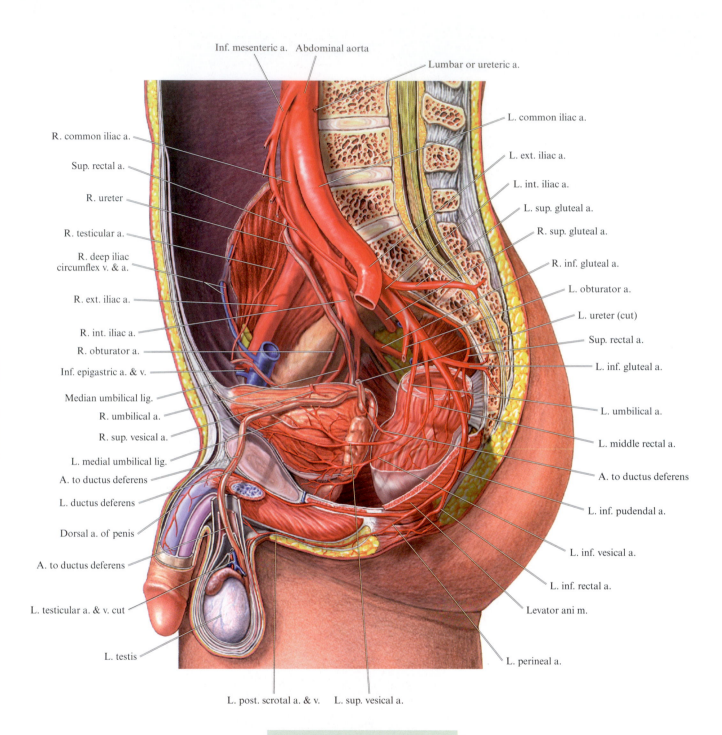

Inf. mesenteric a.   Abdominal aorta

Lumbar or ureteric a.

R. common iliac a.

Sup. rectal a.

R. ureter

R. testicular a.

R. deep iliac circumflex v. & a.

R. ext. iliac a.

R. int. iliac a.

R. obturator a.

Inf. epigastric a. & v.

Median umbilical lig.

R. umbilical a.

R. sup. vesical a.

L. medial umbilical lig.

A. to ductus deferens

L. ductus deferens

Dorsal a. of penis

A. to ductus deferens

L. testicular a. & v. cut

L. testis

L. common iliac a.

L. ext. iliac a.

L. int. iliac a.

L. sup. gluteal a.

R. sup. gluteal a.

R. inf. gluteal a.

L. obturator a.

L. ureter (cut)

Sup. rectal a.

L. inf. gluteal a.

L. umbilical a.

L. middle rectal a.

A. to ductus deferens

L. inf. pudendal a.

L. inf. vesical a.

L. inf. rectal a.

Levator ani m.

L. perineal a.

L. post. scrotal a. & v.   L. sup. vesical a.

Medial View with Peritoneum Removed

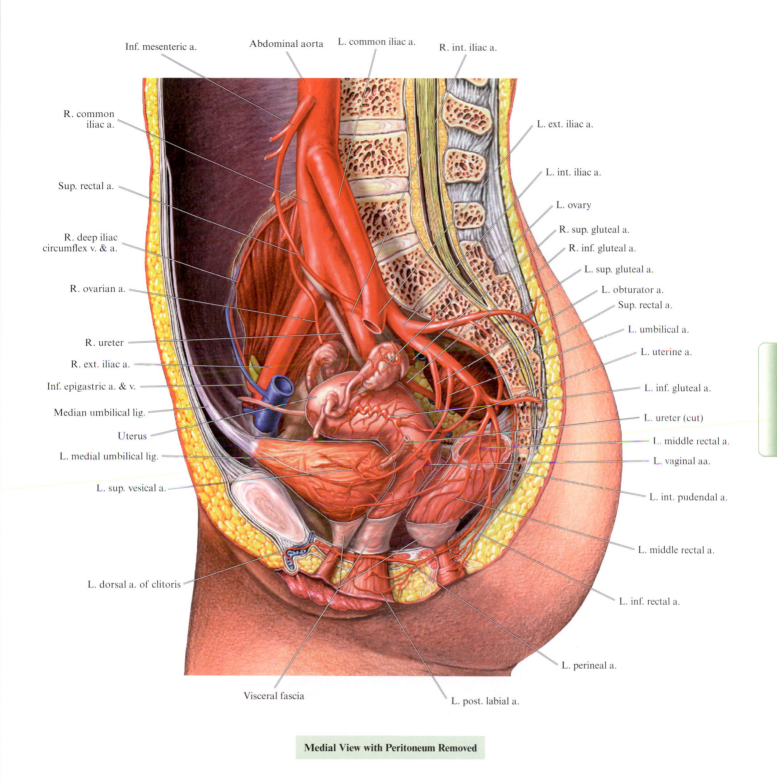

Inf. mesenteric a.

Abdominal aorta

L. common iliac a.

R. int. iliac a.

R. common iliac a.

L. ext. iliac a.

Sup. rectal a.

L. int. iliac a.

L. ovary

R. deep iliac circumflex v. & a.

R. sup. gluteal a.

R. inf. gluteal a.

R. ovarian a.

L. sup. gluteal a.

L. obturator a.

Sup. rectal a.

R. ureter

L. umbilical a.

R. ext. iliac a.

L. uterine a.

Inf. epigastric a. & v.

L. inf. gluteal a.

Median umbilical lig.

L. ureter (cut)

Uterus

L. middle rectal a.

L. medial umbilical lig.

L. vaginal aa.

L. sup. vesical a.

L. int. pudendal a.

L. middle rectal a.

L. dorsal a. of clitoris

L. inf. rectal a.

L. perineal a.

Visceral fascia

L. post. labial a.

Medial View with Peritoneum Removed

PLATE 4.17   DERMATOMES & CUTANEOUS NERVES—MALE

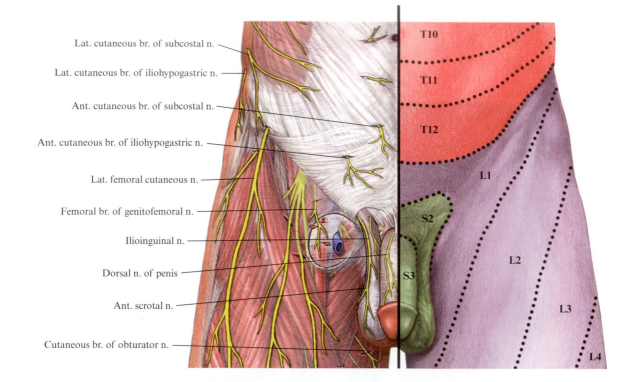

Lat. cutaneous br. of subcostal n.

Lat. cutaneous br. of iliohypogastric n.

Ant. cutaneous br. of subcostal n.

Ant. cutaneous br. of iliohypogastric n.

Lat. femoral cutaneous n.

Femoral br. of genitofemoral n.

Ilioinguinal n.

Dorsal n. of penis

Ant. scrotal n.

Cutaneous br. of obturator n.

T10   T11   T12   L1   S2   S3   L2   L3   L4

Anterior View

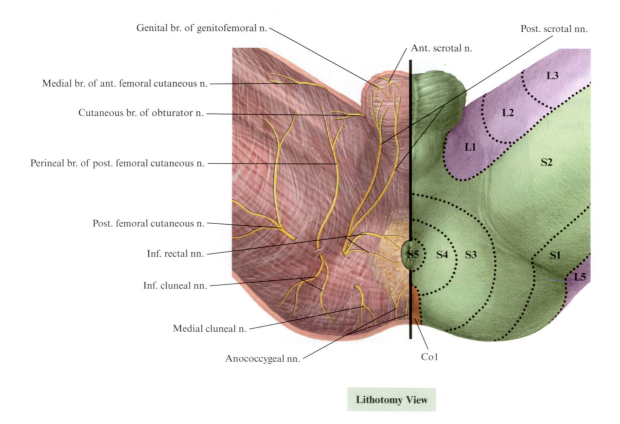

Genital br. of genitofemoral n.

Ant. scrotal n.

Post. scrotal nn.

Medial br. of ant. femoral cutaneous n.

Cutaneous br. of obturator n.

Perineal br. of post. femoral cutaneous n.

Post. femoral cutaneous n.

Inf. rectal nn.

Inf. cluneal nn.

Medial cluneal n.

Anococcygeal nn.

Co1

L3   L2   L1   S2   S5   S4   S3   S1   L5

Lithotomy View

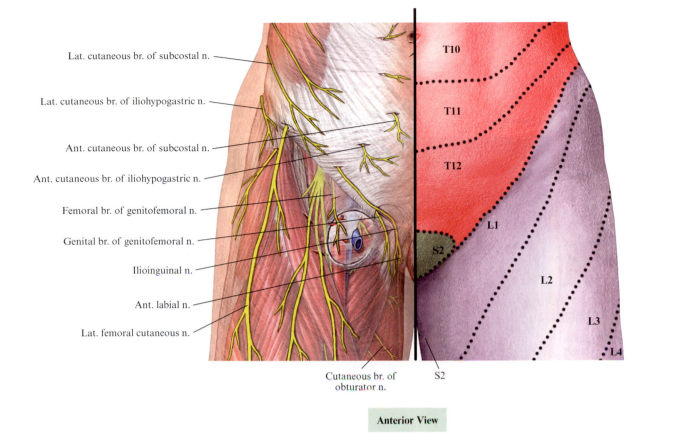

Lat. cutaneous br. of subcostal n.

Lat. cutaneous br. of iliohypogastric n.

Ant. cutaneous br. of subcostal n.

Ant. cutaneous br. of iliohypogastric n.

Femoral br. of genitofemoral n.

Genital br. of genitofemoral n.

Ilioinguinal n.

Ant. labial n.

Lat. femoral cutaneous n.

T10

T11

T12

L1

S2

L2

L3

L4

Cutaneous br. of obturator n.   S2

Anterior View

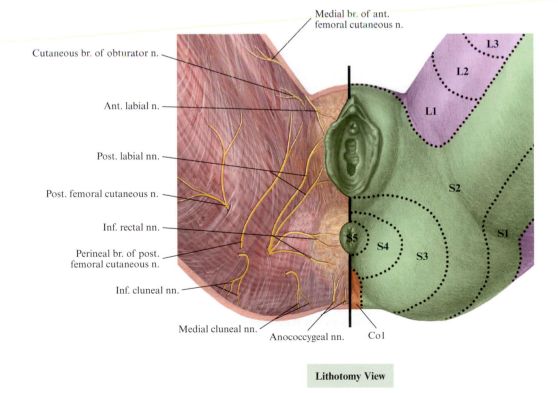

Medial br. of ant. femoral cutaneous n.

Cutaneous br. of obturator n.

Ant. labial n.

Post. labial nn.

Post. femoral cutaneous n.

Inf. rectal nn.

Perineal br. of post. femoral cutaneous n.

Inf. cluneal nn.

Medial cluneal nn.   Anococcygeal nn.   Co1

L3

L2

L1

S2

S5

S4

S3

S1

Lithotomy View

PLATE 4.21   PELVIC AUTONOMIC NERVES—MALE

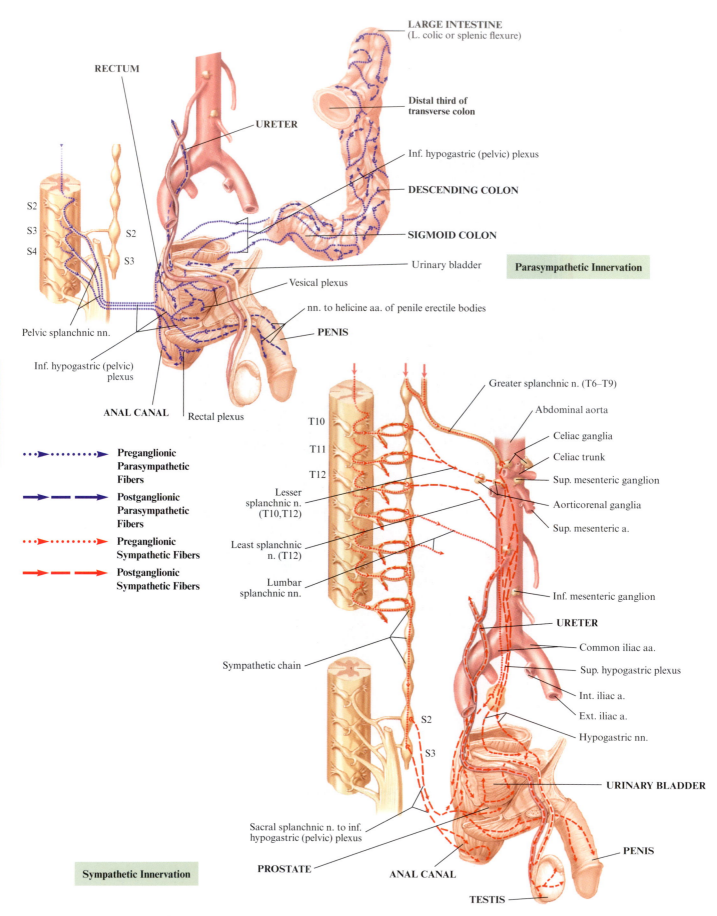

LARGE INTESTINE
(L. colic or splenic flexure)

RECTUM

Distal third of
transverse colon

URETER

Inf. hypogastric (pelvic) plexus

DESCENDING COLON

SIGMOID COLON

Urinary bladder

Parasympathetic Innervation

Vesical plexus

nn. to helicine aa. of penile erectile bodies

PENIS

S2
S3
S4

S2
S3

Pelvic splanchnic nn.

Inf. hypogastric (pelvic)
plexus

ANAL CANAL   Rectal plexus

Greater splanchnic n. (T6–T9)

Abdominal aorta

Celiac ganglia

Celiac trunk

T10

T11

T12

Sup. mesenteric ganglion

Aorticorenal ganglia

Sup. mesenteric a.

Lesser
splanchnic n.
(T10, T12)

Least splanchnic
n. (T12)

Lumbar
splanchnic nn.

Inf. mesenteric ganglion

URETER

Common iliac aa.

Sup. hypogastric plexus

Int. iliac a.

Ext. iliac a.

Hypogastric nn.

- - - ▸ - - - - - - ▸   **Preganglionic
Parasympathetic
Fibers**

━ ▸ ━ ━ ━ ▸   **Postganglionic
Parasympathetic
Fibers**

· · ▸ · · · · · · ▸   **Preganglionic
Sympathetic Fibers**

━ ▸ ━ ━ ━ ▸   **Postganglionic
Sympathetic Fibers**

Sympathetic chain

S2

S3

URINARY BLADDER

PENIS

Sacral splanchnic n. to inf.
hypogastric (pelvic) plexus

Sympathetic Innervation

PROSTATE

ANAL CANAL

TESTIS

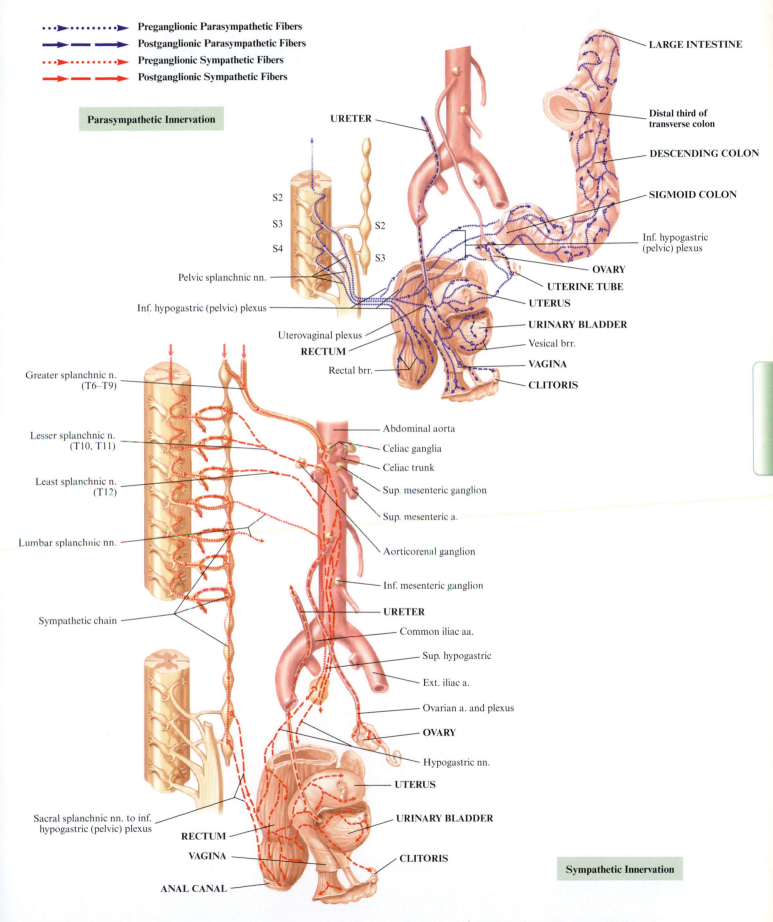

Preganglionic Parasympathetic Fibers
Postganglionic Parasympathetic Fibers
Preganglionic Sympathetic Fibers
Postganglionic Sympathetic Fibers

Parasympathetic Innervation

LARGE INTESTINE

Distal third of transverse colon

DESCENDING COLON

SIGMOID COLON

URETER

S2
S3
S4

S2

S3

Pelvic splanchnic nn.

Inf. hypogastric (pelvic) plexus

Inf. hypogastric (pelvic) plexus

OVARY

UTERINE TUBE

UTERUS

URINARY BLADDER

Vesical brr.

Uterovaginal plexus

RECTUM

Rectal brr.

VAGINA

CLITORIS

Greater splanchnic n. (T6–T9)

Abdominal aorta

Celiac ganglia

Celiac trunk

Lesser splanchnic n. (T10, T11)

Sup. mesenteric ganglion

Sup. mesenteric a.

Least splanchnic n. (T12)

Aorticorenal ganglion

Lumbar splanchnic nn.

Inf. mesenteric ganglion

URETER

Common iliac aa.

Sympathetic chain

Sup. hypogastric

Ext. iliac a.

Ovarian a. and plexus

OVARY

Hypogastric nn.

UTERUS

URINARY BLADDER

Sacral splanchnic nn. to inf. hypogastric (pelvic) plexus

RECTUM

VAGINA

CLITORIS

ANAL CANAL

Sympathetic Innervation

PLATE 4.23   SUPERFICIAL LYMPHATICS

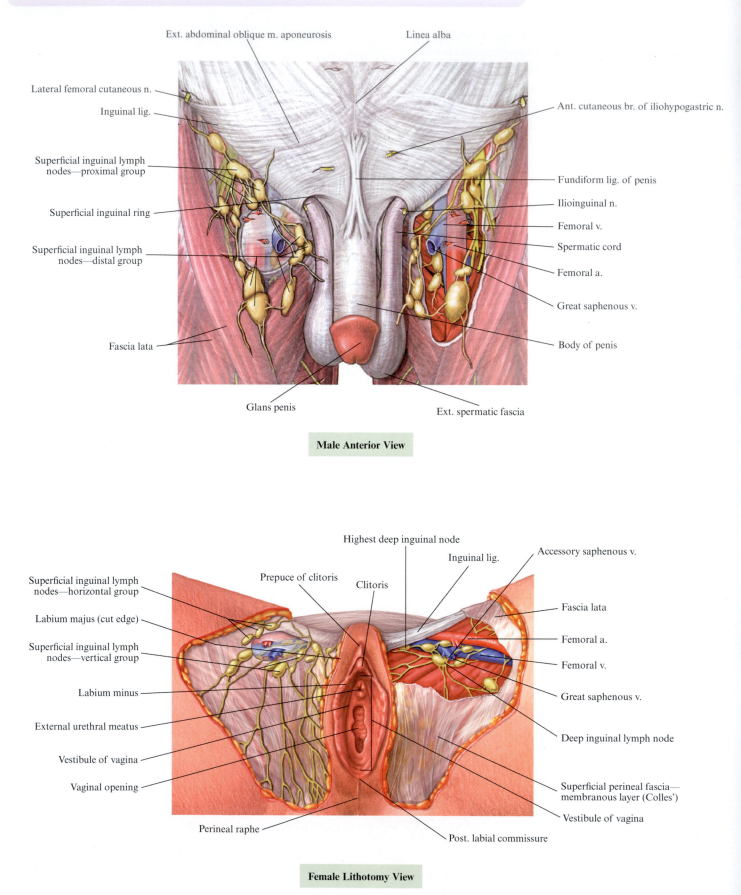

Ext. abdominal oblique m. aponeurosis

Linea alba

Lateral femoral cutaneous n.

Inguinal lig.

Superficial inguinal lymph nodes—proximal group

Superficial inguinal ring

Superficial inguinal lymph nodes—distal group

Fascia lata

Glans penis

Ant. cutaneous br. of iliohypogastric n.

Fundiform lig. of penis

Ilioinguinal n.

Femoral v.

Spermatic cord

Femoral a.

Great saphenous v.

Body of penis

Ext. spermatic fascia

Male Anterior View

Highest deep inguinal node

Prepuce of clitoris   Clitoris

Inguinal lig.

Accessory saphenous v.

Superficial inguinal lymph nodes—horizontal group

Labium majus (cut edge)

Superficial inguinal lymph nodes—vertical group

Labium minus

External urethral meatus

Vestibule of vagina

Vaginal opening

Fascia lata

Femoral a.

Femoral v.

Great saphenous v.

Deep inguinal lymph node

Superficial perineal fascia—membranous layer (Colles')

Vestibule of vagina

Perineal raphe

Post. labial commissure

Female Lithotomy View

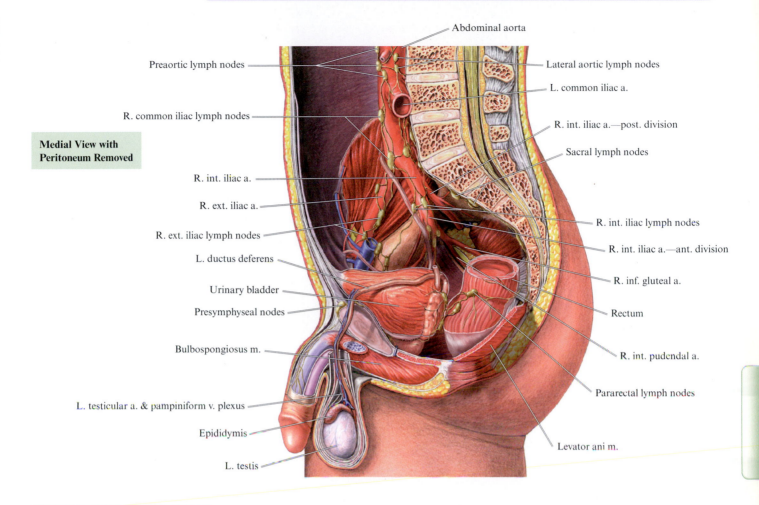

Medial View with Peritoneum Removed

Abdominal aorta

Preaortic lymph nodes

Lateral aortic lymph nodes

L. common iliac a.

R. common iliac lymph nodes

R. int. iliac a.—post. division

Sacral lymph nodes

R. int. iliac a.

R. ext. iliac a.

R. int. iliac lymph nodes

R. ext. iliac lymph nodes

R. int. iliac a.—ant. division

L. ductus deferens

R. inf. gluteal a.

Urinary bladder

Presymphyseal nodes

Rectum

Bulbospongiosus m.

R. int. pudendal a.

Pararectal lymph nodes

L. testicular a. & pampiniform v. plexus

Epididymis

Levator ani m.

L. testis

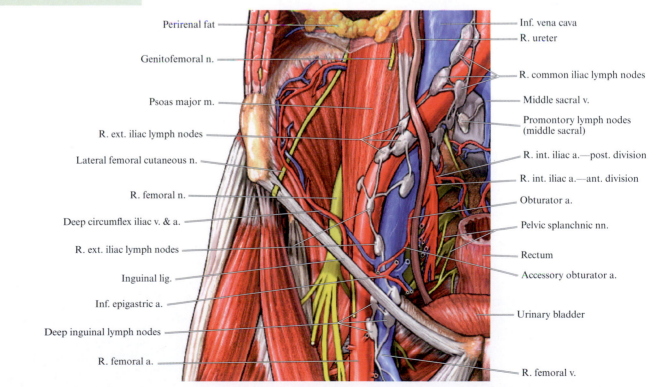

Right Half of Pelvis—Anterior View

Perirenal fat

Inf. vena cava

R. ureter

Genitofemoral n.

R. common iliac lymph nodes

Psoas major m.

Middle sacral v.

R. ext. iliac lymph nodes

Promontory lymph nodes (middle sacral)

Lateral femoral cutaneous n.

R. int. iliac a.—post. division

R. int. iliac a.—ant. division

R. femoral n.

Obturator a.

Deep circumflex iliac v. & a.

Pelvic splanchnic nn.

R. ext. iliac lymph nodes

Rectum

Inguinal lig.

Accessory obturator a.

Inf. epigastric a.

Urinary bladder

Deep inguinal lymph nodes

R. femoral a.

R. femoral v.

PLATE 4.25   UROGENITAL TRACT—FEMALE

♀ = **Characteristic Female Structures**

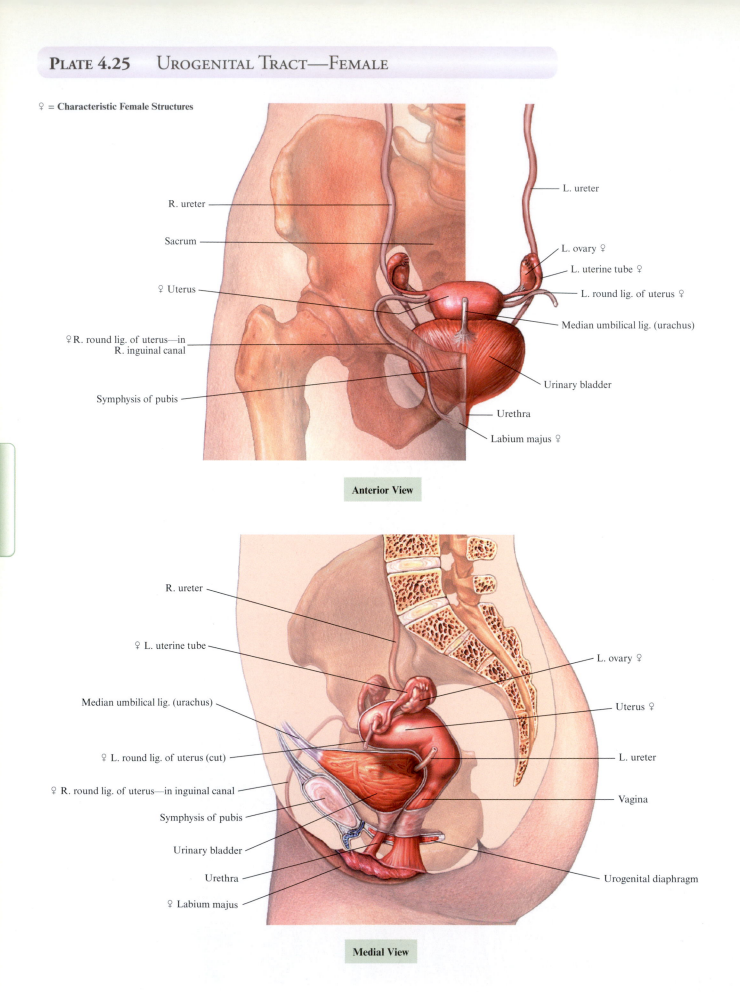

R. ureter

Sacrum

♀ Uterus

♀ R. round lig. of uterus—in
R. inguinal canal

Symphysis of pubis

L. ureter

L. ovary ♀

L. uterine tube ♀

L. round lig. of uterus ♀

Median umbilical lig. (urachus)

Urinary bladder

Urethra

Labium majus ♀

Anterior View

R. ureter

♀ L. uterine tube

Median umbilical lig. (urachus)

♀ L. round lig. of uterus (cut)

♀ R. round lig. of uterus—in inguinal canal

Symphysis of pubis

Urinary bladder

Urethra

♀ Labium majus

L. ovary ♀

Uterus ♀

L. ureter

Vagina

Urogenital diaphragm

Medial View

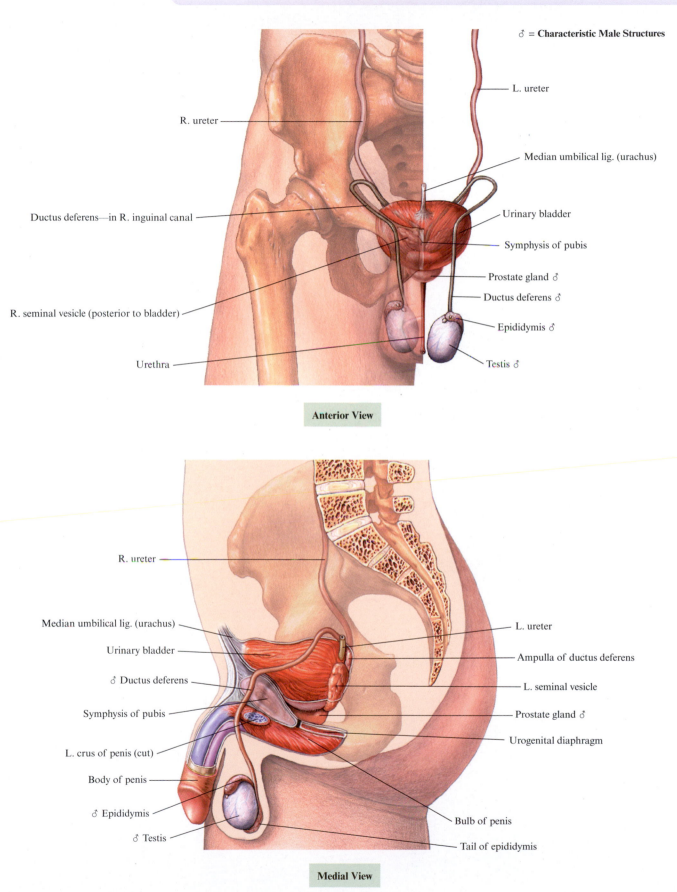

♂ = **Characteristic Male Structures**

L. ureter

R. ureter

Median umbilical lig. (urachus)

Ductus deferens—in R. inguinal canal

Urinary bladder

Symphysis of pubis

Prostate gland ♂

Ductus deferens ♂

R. seminal vesicle (posterior to bladder)

Epididymis ♂

Urethra

Testis ♂

Anterior View

R. ureter

Median umbilical lig. (urachus)

L. ureter

Urinary bladder

Ampulla of ductus deferens

♂ Ductus deferens

L. seminal vesicle

Symphysis of pubis

Prostate gland ♂

Urogenital diaphragm

L. crus of penis (cut)

Body of penis

♂ Epididymis

Bulb of penis

♂ Testis

Tail of epididymis

Medial View

PLATE 4.27   PELVIC CONTENTS—FEMALE

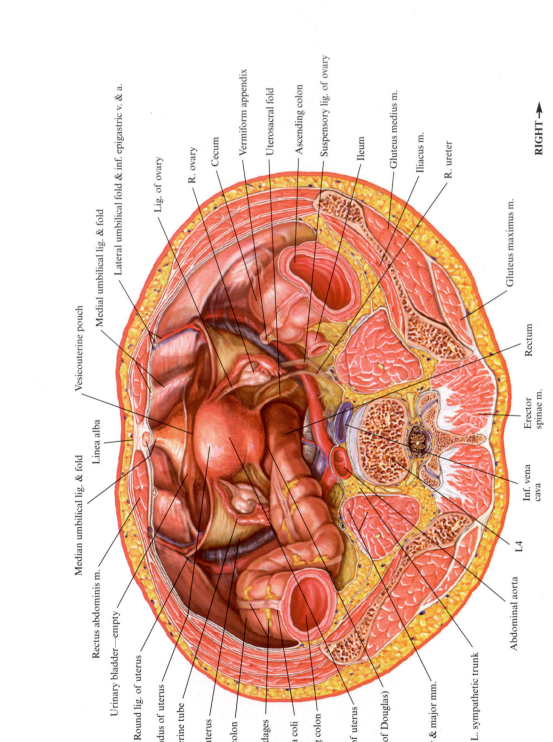

Lateral umbilical fold & inf. epigastric v. & a.

Medial umbilical lig. & fold

Vesicouterine pouch

Lig. of ovary

R. ovary

Cecum

Vermiform appendix

Uterosacral fold

Ascending colon

Suspensory lig. of ovary

Ileum

Gluteus medius m.

Iliacus m.

R. ureter

Gluteus maximus m.

Rectum

Erector spinae m.

Inf. vena cava

L4

Abdominal aorta

L. sympathetic trunk

Psoas minor & major mm.

Rectouterine pouch (of Douglas)

Body of uterus

Descending colon

Tenia coli

Omental [epiploic] appendages

Sigmoid colon

Broad lig. of uterus

Uterine tube

Fundus of uterus

Round lig. of uterus

Urinary bladder—empty

Median umbilical lig. & fold

Rectus abdominis m.

Linea alba

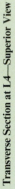

Transverse Section at L4—Superior View

RIGHT →

← LEFT

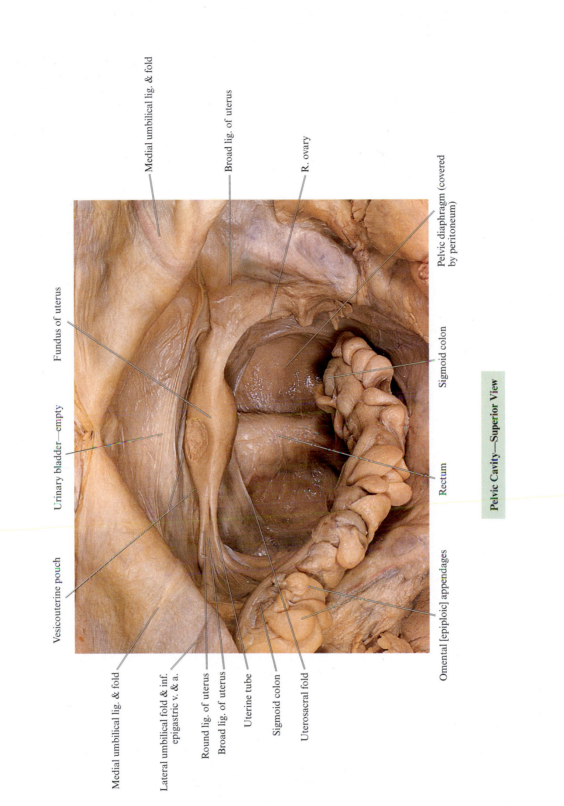

Medial umbilical lig. & fold

Broad lig. of uterus

R. ovary

Pelvic diaphragm (covered by peritoneum)

Fundus of uterus

Sigmoid colon

Urinary bladder—empty

Rectum

Vesicouterine pouch

Pelvic Cavity—Superior View

Omental [epiploic] appendages

Medial umbilical lig. & fold

Lateral umbilical fold & inf. epigastric v. & a.

Round lig. of uterus

Broad lig. of uterus

Uterine tube

Sigmoid colon

Uterosacral fold

PLATE 4.29 PELVIC CONTENTS—FEMALE

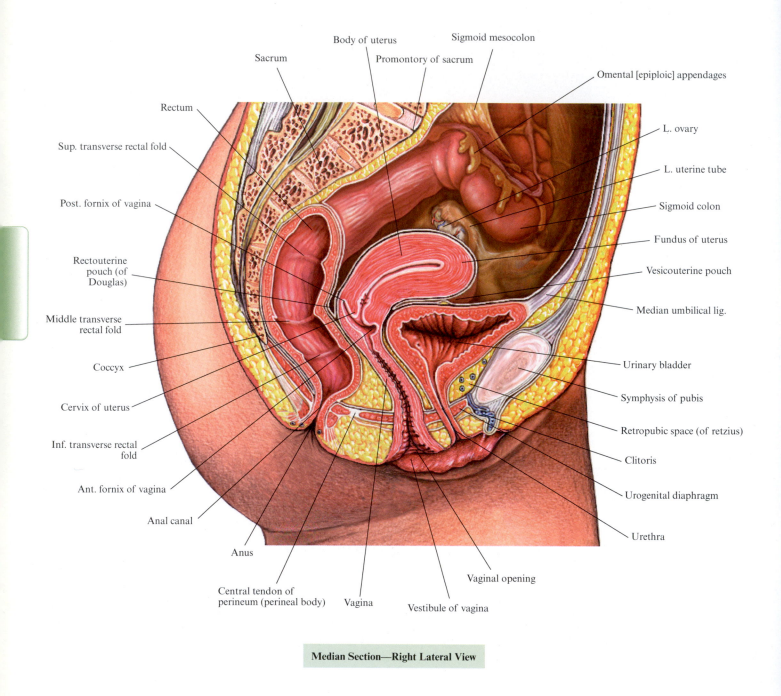

Sacrum

Body of uterus

Promontory of sacrum

Sigmoid mesocolon

Omental [epiploic] appendages

Rectum

Sup. transverse rectal fold

Post. fornix of vagina

Rectouterine pouch (of Douglas)

Middle transverse rectal fold

Coccyx

Cervix of uterus

Inf. transverse rectal fold

Ant. fornix of vagina

Anal canal

Anus

Central tendon of perineum (perineal body)

Vagina

Vestibule of vagina

Vaginal opening

L. ovary

L. uterine tube

Sigmoid colon

Fundus of uterus

Vesicouterine pouch

Median umbilical lig.

Urinary bladder

Symphysis of pubis

Retropubic space (of retzius)

Clitoris

Urogenital diaphragm

Urethra

Median Section—Right Lateral View

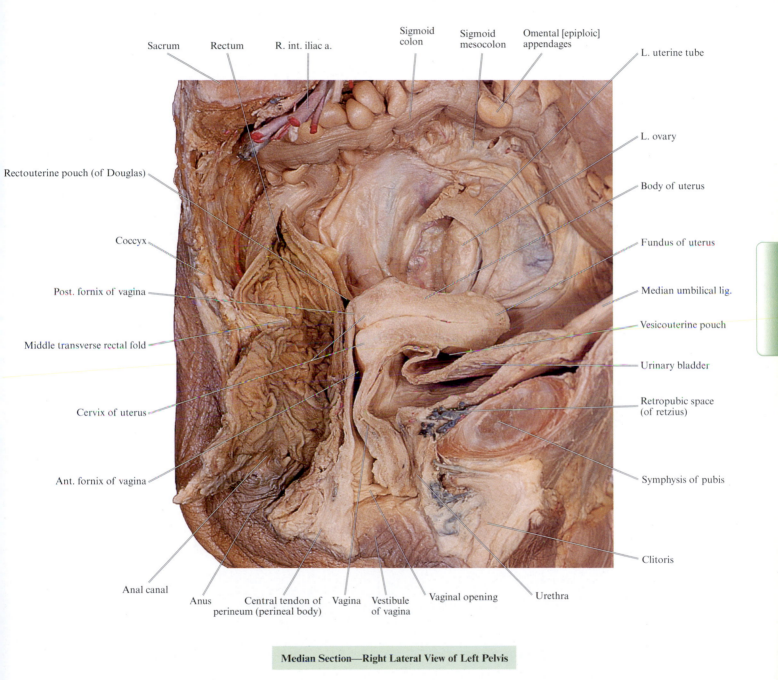

Sacrum   Rectum   R. int. iliac a.   Sigmoid colon   Sigmoid mesocolon   Omental [epiploic] appendages   L. uterine tube

Rectouterine pouch (of Douglas)

L. ovary

Body of uterus

Coccyx

Fundus of uterus

Post. fornix of vagina

Median umbilical lig.

Middle transverse rectal fold

Vesicouterine pouch

Urinary bladder

Retropubic space (of retzius)

Cervix of uterus

Ant. fornix of vagina

Symphysis of pubis

Clitoris

Anal canal   Anus   Central tendon of perineum (perineal body)   Vagina   Vestibule of vagina   Vaginal opening   Urethra

Median Section—Right Lateral View of Left Pelvis

PLATE 4.31   PELVIC CONTENTS—FEMALE

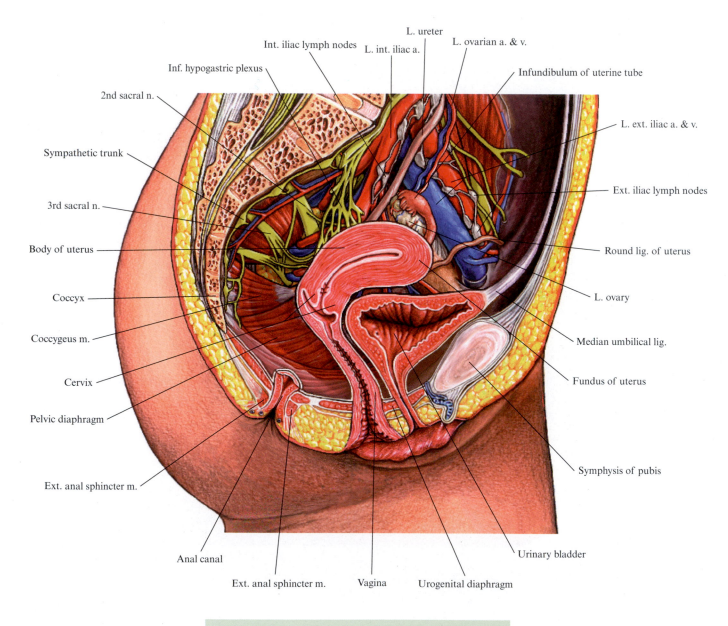

L. ureter

Int. iliac lymph nodes   L. int. iliac a.   L. ovarian a. & v.

Inf. hypogastric plexus   Infundibulum of uterine tube

2nd sacral n.

L. ext. iliac a. & v.

Sympathetic trunk

Ext. iliac lymph nodes

3rd sacral n.

Body of uterus   Round lig. of uterus

Coccyx   L. ovary

Coccygeus m.   Median umbilical lig.

Cervix   Fundus of uterus

Pelvic diaphragm

Ext. anal sphincter m.   Symphysis of pubis

Anal canal   Urinary bladder

Ext. anal sphincter m.   Vagina   Urogenital diaphragm

Median Section—Right Lateral View with Peritoneum Removed

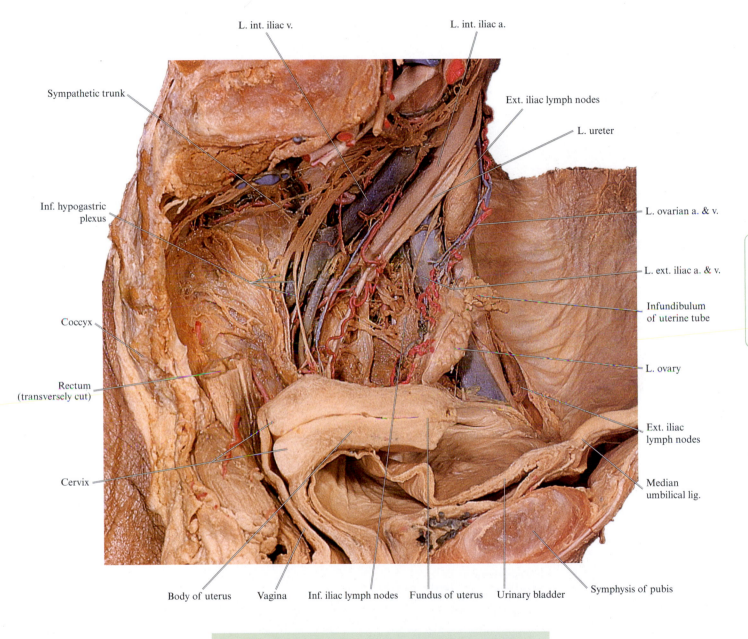

L. int. iliac v.

L. int. iliac a.

Sympathetic trunk

Ext. iliac lymph nodes

L. ureter

Inf. hypogastric plexus

L. ovarian a. & v.

L. ext. iliac a. & v.

Infundibulum of uterine tube

Coccyx

L. ovary

Rectum (transversely cut)

Ext. iliac lymph nodes

Cervix

Median umbilical lig.

Body of uterus   Vagina   Inf. iliac lymph nodes   Fundus of uterus   Urinary bladder   Symphysis of pubis

Left Half of Hemisected Pelvis—Medial View with Peritoneum Removed

PLATE 4.33   PELVIC CONTENTS—FEMALE

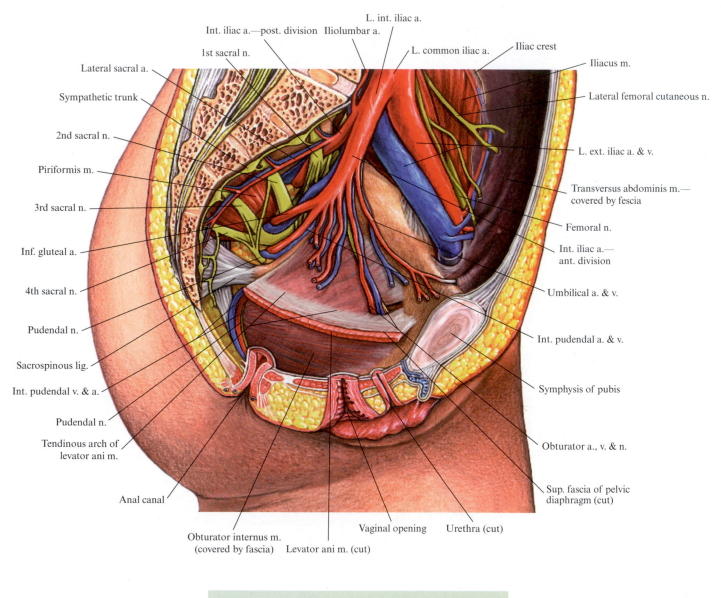

Int. iliac a.—post. division   Iliolumbar a.

L. int. iliac a.

1st sacral n.

L. common iliac a.

Iliac crest

Lateral sacral a.

Iliacus m.

Sympathetic trunk

Lateral femoral cutaneous n.

2nd sacral n.

Piriformis m.

L. ext. iliac a. & v.

Transversus abdominis m.—covered by fescia

3rd sacral n.

Femoral n.

Inf. gluteal a.

Int. iliac a.—ant. division

4th sacral n.

Umbilical a. & v.

Pudendal n.

Int. pudendal a. & v.

Sacrospinous lig.

Int. pudendal v. & a.

Symphysis of pubis

Pudendal n.

Tendinous arch of levator ani m.

Obturator a., v. & n.

Anal canal

Sup. fascia of pelvic diaphragm (cut)

Obturator internus m. (covered by fascia)   Levator ani m. (cut)   Vaginal opening   Urethra (cut)

Median Section—Right Lateral View with Peritoneum Removed

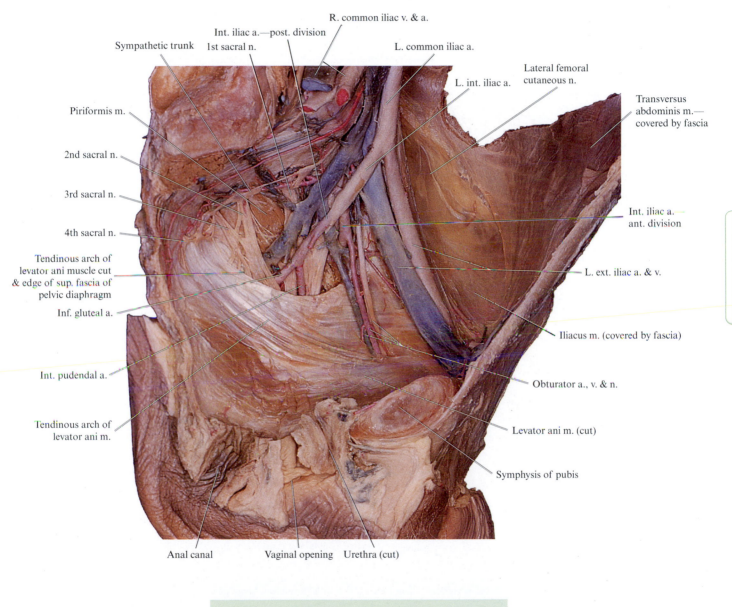

R. common iliac v. & a.

Int. iliac a.—post. division

1st sacral n.

L. common iliac a.

Sympathetic trunk

Lateral femoral
cutaneous n.

L. int. iliac a.

Piriformis m.

Transversus
abdominis m.—
covered by fascia

2nd sacral n.

3rd sacral n.

Int. iliac a.—
ant. division

4th sacral n.

Tendinous arch of
levator ani muscle cut
& edge of sup. fascia of
pelvic diaphragm

L. ext. iliac a. & v.

Inf. gluteal a.

Iliacus m. (covered by fascia)

Int. pudendal a.

Obturator a., v. & n.

Tendinous arch of
levator ani m.

Levator ani m. (cut)

Symphysis of pubis

Anal canal   Vaginal opening   Urethra (cut)

Median Section—Right Lateral View with Peritoneum Removed

PLATE 4.35   LATERAL PELVIC WALL—FEMALE

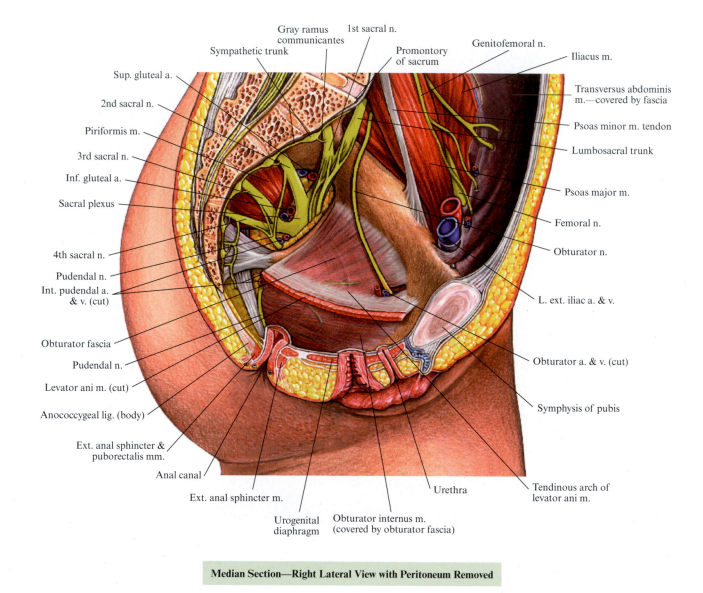

Gray ramus communicantes

1st sacral n.

Sympathetic trunk

Promontory of sacrum

Genitofemoral n.

Iliacus m.

Sup. gluteal a.

Transversus abdominis m.—covered by fascia

2nd sacral n.

Psoas minor m. tendon

Piriformis m.

Lumbosacral trunk

3rd sacral n.

Inf. gluteal a.

Psoas major m.

Sacral plexus

Femoral n.

Obturator n.

4th sacral n.

Pudendal n.

Int. pudendal a. & v. (cut)

L. ext. iliac a. & v.

Obturator fascia

Pudendal n.

Obturator a. & v. (cut)

Levator ani m. (cut)

Anococcygeal lig. (body)

Symphysis of pubis

Ext. anal sphincter & puborectalis mm.

Anal canal

Tendinous arch of levator ani m.

Ext. anal sphincter m.

Urethra

Urogenital diaphragm

Obturator internus m. (covered by obturator fascia)

Median Section—Right Lateral View with Peritoneum Removed

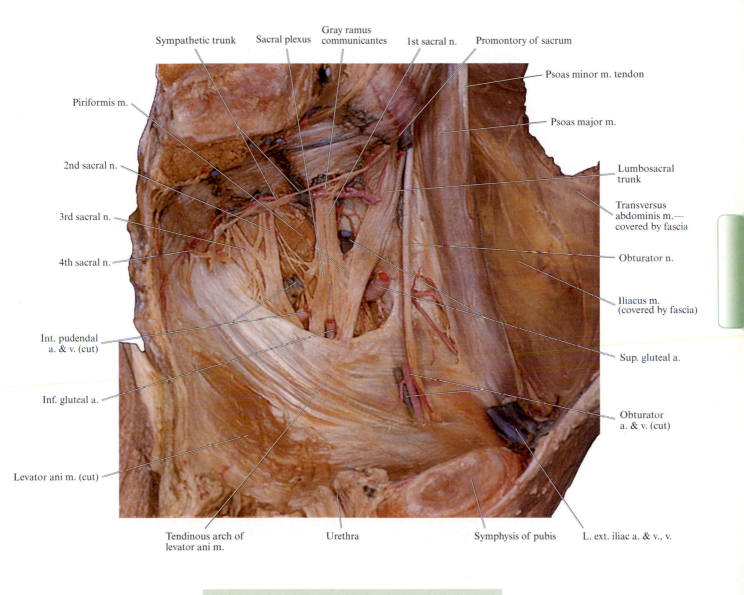

Sympathetic trunk

Sacral plexus

Gray ramus communicantes

1st sacral n.

Promontory of sacrum

Psoas minor m. tendon

Piriformis m.

Psoas major m.

2nd sacral n.

Lumbosacral trunk

Transversus abdominis m.— covered by fascia

3rd sacral n.

Obturator n.

4th sacral n.

Iliacus m. (covered by fascia)

Int. pudendal a. & v. (cut)

Sup. gluteal a.

Inf. gluteal a.

Obturator a. & v. (cut)

Levator ani m. (cut)

Tendinous arch of levator ani m.

Urethra

Symphysis of pubis

L. ext. iliac a. & v., v.

Median Section—Right Lateral View with Peritoneum Removed

PLATE 4.37   PELVIC CONTENTS—MALE

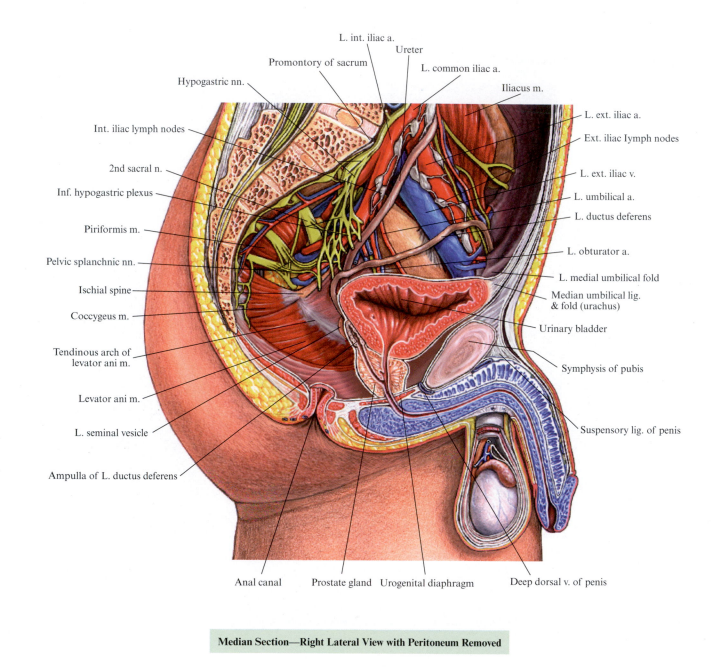

L. int. iliac a.

Ureter

Promontory of sacrum

L. common iliac a.

Hypogastric nn.

Iliacus m.

Int. iliac lymph nodes

L. ext. iliac a.

Ext. iliac lymph nodes

2nd sacral n.

L. ext. iliac v.

Inf. hypogastric plexus

L. umbilical a.

L. ductus deferens

Piriformis m.

L. obturator a.

Pelvic splanchnic nn.

L. medial umbilical fold

Ischial spine

Median umbilical lig. & fold (urachus)

Coccygeus m.

Urinary bladder

Tendinous arch of levator ani m.

Symphysis of pubis

Levator ani m.

L. seminal vesicle

Suspensory lig. of penis

Ampulla of L. ductus deferens

Anal canal   Prostate gland   Urogenital diaphragm   Deep dorsal v. of penis

Median Section—Right Lateral View with Peritoneum Removed

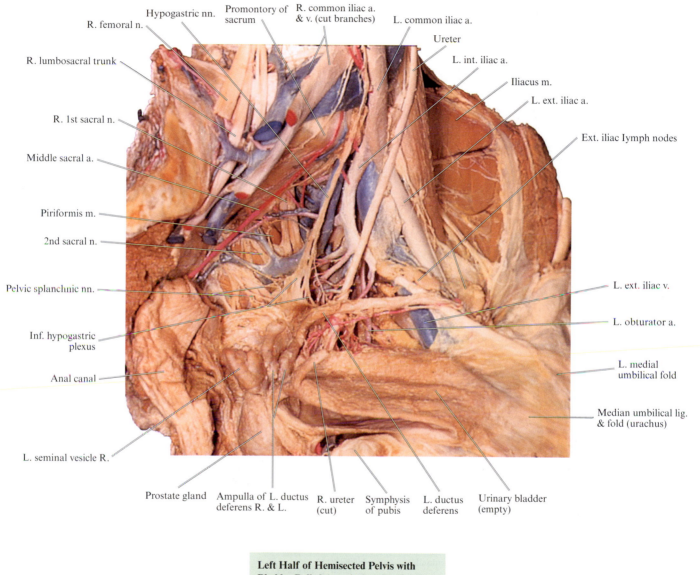

R. femoral n.

Hypogastric nn.

Promontory of sacrum

R. common iliac a. & v. (cut branches)

L. common iliac a.

Ureter

R. lumbosacral trunk

L. int. iliac a.

Iliacus m.

L. ext. iliac a.

R. 1st sacral n.

Ext. iliac lymph nodes

Middle sacral a.

Piriformis m.

2nd sacral n.

Pelvic splanchnic nn.

L. ext. iliac v.

L. obturator a.

Inf. hypogastric plexus

L. medial umbilical fold

Anal canal

Median umbilical lig. & fold (urachus)

L. seminal vesicle R.

Prostate gland

Ampulla of L. ductus deferens R. & L.

R. ureter (cut)

Symphysis of pubis

L. ductus deferens

Urinary bladder (empty)

Left Half of Hemisected Pelvis with Bladder Pulled Anteriorly—Medial View

PLATE 4.41   PERINEUM—FEMALE I

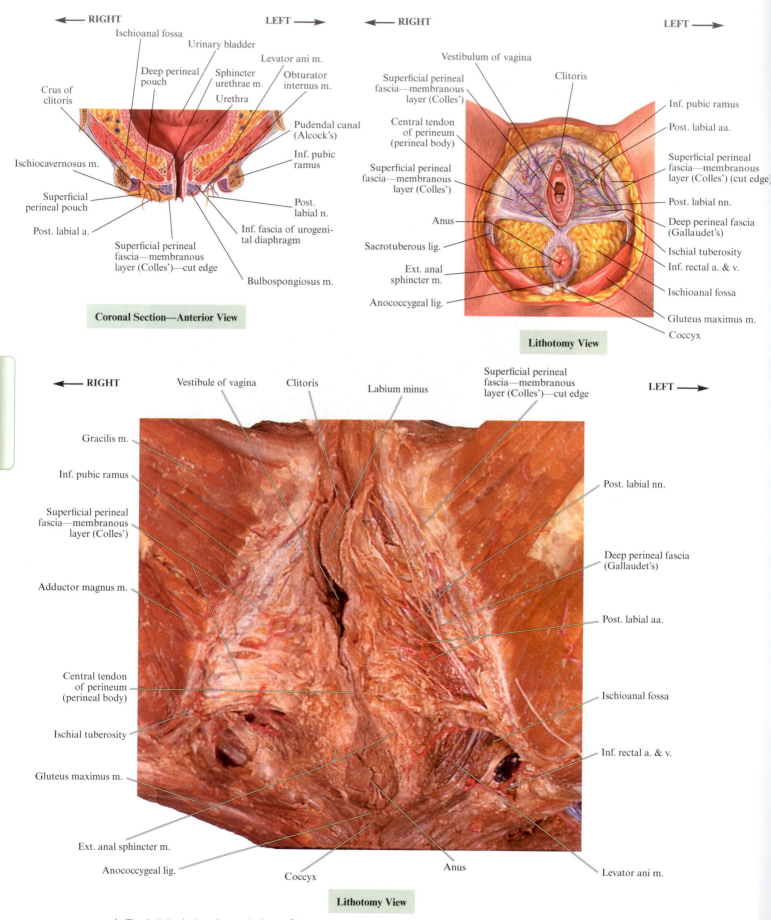

RIGHT → | ← LEFT   RIGHT → | ← LEFT

Ischioanal fossa
Urinary bladder
Deep perineal pouch
Sphincter urethrae m.
Levator ani m.
Obturator internus m.
Crus of clitoris
Urethra
Pudendal canal (Alcock's)
Inf. pubic ramus
Ischiocavernosus m.
Superficial perineal pouch
Post. labial n.
Post. labial a.
Inf. fascia of urogenital diaphragm
Superficial perineal fascia—membranous layer (Colles')—cut edge
Bulbospongiosus m.

Coronal Section—Anterior View

Vestibulum of vagina
Clitoris
Superficial perineal fascia—membranous layer (Colles')
Central tendon of perineum (perineal body)
Inf. pubic ramus
Post. labial aa.
Superficial perineal fascia—membranous layer (Colles')
Superficial perineal fascia—membranous layer (Colles') (cut edge)
Anus
Post. labial nn.
Sacrotuberous lig.
Deep perineal fascia (Gallaudet's)
Ischial tuberosity
Ext. anal sphincter m.
Inf. rectal a. & v.
Anococcygeal lig.
Ischioanal fossa
Gluteus maximus m.
Coccyx

Lithotomy View

RIGHT →
Vestibule of vagina
Clitoris
Labium minus
Superficial perineal fascia—membranous layer (Colles')—cut edge
LEFT →
Gracilis m.
Inf. pubic ramus
Superficial perineal fascia—membranous layer (Colles')
Adductor magnus m.
Post. labial nn.
Deep perineal fascia (Gallaudet's)
Post. labial aa.
Central tendon of perineum (perineal body)
Ischioanal fossa
Ischial tuberosity
Inf. rectal a. & v.
Gluteus maximus m.
Ext. anal sphincter m.
Anococcygeal lig.
Coccyx
Anus
Levator ani m.

Lithotomy View

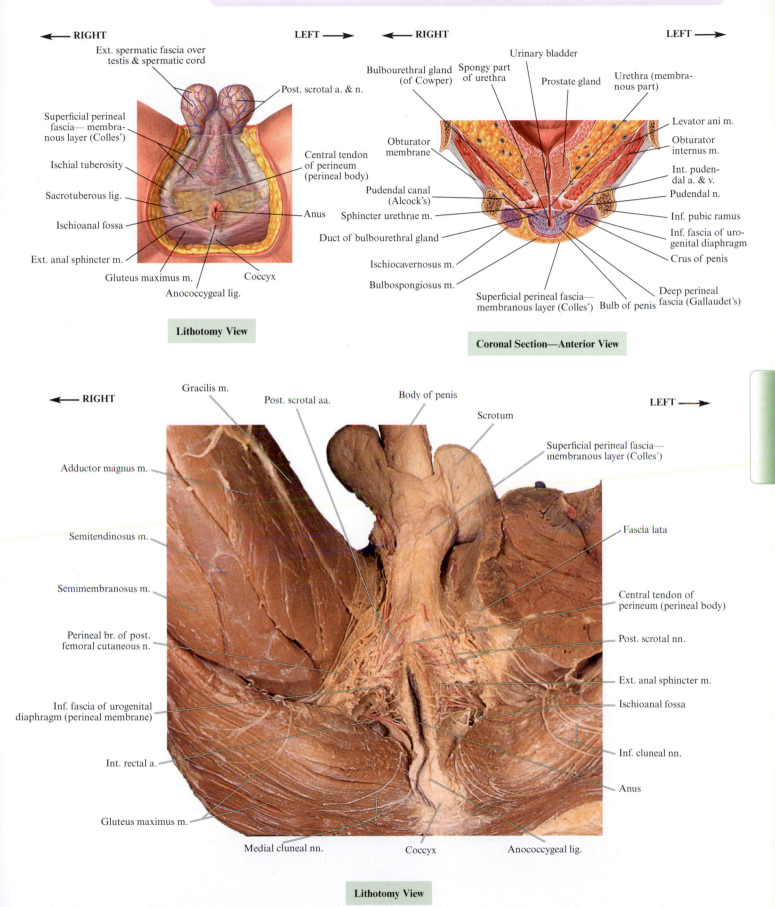

Lithotomy View

← RIGHT   LEFT →

Ext. spermatic fascia over testis & spermatic cord

Post. scrotal a. & n.

Superficial perineal fascia— membranous layer (Colles')

Central tendon of perineum (perineal body)

Ischial tuberosity

Sacrotuberous lig.

Anus

Ischioanal fossa

Ext. anal sphincter m.

Gluteus maximus m.   Coccyx

Anococcygeal lig.

← RIGHT   LEFT →

Bulbourethral gland (of Cowper)   Spongy part of urethra   Urinary bladder   Prostate gland   Urethra (membra- nous part)

Obturator membrane

Levator ani m.

Obturator internus m.

Pudendal canal (Alcock's)   Int. puden- dal a. & v.

Sphincter urethrae m.   Pudendal n.

Duct of bulbourethral gland   Inf. pubic ramus

Inf. fascia of uro- genital diaphragm

Ischiocavernosus m.   Crus of penis

Bulbospongiosus m.   Deep perineal fascia (Gallaudet's)

Superficial perineal fascia— membranous layer (Colles')   Bulb of penis

Coronal Section—Anterior View

← RIGHT   LEFT →

Gracilis m.   Post. scrotal aa.   Body of penis   Scrotum

Superficial perineal fascia— membranous layer (Colles')

Adductor magnus m.

Semitendinosus m.

Fascia lata

Semimembranosus m.

Central tendon of perineum (perineal body)

Perineal br. of post. femoral cutaneous n.

Post. scrotal nn.

Ext. anal sphincter m.

Ischioanal fossa

Inf. fascia of urogenital diaphragm (perineal membrane)

Int. rectal a.

Inf. cluneal nn.

Anus

Gluteus maximus m.

Medial cluneal nn.   Coccyx   Anococcygeal lig.

Lithotomy View

PLATE 4.43   PERINEUM—FEMALE II

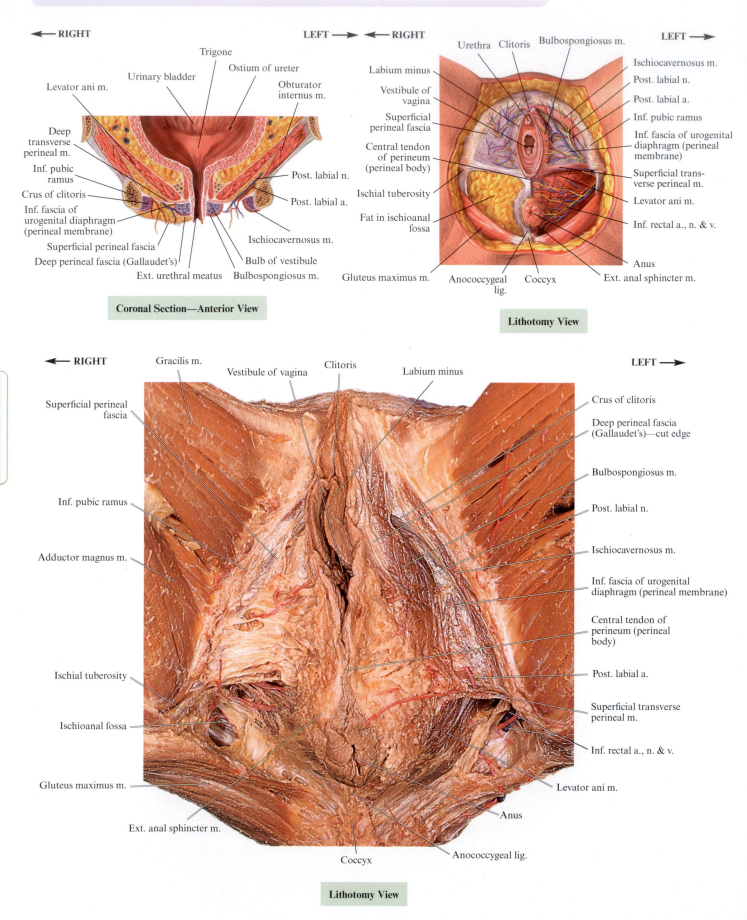

← **RIGHT**   **LEFT** →   ← **RIGHT**   **LEFT** →

Trigone
Urinary bladder
Ostium of ureter
Levator ani m.
Obturator internus m.
Deep transverse perineal m.
Inf. pubic ramus
Crus of clitoris
Inf. fascia of urogenital diaphragm (perineal membrane)
Superficial perineal fascia
Deep perineal fascia (Gallaudet's)
Ext. urethral meatus
Post. labial n.
Post. labial a.
Ischiocavernosus m.
Bulb of vestibule
Bulbospongiosus m.

Coronal Section—Anterior View

Urethra   Clitoris   Bulbospongiosus m.
Labium minus
Vestibule of vagina
Superficial perineal fascia
Central tendon of perineum (perineal body)
Ischial tuberosity
Fat in ischioanal fossa
Gluteus maximus m.
Anococcygeal lig.
Coccyx
Ischiocavernosus m.
Post. labial n.
Post. labial a.
Inf. pubic ramus
Inf. fascia of urogenital diaphragm (perineal membrane)
Superficial transverse perineal m.
Levator ani m.
Inf. rectal a., n. & v.
Anus
Ext. anal sphincter m.

Lithotomy View

← **RIGHT**   **LEFT** →

Gracilis m.
Vestibule of vagina   Clitoris   Labium minus
Superficial perineal fascia
Inf. pubic ramus
Adductor magnus m.
Ischial tuberosity
Ischioanal fossa
Gluteus maximus m.
Ext. anal sphincter m.
Coccyx
Anococcygeal lig.
Crus of clitoris
Deep perineal fascia (Gallaudet's)—cut edge
Bulbospongiosus m.
Post. labial n.
Ischiocavernosus m.
Inf. fascia of urogenital diaphragm (perineal membrane)
Central tendon of perineum (perineal body)
Post. labial a.
Superficial transverse perineal m.
Inf. rectal a., n. & v.
Levator ani m.
Anus

Lithotomy View

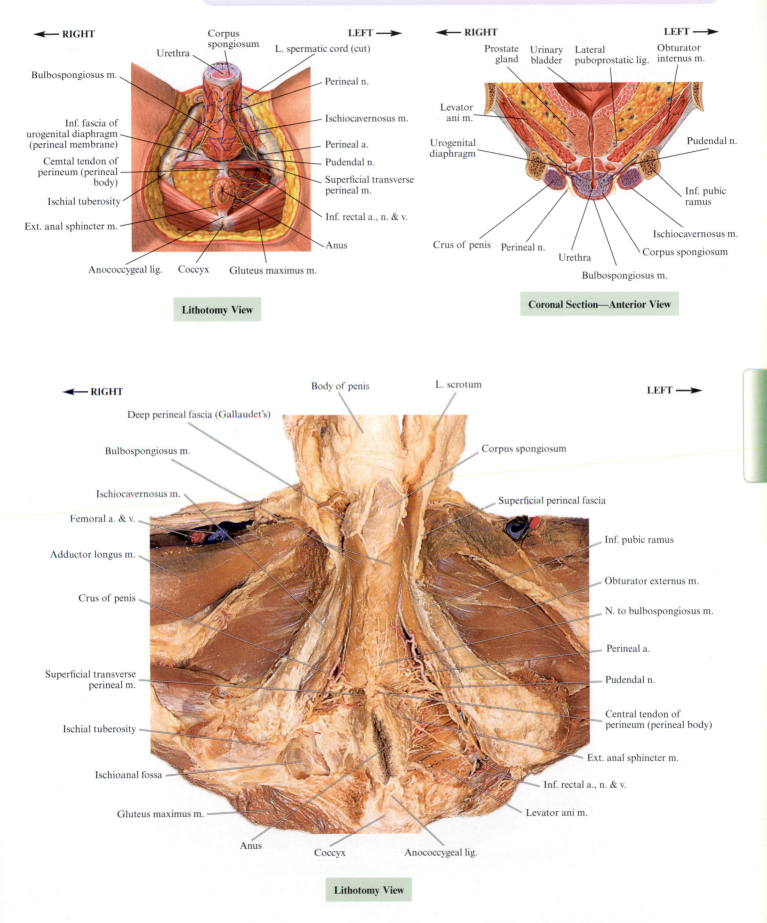

← RIGHT   LEFT →

Urethra
Corpus spongiosum
L. spermatic cord (cut)
Bulbospongiosus m.
Perineal n.
Ischiocavernosus m.
Inf. fascia of urogenital diaphragm (perineal membrane)
Perineal a.
Pudendal n.
Cemtal tendon of perineum (perineal body)
Superficial transverse perineal m.
Ischial tuberosity
Ext. anal sphincter m.
Inf. rectal a., n. & v.
Anus
Anococcygeal lig.   Coccyx   Gluteus maximus m.

Lithotomy View

← RIGHT   LEFT →

Prostate gland
Urinary bladder
Lateral puboprostatic lig.
Obturator internus m.
Levator ani m.
Urogenital diaphragm
Pudendal n.
Inf. pubic ramus
Crus of penis   Perineal n.   Urethra   Ischiocavernosus m.
Bulbospongiosus m.   Corpus spongiosum

Coronal Section—Anterior View

← RIGHT   LEFT →

Body of penis   L. scrotum

Deep perineal fascia (Gallaudet's)
Corpus spongiosum
Bulbospongiosus m.
Superficial perineal fascia
Ischiocavernosus m.
Femoral a. & v.
Inf. pubic ramus
Adductor longus m.
Obturator externus m.
Crus of penis
N. to bulbospongiosus m.
Perineal a.
Pudendal n.
Superficial transverse perineal m.
Central tendon of perineum (perineal body)
Ischial tuberosity
Ext. anal sphincter m.
Ischioanal fossa
Inf. rectal a., n. & v.
Gluteus maximus m.
Levator ani m.
Anus   Coccyx   Anococcygeal lig.

Lithotomy View

PLATE 4.45   PERINEUM—FEMALE III

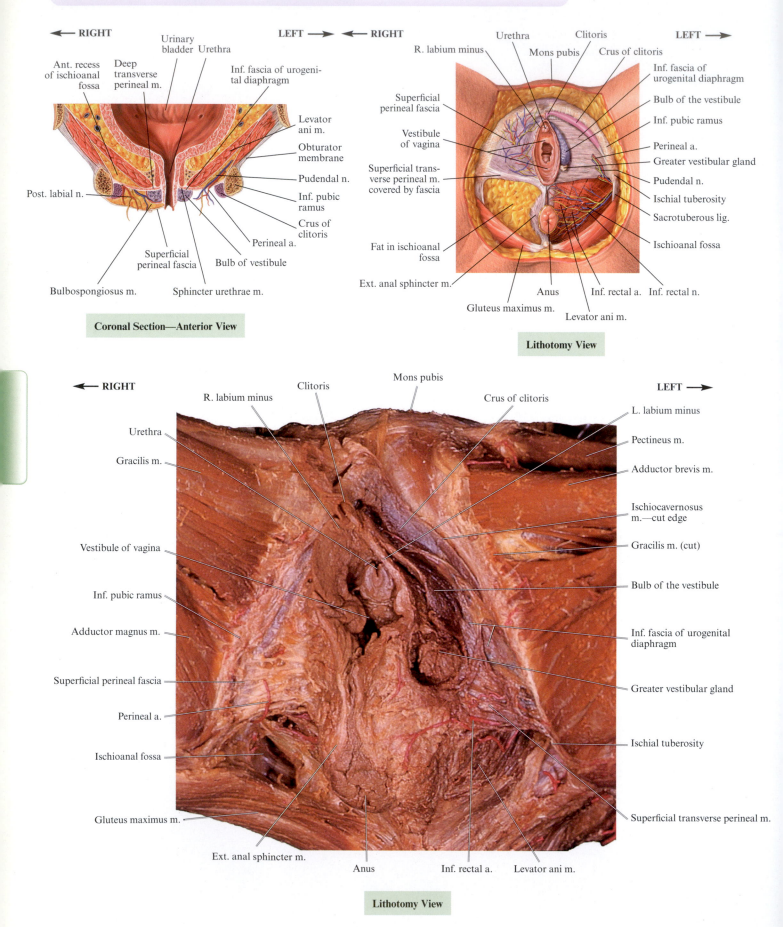

RIGHT ←   **LEFT** →   ← **RIGHT**

Ant. recess
of ischioanal
fossa

Deep
transverse
perineal m.

Urinary
bladder

Urethra

Inf. fascia of urogeni-
tal diaphragm

Levator
ani m.

Obturator
membrane

Pudendal n.

Inf. pubic
ramus

Post. labial n.

Crus of
clitoris

Perineal a.

Bulbospongiosus m.

Superficial
perineal fascia

Bulb of vestibule

Sphincter urethrae m.

Coronal Section—Anterior View

Urethra

Clitoris

R. labium minus

Mons pubis

Crus of clitoris

LEFT →

Inf. fascia of
urogenital diaphragm

Superficial
perineal fascia

Bulb of the vestibule

Inf. pubic ramus

Vestibule
of vagina

Perineal a.

Greater vestibular gland

Superficial trans-
verse perineal m.
covered by fascia

Pudendal n.

Ischial tuberosity

Sacrotuberous lig.

Fat in ischioanal
fossa

Ischioanal fossa

Ext. anal sphincter m.

Anus

Inf. rectal a.

Inf. rectal n.

Gluteus maximus m.

Levator ani m.

Lithotomy View

RIGHT ←

R. labium minus

Clitoris

Mons pubis

Crus of clitoris

LEFT →

L. labium minus

Urethra

Pectineus m.

Gracilis m.

Adductor brevis m.

Ischiocavernosus
m.—cut edge

Gracilis m. (cut)

Vestibule of vagina

Bulb of the vestibule

Inf. pubic ramus

Adductor magnus m.

Inf. fascia of urogenital
diaphragm

Superficial perineal fascia

Greater vestibular gland

Perineal a.

Ischioanal fossa

Ischial tuberosity

Gluteus maximus m.

Superficial transverse perineal m.

Ext. anal sphincter m.

Anus

Inf. rectal a.

Levator ani m.

Lithotomy View

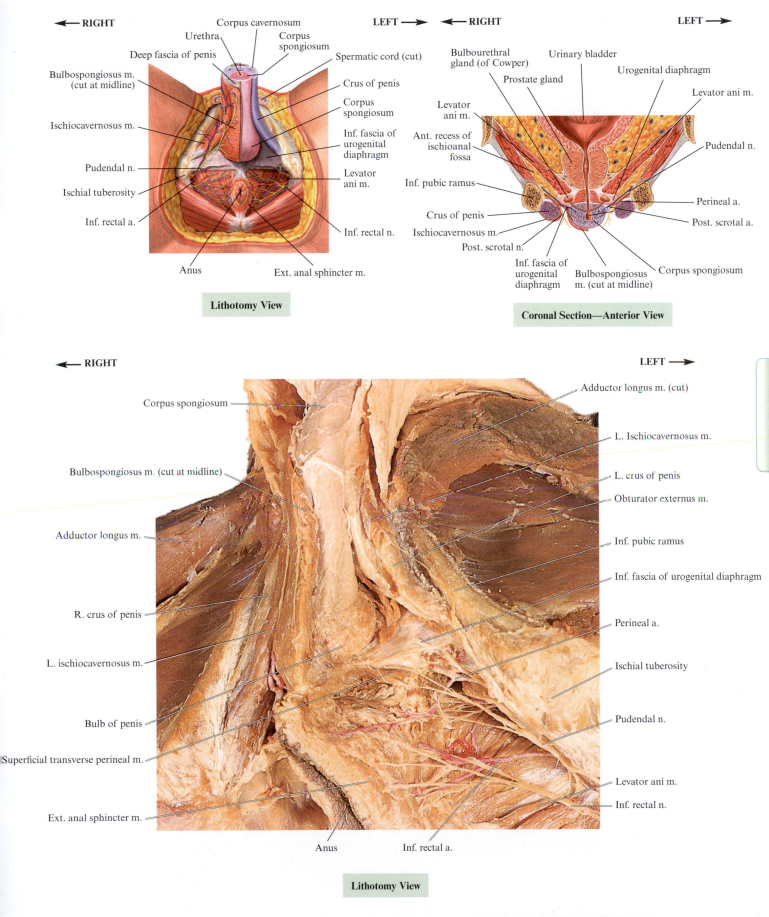

← RIGHT   LEFT →   ← RIGHT   LEFT →

Corpus cavernosum

Urethra   Corpus
Deep fascia of penis   spongiosum

Spermatic cord (cut)

Bulbospongiosus m.
(cut at midline)

Crus of penis

Ischiocavernosus m.

Corpus
spongiosum

Pudendal n.

Inf. fascia of
urogenital
diaphragm

Ischial tuberosity

Levator
ani m.

Inf. rectal a.

Inf. rectal n.

Anus   Ext. anal sphincter m.

Lithotomy View

Bulbourethral   Urinary bladder
gland (of Cowper)

Prostate gland   Urogenital diaphragm

Levator   Levator ani m.
ani m.

Ant. recess of
ischioanal
fossa   Pudendal n.

Inf. pubic ramus

Crus of penis   Perineal a.

Ischiocavernosus m.   Post. scrotal a.

Post. scrotal n.

Inf. fascia of   Bulbospongiosus   Corpus spongiosum
urogenital   m. (cut at midline)
diaphragm

Coronal Section—Anterior View

← RIGHT   LEFT →

Corpus spongiosum   Adductor longus m. (cut)

L. Ischiocavernosus m.

Bulbospongiosus m. (cut at midline)   L. crus of penis

Obturator externus m.

Adductor longus m.   Inf. pubic ramus

Inf. fascia of urogenital diaphragm

R. crus of penis   Perineal a.

L. ischiocavernosus m.   Ischial tuberosity

Bulb of penis   Pudendal n.

Superficial transverse perineal m.   Levator ani m.

Inf. rectal n.

Ext. anal sphincter m.

Anus   Inf. rectal a.

Lithotomy View

CHAPTER 4 | **PELVIS AND PERINEUM**   197

PLATE 4.47   PERINEUM—FEMALE IV

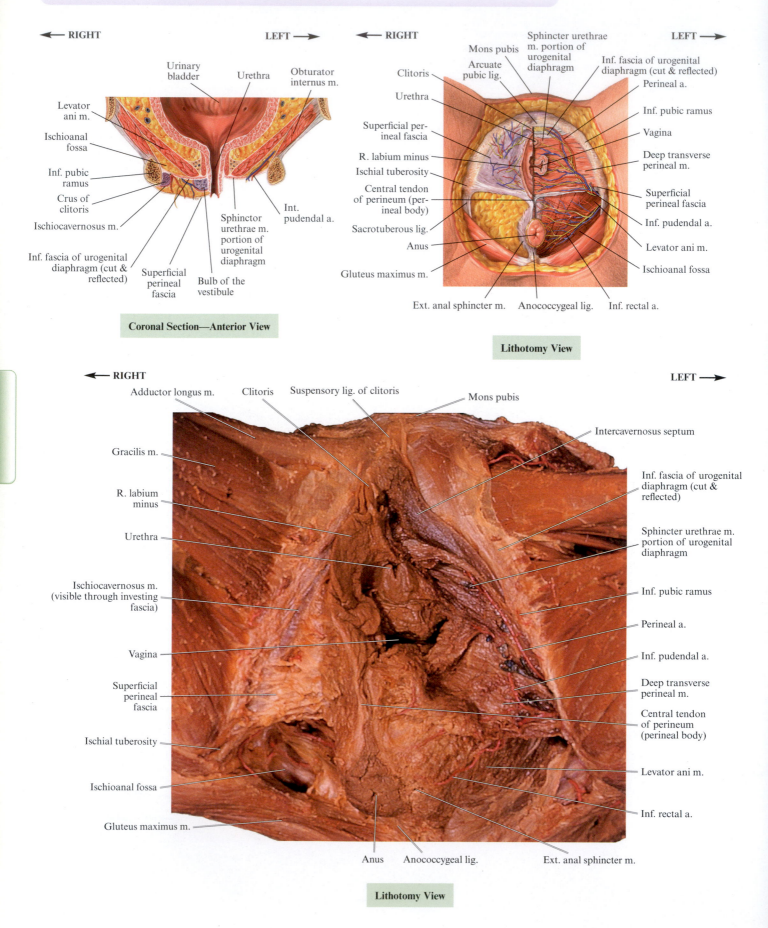

← RIGHT   LEFT →

Urinary bladder
Urethra
Obturator internus m.

Levator ani m.

Ischioanal fossa

Inf. pubic ramus

Crus of clitoris

Ischiocavernosus m.

Inf. fascia of urogenital diaphragm (cut & reflected)

Superficial perineal fascia

Sphinctor urethrae m. portion of urogenital diaphragm

Bulb of the vestibule

Int. pudendal a.

Coronal Section—Anterior View

← RIGHT   LEFT →

Mons pubis
Arcuate pubic lig.
Clitoris
Urethra
Superficial per- ineal fascia
R. labium minus
Ischial tuberosity
Central tendon of perineum (per- ineal body)
Sacrotuberous lig.
Anus
Gluteus maximus m.

Sphincter urethrae m. portion of urogenital diaphragm
Inf. fascia of urogenital diaphragm (cut & reflected)
Perineal a.
Inf. pubic ramus
Vagina
Deep transverse perineal m.
Superficial perineal fascia
Inf. pudendal a.
Levator ani m.
Ischioanal fossa

Ext. anal sphincter m.   Anococcygeal lig.   Inf. rectal a.

Lithotomy View

← RIGHT   LEFT →

Adductor longus m.
Clitoris
Suspensory lig. of clitoris
Mons pubis

Gracilis m.

R. labium minus

Urethra

Ischiocavernosus m. (visible through investing fascia)

Vagina

Superficial perineal fascia

Ischial tuberosity

Ischioanal fossa

Gluteus maximus m.

Intercavernosus septum

Inf. fascia of urogenital diaphragm (cut & reflected)

Sphincter urethrae m. portion of urogenital diaphragm

Inf. pubic ramus

Perineal a.

Inf. pudendal a.

Deep transverse perineal m.

Central tendon of perineum (perineal body)

Levator ani m.

Inf. rectal a.

Anus   Anococcygeal lig.   Ext. anal sphincter m.

Lithotomy View

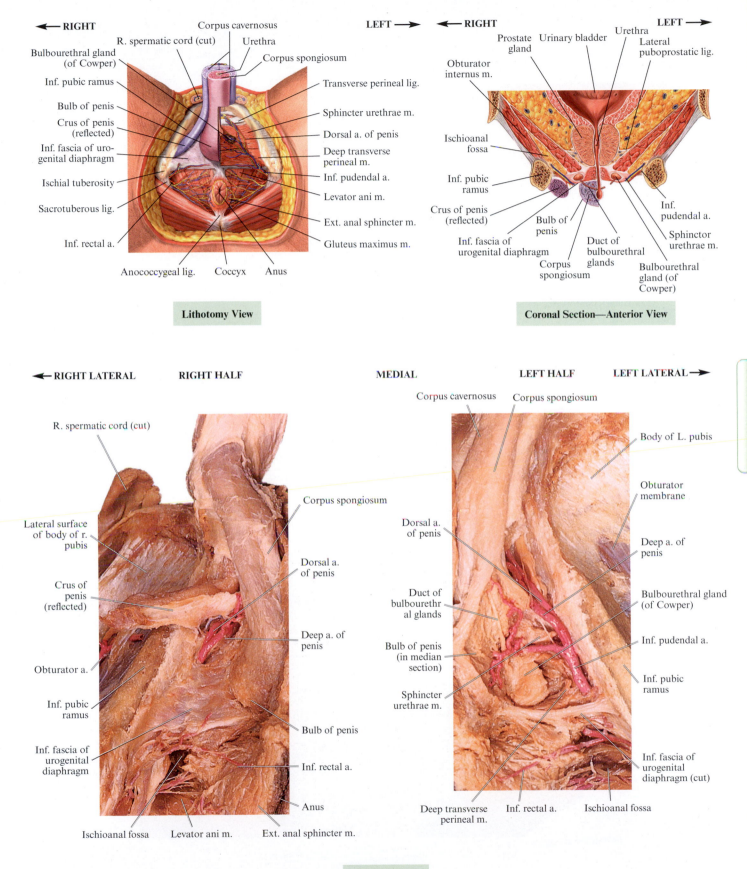

Lithotomy View

← RIGHT   LEFT →

Corpus cavernosus
R. spermatic cord (cut)   Urethra
Corpus spongiosum
Bulbourethral gland (of Cowper)
Transverse perineal lig.
Inf. pubic ramus
Sphincter urethrae m.
Bulb of penis
Crus of penis (reflected)
Dorsal a. of penis
Inf. fascia of uro-genital diaphragm
Deep transverse perineal m.
Ischial tuberosity
Inf. pudendal a.
Sacrotuberous lig.
Levator ani m.
Inf. rectal a.
Ext. anal sphincter m.
Gluteus maximus m.
Anococcygeal lig.   Coccyx   Anus

Coronal Section—Anterior View

← RIGHT   LEFT →

Prostate gland   Urinary bladder
Urethra
Lateral puboprostatic lig.
Obturator internus m.
Ischioanal fossa
Inf. pubic ramus
Crus of penis (reflected)
Bulb of penis
Inf. fascia of urogenital diaphragm
Corpus spongiosum
Duct of bulbourethral glands
Inf. pudendal a.
Sphincter urethrae m.
Bulbourethral gland (of Cowper)

← RIGHT LATERAL   RIGHT HALF   MEDIAL   LEFT HALF   LEFT LATERAL →

Corpus cavernosus   Corpus spongiosum
R. spermatic cord (cut)
Body of L. pubis
Lateral surface of body of r. pubis
Corpus spongiosum
Obturator membrane
Dorsal a. of penis
Dorsal a. of penis
Deep a. of penis
Crus of penis (reflected)
Deep a. of penis
Duct of bulbourethral glands
Bulbourethral gland (of Cowper)
Obturator a.
Deep a. of penis
Inf. pudendal a.
Inf. pubic ramus
Bulb of penis (in median section)
Inf. pubic ramus
Inf. fascia of urogenital diaphragm
Bulb of penis
Sphincter urethrae m.
Inf. rectal a.
Inf. fascia of urogenital diaphragm (cut)
Anus
Ischioanal fossa   Levator ani m.   Ext. anal sphincter m.
Deep transverse perineal m.   Inf. rectal a.   Ischioanal fossa

Lithotomy View

PLATE 4.49   PERINEUM—FEMALE V

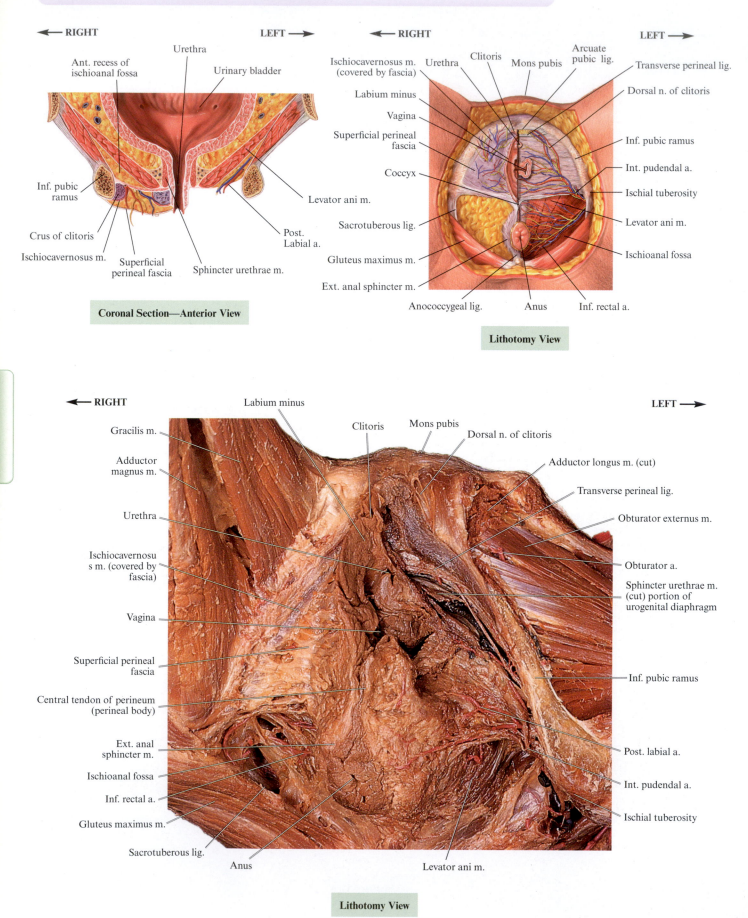

← RIGHT   LEFT →

Urethra

Ant. recess of
ischioanal fossa

Urinary bladder

Inf. pubic
ramus

Crus of clitoris

Ischiocavernosus m.

Superficial
perineal fascia

Sphincter urethrae m.

Levator ani m.

Post.
Labial a.

Coronal Section—Anterior View

← RIGHT   LEFT →

Ischiocavernosus m.
(covered by fascia)

Urethra   Clitoris   Mons pubis

Arcuate
pubic lig.

Transverse perineal lig.

Labium minus

Dorsal n. of clitoris

Vagina

Inf. pubic ramus

Superficial perineal
fascia

Int. pudendal a.

Coccyx

Ischial tuberosity

Sacrotuberous lig.

Levator ani m.

Gluteus maximus m.

Ischioanal fossa

Ext. anal sphincter m.

Anococcygeal lig.   Anus   Inf. rectal a.

Lithotomy View

← RIGHT   Labium minus   LEFT →

Gracilis m.

Clitoris   Mons pubis

Dorsal n. of clitoris

Adductor
magnus m.

Adductor longus m. (cut)

Urethra

Transverse perineal lig.

Ischiocavernosu
s m. (covered by
fascia)

Obturator externus m.

Obturator a.

Vagina

Sphincter urethrae m.
(cut) portion of
urogenital diaphragm

Superficial perineal
fascia

Central tendon of perineum
(perineal body)

Inf. pubic ramus

Ext. anal
sphincter m.

Ischioanal fossa

Post. labial a.

Inf. rectal a.

Int. pudendal a.

Gluteus maximus m.

Ischial tuberosity

Sacrotuberous lig.

Anus   Levator ani m.

Lithotomy View

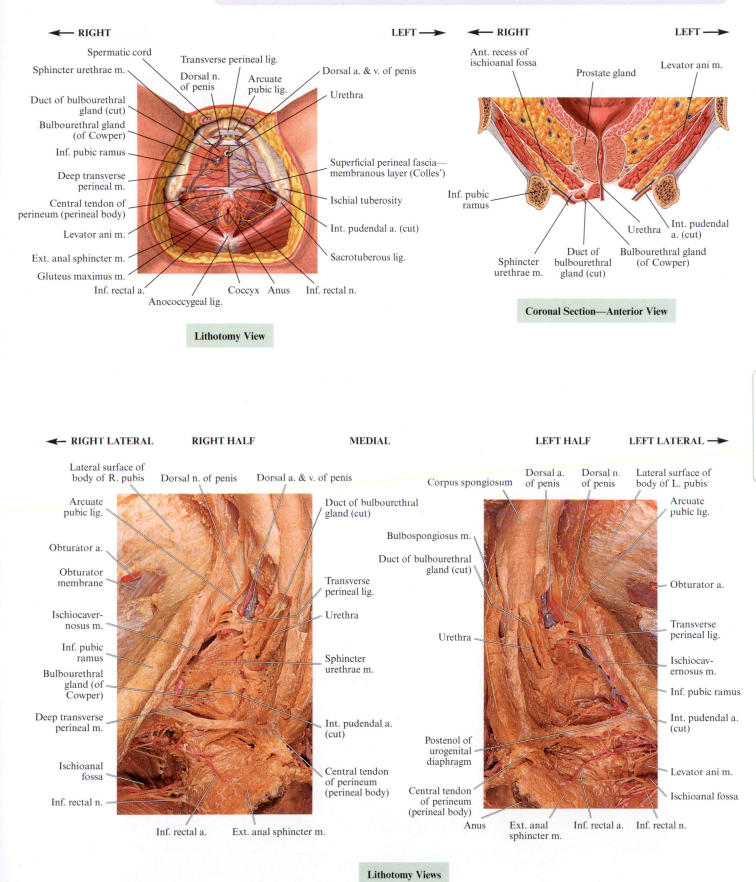

← RIGHT **LEFT →** **← RIGHT** **LEFT →**

Spermatic cord

Sphincter urethrae m.

Transverse perineal lig.

Dorsal n. of penis

Arcuate pubic lig.

Dorsal a. & v. of penis

Duct of bulbourethral gland (cut)

Bulbourethral gland (of Cowper)

Inf. pubic ramus

Deep transverse perineal m.

Central tendon of perineum (perineal body)

Levator ani m.

Ext. anal sphincter m.

Gluteus maximus m.

Inf. rectal a.

Anococcygeal lig.

Urethra

Superficial perineal fascia—membranous layer (Colles')

Ischial tuberosity

Int. pudendal a. (cut)

Sacrotuberous lig.

Coccyx   Anus   Inf. rectal n.

Lithotomy View

Ant. recess of ischioanal fossa

Prostate gland

Levator ani m.

Inf. pubic ramus

Sphincter urethrae m.

Duct of bulbourethral gland (cut)

Bulbourethral gland (of Cowper)

Urethra

Int. pudendal a. (cut)

Coronal Section—Anterior View

← RIGHT LATERAL   RIGHT HALF   MEDIAL   LEFT HALF   LEFT LATERAL →

Lateral surface of body of R. pubis

Dorsal n. of penis

Dorsal a. & v. of penis

Arcuate pubic lig.

Obturator a.

Obturator membrane

Ischiocavernosus m.

Inf. pubic ramus

Bulbourethral gland (of Cowper)

Deep transverse perineal m.

Ischioanal fossa

Inf. rectal n.

Inf. rectal a.   Ext. anal sphincter m.

Duct of bulbourethral gland (cut)

Transverse perineal lig.

Urethra

Sphincter urethrae m.

Int. pudendal a. (cut)

Central tendon of perineum (perineal body)

Corpus spongiosum

Dorsal a. of penis

Dorsal n. of penis

Lateral surface of body of L. pubis

Arcuate pubic lig.

Bulbospongiosus m.

Duct of bulbourethral gland (cut)

Urethra

Postenol of urogenital diaphragm

Central tendon of perineum (perineal body)

Anus   Ext. anal sphincter m.   Inf. rectal a.   Inf. rectal n.

Obturator a.

Transverse perineal lig.

Ischiocavernosus m.

Inf. pubic ramus

Int. pudendal a. (cut)

Levator ani m.

Ischioanal fossa

Lithotomy Views

PLATE 4.51   PERINEUM—FEMALE VI

← RIGHT   LEFT →

Levator ani m.

Ant. recess of
ischioanal fossa

Urinary bladder

Sup. fascia of
pelvic diaphragm

Obturator
internus m.

Urethra

Inf. pubic ramus

Inf. fascia of pelvic
diaphragm

Ischiocavernosus m.

Superficial
perineal fascia

Coronal Section—Anterior View

← RIGHT   LEFT →

Urethra   Clitoris

Labium minus   Arcuate pubic lig.

Ischiocavernosus m.—
covered by fascia   Inf. pubic ramus

Vagina   Levator ani m.

Superficial
perineal fascia   Ischial tuberosity

Ischial tuberosity   Inf. rectal a.

Sacrotuberous lig.   Ischioanal fossa

Central tendon of perineum
(perineal body)   Inf. rectal n.

Fat in ischioanal fossa   Gluteus maximus m.

Ext. anal sphincter m.   Anococcygeal lig.

Anus   Coccyx

Lithotomy View

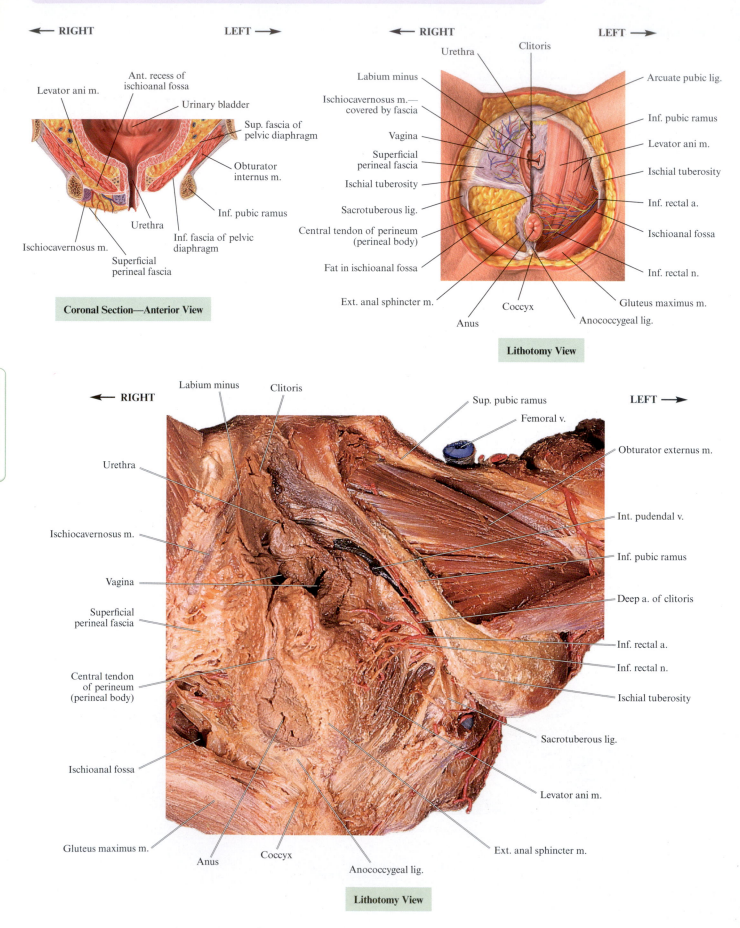

← RIGHT   LEFT →

Labium minus   Clitoris   Sup. pubic ramus

Femoral v.

Obturator externus m.

Urethra

Int. pudendal v.

Ischiocavernosus m.   Inf. pubic ramus

Vagina   Deep a. of clitoris

Superficial
perineal fascia   Inf. rectal a.

Central tendon
of perineum
(perineal body)   Inf. rectal n.

Ischial tuberosity

Sacrotuberous lig.

Ischioanal fossa

Levator ani m.

Gluteus maximus m.   Ext. anal sphincter m.

Anus   Coccyx

Anococcygeal lig.

Lithotomy View

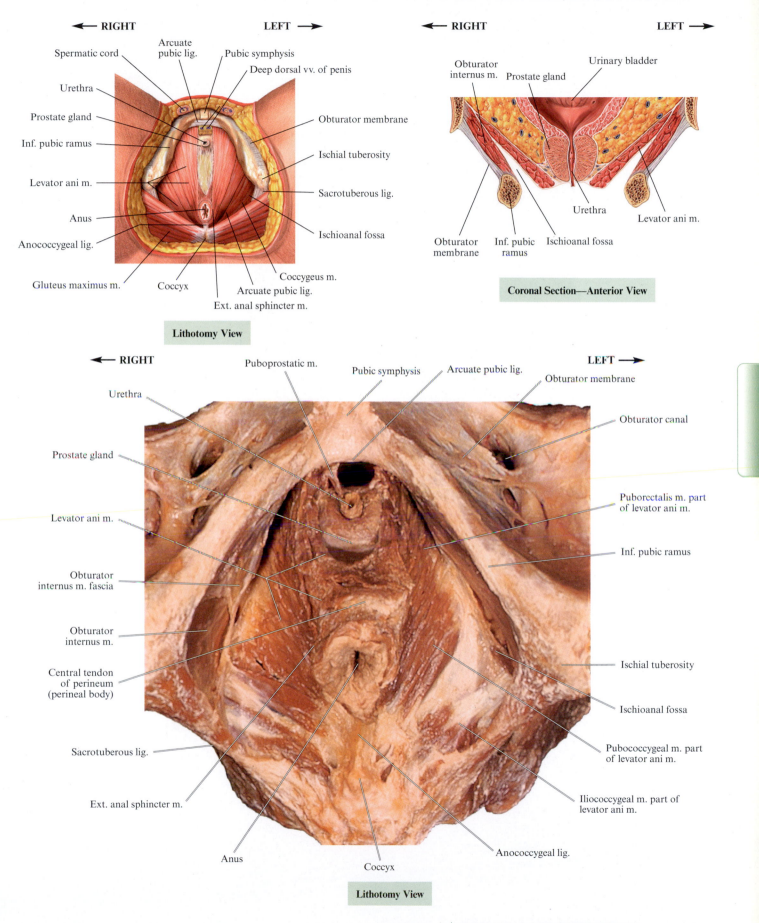

← RIGHT   **LEFT →**

Spermatic cord
Arcuate pubic lig.
Pubic symphysis
Deep dorsal vv. of penis
Urethra
Prostate gland
Inf. pubic ramus
Levator ani m.
Anus
Anococcygeal lig.
Obturator membrane
Ischial tuberosity
Sacrotuberous lig.
Ischioanal fossa
Gluteus maximus m.
Coccyx
Arcuate pubic lig.
Coccygeus m.
Ext. anal sphincter m.

Lithotomy View

← RIGHT   **LEFT →**

Obturator internus m.
Prostate gland
Urinary bladder
Obturator membrane
Inf. pubic ramus
Urethra
Ischioanal fossa
Levator ani m.

Coronal Section—Anterior View

← RIGHT   **LEFT →**

Puboprostatic m.
Pubic symphysis
Arcuate pubic lig.
Obturator membrane
Urethra
Obturator canal
Prostate gland
Puborectalis m. part of levator ani m.
Levator ani m.
Inf. pubic ramus
Obturator internus m. fascia
Obturator internus m.
Central tendon of perineum (perineal body)
Ischial tuberosity
Ischioanal fossa
Sacrotuberous lig.
Pubococcygeal m. part of levator ani m.
Ext. anal sphincter m.
Iliococcygeal m. part of levator ani m.
Anococcygeal lig.
Anus
Coccyx

Lithotomy View

PLATE 4.53   PUDENDAL STRUCTURES

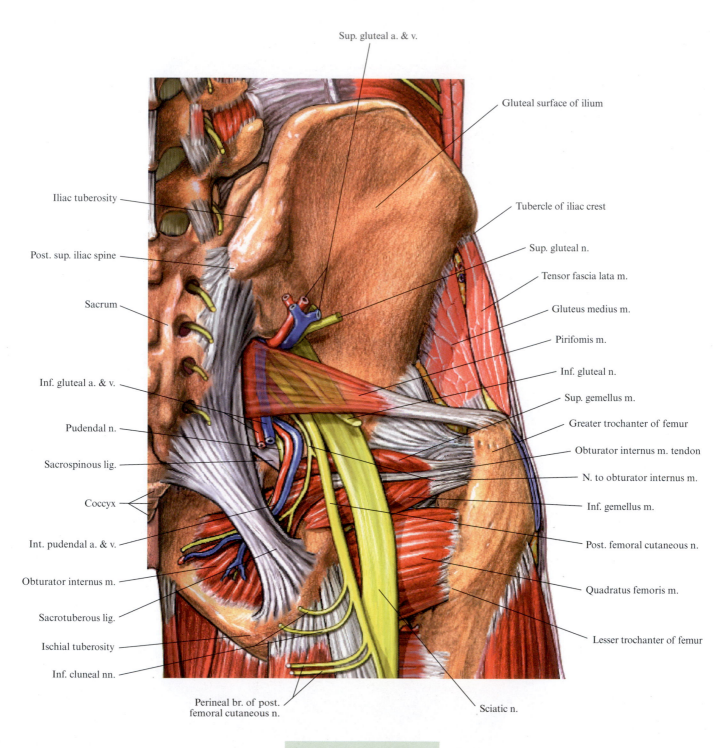

Sup. gluteal a. & v.

Gluteal surface of ilium

Iliac tuberosity

Tubercle of iliac crest

Post. sup. iliac spine

Sup. gluteal n.

Tensor fascia lata m.

Sacrum

Gluteus medius m.

Pirifomis m.

Inf. gluteal n.

Inf. gluteal a. & v.

Sup. gemellus m.

Greater trochanter of femur

Pudendal n.

Obturator internus m. tendon

Sacrospinous lig.

N. to obturator internus m.

Coccyx

Inf. gemellus m.

Int. pudendal a. & v.

Post. femoral cutaneous n.

Obturator internus m.

Quadratus femoris m.

Sacrotuberous lig.

Ischial tuberosity

Lesser trochanter of femur

Inf. cluneal nn.

Perineal br. of post. femoral cutaneous n.

Sciatic n.

Gluteal Region—Posterior View

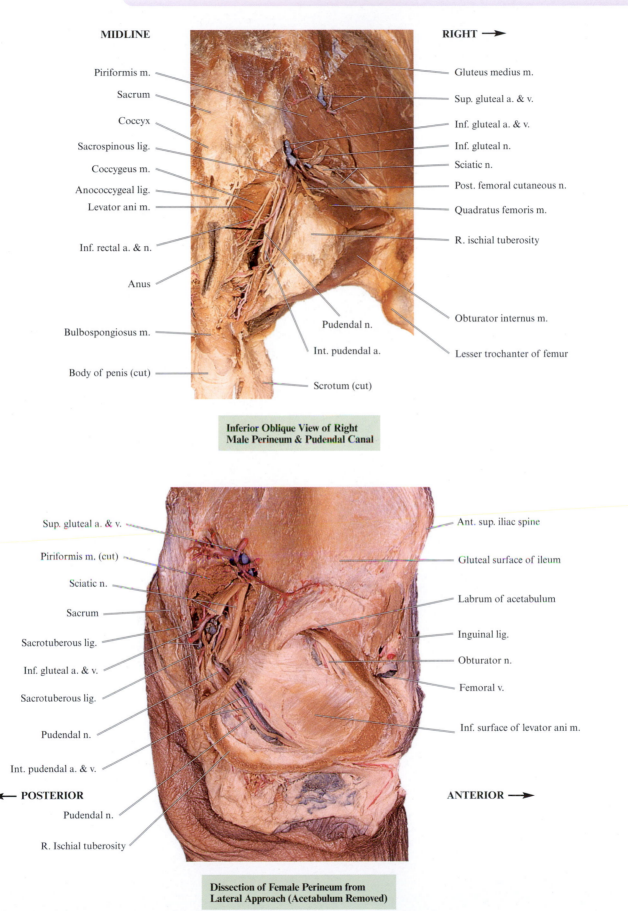

MIDLINE   **RIGHT →**

Piriformis m.   Gluteus medius m.

Sacrum   Sup. gluteal a. & v.

Coccyx   Inf. gluteal a. & v.

Sacrospinous lig.   Inf. gluteal n.

Coccygeus m.   Sciatic n.

Anococcygeal lig.   Post. femoral cutaneous n.

Levator ani m.   Quadratus femoris m.

Inf. rectal a. & n.   R. ischial tuberosity

Anus

Bulbospongiosus m.   Obturator internus m.

                                Pudendal n.

Body of penis (cut)   Int. pudendal a.   Lesser trochanter of femur

                                Scrotum (cut)

**Inferior Oblique View of Right
Male Perineum & Pudendal Canal**

Sup. gluteal a. & v.   Ant. sup. iliac spine

Piriformis m. (cut)   Gluteal surface of ileum

Sciatic n.   Labrum of acetabulum

Sacrum

Sacrotuberous lig.   Inguinal lig.

Inf. gluteal a. & v.   Obturator n.

Sacrotuberous lig.   Femoral v.

Pudendal n.   Inf. surface of levator ani m.

Int. pudendal a. & v.

← POSTERIOR   **ANTERIOR →**

Pudendal n.

R. Ischial tuberosity

**Dissection of Female Perineum from
Lateral Approach (Acetabulum Removed)**

CHAPTER 4 | **PELVIS AND PERINEUM**   205

PLATE 4.55 **RECTUM & ANAL CANAL—ARTERIES**

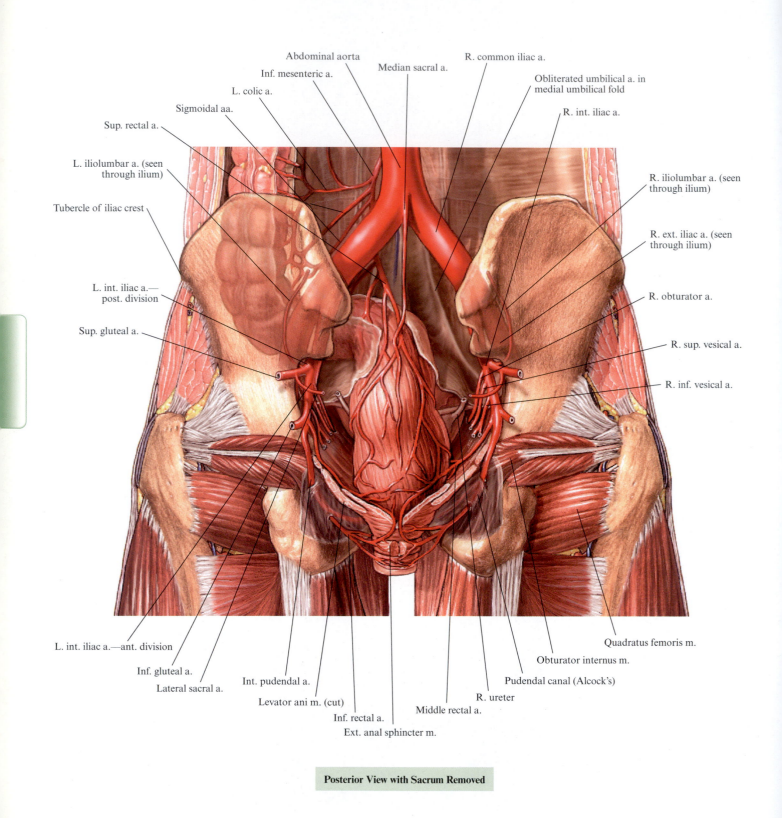

Abdominal aorta

Inf. mesenteric a.

Median sacral a.

R. common iliac a.

L. colic a.

Obliterated umbilical a. in medial umbilical fold

Sigmoidal aa.

R. int. iliac a.

Sup. rectal a.

L. iliolumbar a. (seen through ilium)

R. iliolumbar a. (seen through ilium)

Tubercle of iliac crest

R. ext. iliac a. (seen through ilium)

L. int. iliac a.— post. division

R. obturator a.

Sup. gluteal a.

R. sup. vesical a.

R. inf. vesical a.

L. int. iliac a.—ant. division

Quadratus femoris m.

Inf. gluteal a.

Obturator internus m.

Lateral sacral a.

Pudendal canal (Alcock's)

Int. pudendal a.

R. ureter

Levator ani m. (cut)

Middle rectal a.

Inf. rectal a.

Ext. anal sphincter m.

Posterior View with Sacrum Removed

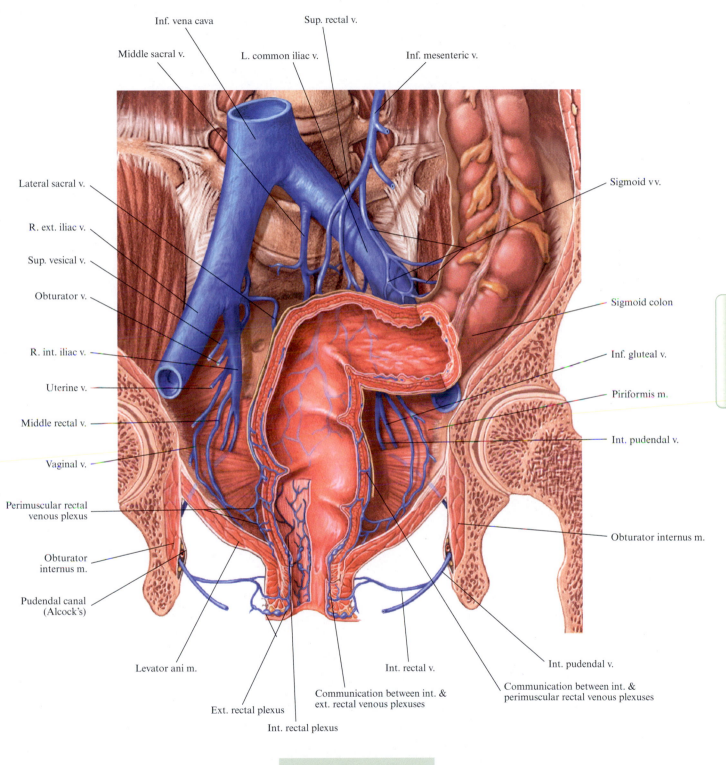

Inf. vena cava

Sup. rectal v.

Middle sacral v.

L. common iliac v.

Inf. mesenteric v.

Lateral sacral v.

Sigmoid v v.

R. ext. iliac v.

Sup. vesical v.

Obturator v.

Sigmoid colon

R. int. iliac v.

Inf. gluteal v.

Uterine v.

Piriformis m.

Middle rectal v.

Int. pudendal v.

Vaginal v.

Perimuscular rectal
venous plexus

Obturator internus m.

Obturator
internus m.

Pudendal canal
(Alcock's)

Levator ani m.

Int. pudendal v.

Communication between int. &
perimuscular rectal venous plexuses

Ext. rectal plexus

Int. rectal v.

Communication between int. &
ext. rectal venous plexuses

Int. rectal plexus

Coronal Section—Anterior View

PLATE 4.57   RECTUM & ANAL CANAL

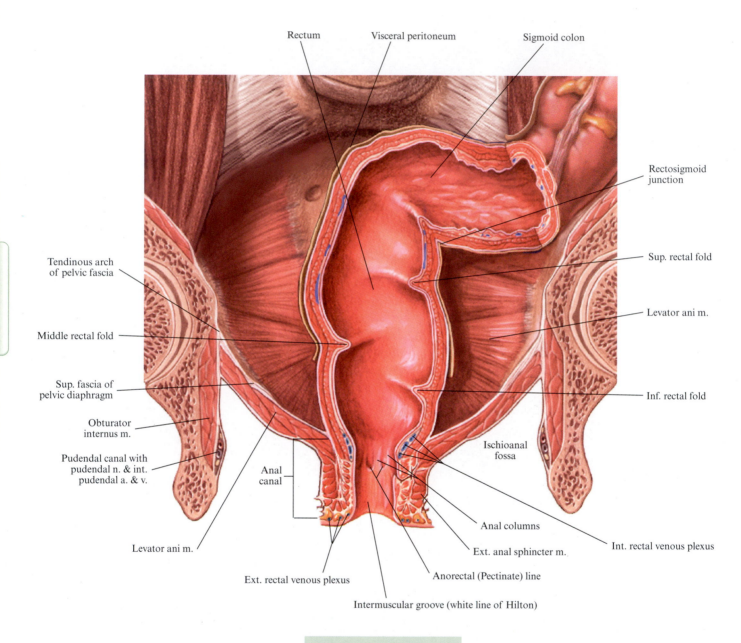

Rectum

Visceral peritoneum

Sigmoid colon

Rectosigmoid junction

Sup. rectal fold

Levator ani m.

Tendinous arch of pelvic fascia

Middle rectal fold

Sup. fascia of pelvic diaphragm

Inf. rectal fold

Obturator internus m.

Pudendal canal with pudendal n. & int. pudendal a. & v.

Anal canal

Ischioanal fossa

Levator ani m.

Anal columns

Ext. anal sphincter m.

Int. rectal venous plexus

Ext. rectal venous plexus

Anorectal (Pectinate) line

Intermuscular groove (white line of Hilton)

Coronal Section—Anterior View

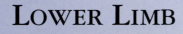

5 LOWER LIMB

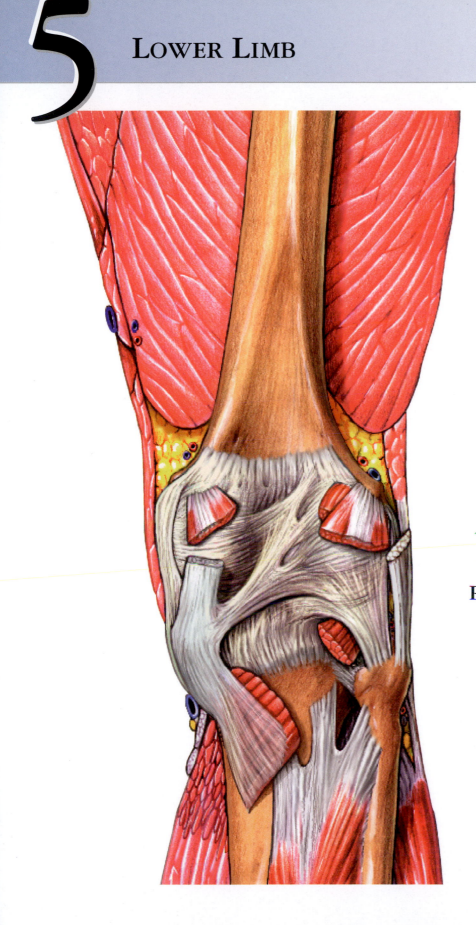

PLATE 5.1   SURFACE ANATOMY

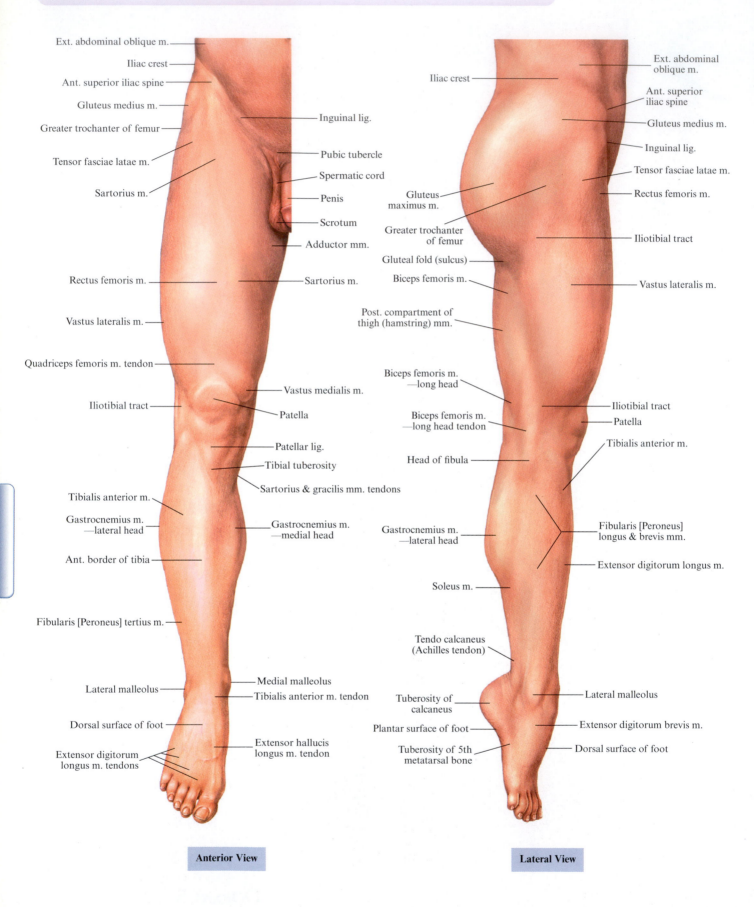

Ext. abdominal oblique m.
Iliac crest
Ant. superior iliac spine
Gluteus medius m.
Greater trochanter of femur
Tensor fasciae latae m.
Sartorius m.

Rectus femoris m.

Vastus lateralis m.

Quadriceps femoris m. tendon

Iliotibial tract

Tibialis anterior m.
Gastrocnemius m. —lateral head
Ant. border of tibia

Fibularis [Peroneus] tertius m.

Lateral malleolus

Dorsal surface of foot

Extensor digitorum longus m. tendons

Inguinal lig.

Pubic tubercle
Spermatic cord
Penis
Scrotum
Adductor mm.

Sartorius m.

Vastus medialis m.
Patella
Patellar lig.
Tibial tuberosity
Sartorius & gracilis mm. tendons

Gastrocnemius m. —medial head

Medial malleolus
Tibialis anterior m. tendon

Extensor hallucis longus m. tendon

Anterior View

Iliac crest

Ext. abdominal oblique m.
Ant. superior iliac spine
Gluteus medius m.
Inguinal lig.
Tensor fasciae latae m.
Rectus femoris m.

Iliotibial tract

Gluteus maximus m.
Greater trochanter of femur
Gluteal fold (sulcus)
Biceps femoris m.

Post. compartment of thigh (hamstring) mm.

Biceps femoris m. —long head

Biceps femoris m. —long head tendon

Head of fibula

Gastrocnemius m. —lateral head

Soleus m.

Tendo calcaneus (Achilles tendon)

Tuberosity of calcaneus

Plantar surface of foot
Tuberosity of 5th metatarsal bone

Vastus lateralis m.

Iliotibial tract
Patella
Tibialis anterior m.

Fibularis [Peroneus] longus & brevis mm.
Extensor digitorum longus m.

Lateral malleolus
Extensor digitorum brevis m.
Dorsal surface of foot

Lateral View

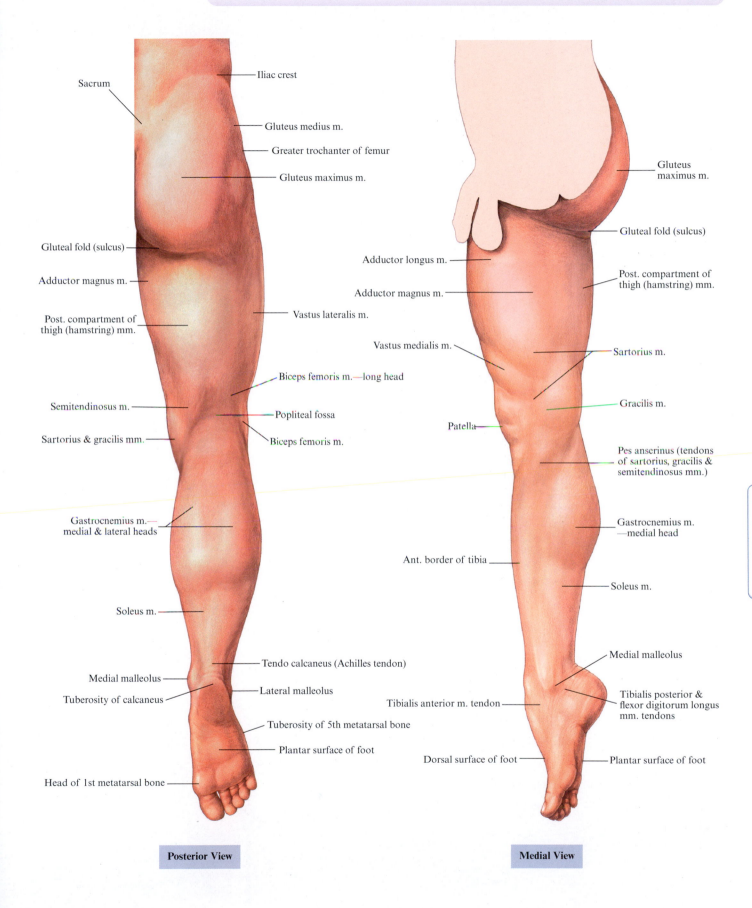

Sacrum

Iliac crest

Gluteus medius m.

Greater trochanter of femur

Gluteus maximus m.

Gluteus maximus m.

Gluteal fold (sulcus)

Gluteal fold (sulcus)

Adductor magnus m.

Adductor longus m.

Post. compartment of thigh (hamstring) mm.

Post. compartment of thigh (hamstring) mm.

Adductor magnus m.

Vastus lateralis m.

Vastus medialis m.

Sartorius m.

Biceps femoris m.—long head

Gracilis m.

Semitendinosus m.

Popliteal fossa

Patella

Sartorius & gracilis mm.

Biceps femoris m.

Pes anserinus (tendons of sartorius, gracilis & semitendinosus mm.)

Gastrocnemius m.— medial & lateral heads

Gastrocnemius m. —medial head

Ant. border of tibia

Soleus m.

Soleus m.

Tendo calcaneus (Achilles tendon)

Medial malleolus

Medial malleolus

Lateral malleolus

Tuberosity of calcaneus

Tibialis posterior & flexor digitorum longus mm. tendons

Tuberosity of 5th metatarsal bone

Tibialis anterior m. tendon

Plantar surface of foot

Head of 1st metatarsal bone

Dorsal surface of foot

Plantar surface of foot

Posterior View

Medial View

PLATE 5.3   SKELETON & MUSCLE ATTACHMENTS

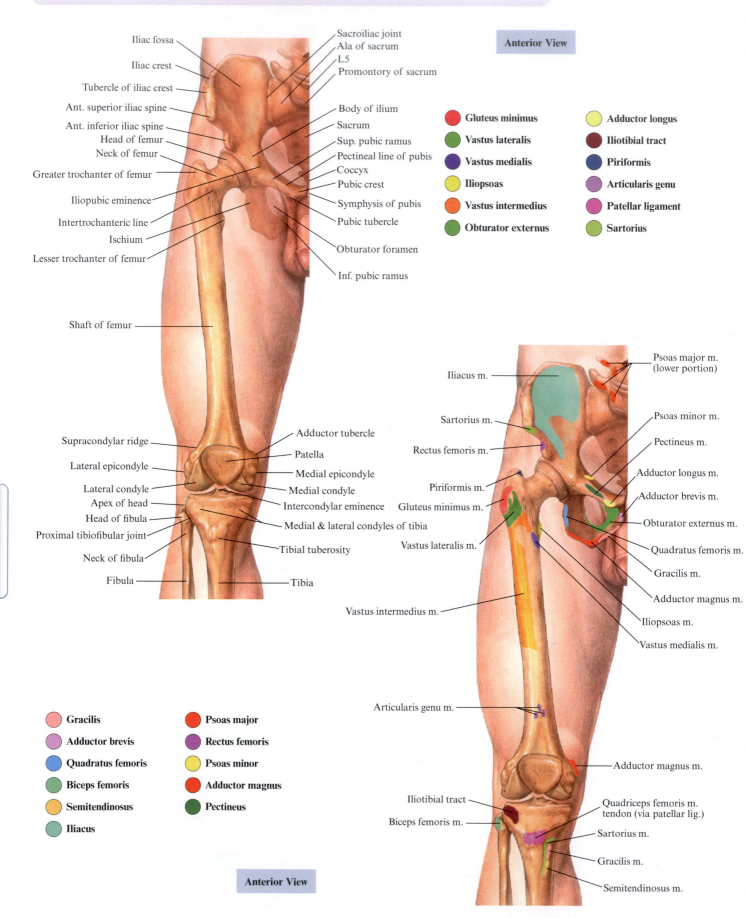

Anterior View

Iliac fossa
Iliac crest
Tubercle of iliac crest
Ant. superior iliac spine
Ant. inferior iliac spine
Head of femur
Neck of femur
Greater trochanter of femur
Iliopubic eminence
Intertrochanteric line
Ischium
Lesser trochanter of femur

Sacroiliac joint
Ala of sacrum
L5
Promontory of sacrum

Body of ilium
Sacrum
Sup. pubic ramus
Pectineal line of pubis
Coccyx
Pubic crest
Symphysis of pubis
Pubic tubercle
Obturator foramen
Inf. pubic ramus

Shaft of femur

● Gluteus minimus
● Vastus lateralis
● Vastus medialis
● Iliopsoas
● Vastus intermedius
● Obturator externus

● Adductor longus
● Iliotibial tract
● Piriformis
● Articularis genu
● Patellar ligament
● Sartorius

Supracondylar ridge
Lateral epicondyle
Lateral condyle
Apex of head
Head of fibula
Proximal tibiofibular joint
Neck of fibula
Fibula

Adductor tubercle
Patella
Medial epicondyle
Medial condyle
Intercondylar eminence
Medial & lateral condyles of tibia
Tibial tuberosity
Tibia

Iliacus m.
Sartorius m.
Rectus femoris m.
Piriformis m.
Gluteus minimus m.
Vastus lateralis m.
Vastus intermedius m.
Articularis genu m.
Iliotibial tract
Biceps femoris m.

Psoas major m. (lower portion)
Psoas minor m.
Pectineus m.
Adductor longus m.
Adductor brevis m.
Obturator externus m.
Quadratus femoris m.
Gracilis m.
Adductor magnus m.
Iliopsoas m.
Vastus medialis m.

Adductor magnus m.
Quadriceps femoris m. tendon (via patellar lig.)
Sartorius m.
Gracilis m.
Semitendinosus m.

● Gracilis
● Adductor brevis
● Quadratus femoris
● Biceps femoris
● Semitendinosus
● Iliacus

● Psoas major
● Rectus femoris
● Psoas minor
● Adductor magnus
● Pectineus

Anterior View

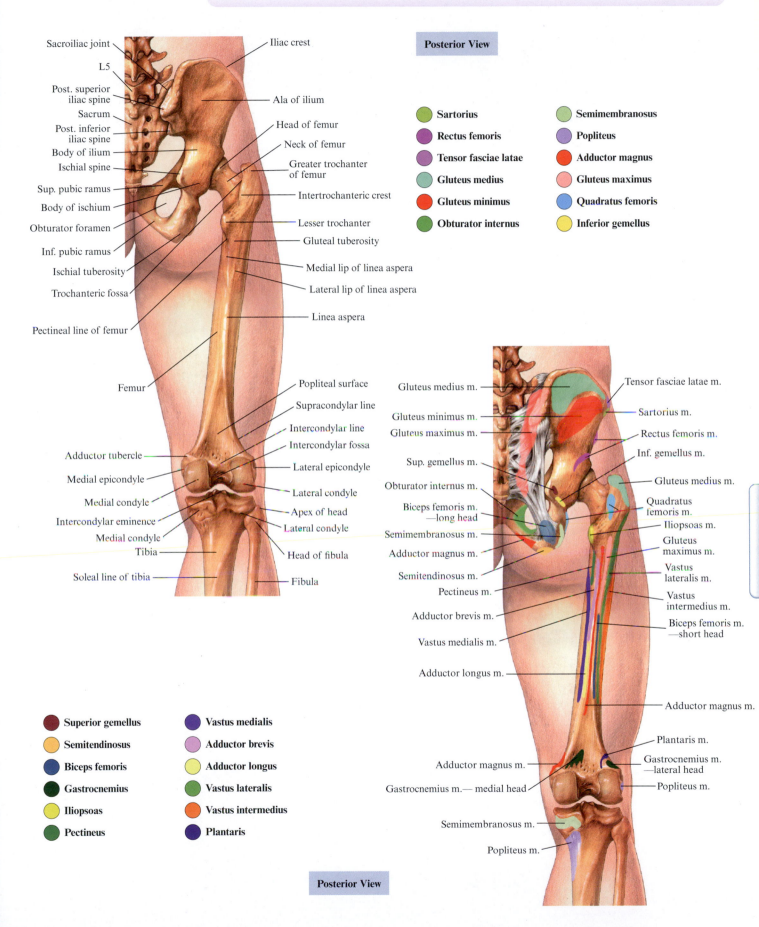

Posterior View

Sacroiliac joint
L5
Post. superior iliac spine
Sacrum
Post. inferior iliac spine
Body of ilium
Ischial spine
Sup. pubic ramus
Body of ischium
Obturator foramen
Inf. pubic ramus
Ischial tuberosity
Trochanteric fossa
Pectineal line of femur
Femur
Adductor tubercle
Medial epicondyle
Medial condyle
Intercondylar eminence
Medial condyle
Tibia
Soleal line of tibia

Iliac crest
Ala of ilium
Head of femur
Neck of femur
Greater trochanter of femur
Intertrochanteric crest
Lesser trochanter
Gluteal tuberosity
Medial lip of linea aspera
Lateral lip of linea aspera
Linea aspera
Popliteal surface
Supracondylar line
Intercondylar line
Intercondylar fossa
Lateral epicondyle
Lateral condyle
Apex of head
Lateral condyle
Head of fibula
Fibula

● **Sartorius**
● **Rectus femoris**
● **Tensor fasciae latae**
● **Gluteus medius**
● **Gluteus minimus**
● **Obturator internus**

● **Semimembranosus**
● **Popliteus**
● **Adductor magnus**
● **Gluteus maximus**
● **Quadratus femoris**
● **Inferior gemellus**

Gluteus medius m.
Gluteus minimus m.
Gluteus maximus m.
Sup. gemellus m.
Obturator internus m.
Biceps femoris m. —long head
Semimembranosus m.
Adductor magnus m.
Semitendinosus m.
Pectineus m.
Adductor brevis m.
Vastus medialis m.
Adductor longus m.

Tensor fasciae latae m.
Sartorius m.
Rectus femoris m.
Inf. gemellus m.
Gluteus medius m.
Quadratus femoris m.
Iliopsoas m.
Gluteus maximus m.
Vastus lateralis m.
Vastus intermedius m.
Biceps femoris m. —short head
Adductor magnus m.
Plantaris m.
Gastrocnemius m. —lateral head
Popliteus m.

Adductor magnus m.
Gastrocnemius m.— medial head
Semimembranosus m.
Popliteus m.

● **Superior gemellus**
● **Semitendinosus**
● **Biceps femoris**
● **Gastrocnemius**
● **Iliopsoas**
● **Pectineus**

● **Vastus medialis**
● **Adductor brevis**
● **Adductor longus**
● **Vastus lateralis**
● **Vastus intermedius**
● **Plantaris**

Posterior View

PLATE 5.5   SKELETON & MUSCLE ATTACHMENTS

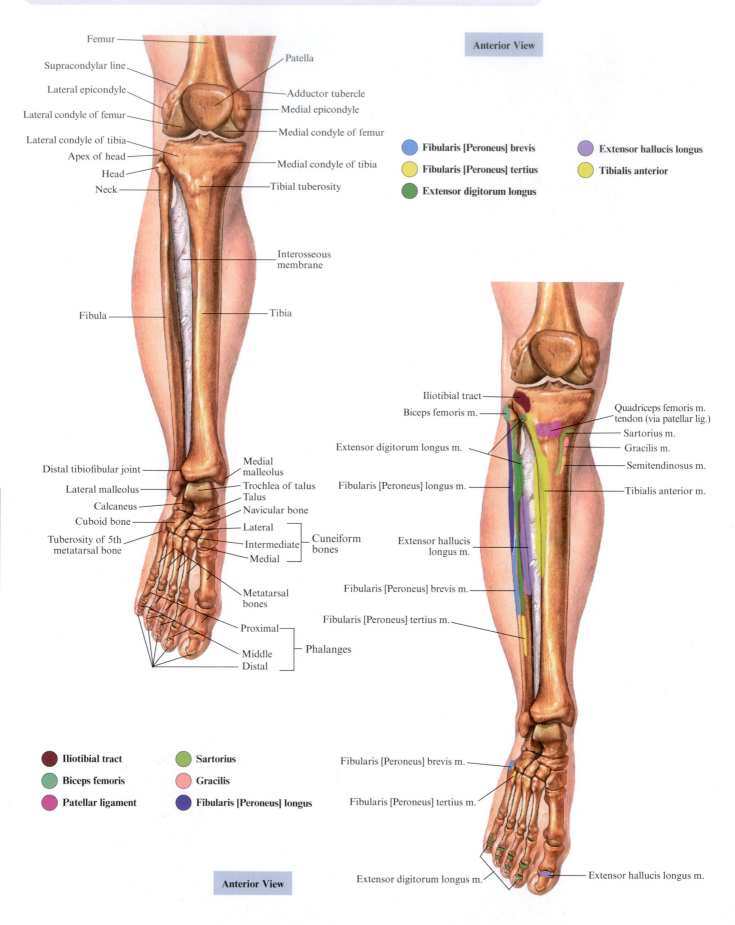

Anterior View

Femur
Supracondylar line
Lateral epicondyle
Lateral condyle of femur
Lateral condyle of tibia
Apex of head
Head
Neck

Patella
Adductor tubercle
Medial epicondyle
Medial condyle of femur
Medial condyle of tibia
Tibial tuberosity

Interosseous membrane

Fibula
Tibia

Distal tibiofibular joint
Lateral malleolus
Calcaneus
Cuboid bone
Tuberosity of 5th metatarsal bone

Medial malleolus
Trochlea of talus
Talus
Navicular bone
Lateral
Intermediate
Medial
} Cuneiform bones

Metatarsal bones
Proximal
Middle
Distal
} Phalanges

● Fibularis [Peroneus] brevis
● Fibularis [Peroneus] tertius
● Extensor digitorum longus

● Extensor hallucis longus
● Tibialis anterior

Iliotibial tract
Biceps femoris m.
Extensor digitorum longus m.
Fibularis [Peroneus] longus m.
Extensor hallucis longus m.
Fibularis [Peroneus] brevis m.
Fibularis [Peroneus] tertius m.

Quadriceps femoris m. tendon (via patellar lig.)
Sartorius m.
Gracilis m.
Semitendinosus m.
Tibialis anterior m.

Fibularis [Peroneus] brevis m.
Fibularis [Peroneus] tertius m.

Extensor digitorum longus m.
Extensor hallucis longus m.

● Iliotibial tract
● Biceps femoris
● Patellar ligament
● Sartorius
● Gracilis
● Fibularis [Peroneus] longus

Anterior View

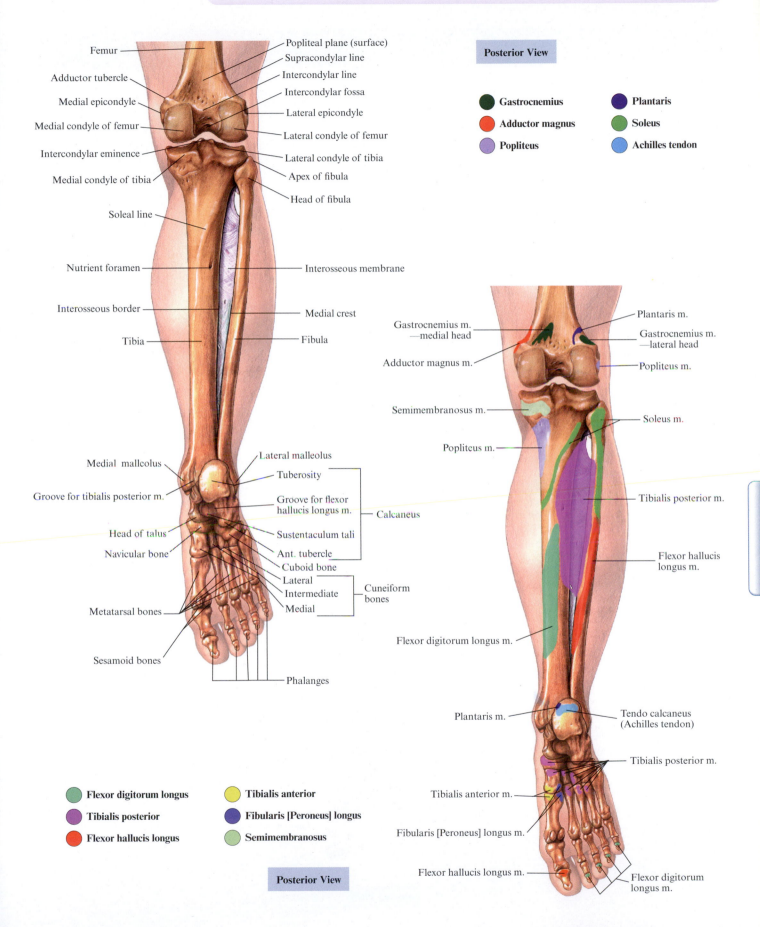

Posterior View

● **Gastrocnemius**   ● **Plantaris**
● **Adductor magnus**   ● **Soleus**
● **Popliteus**   ● **Achilles tendon**

Femur

Adductor tubercle

Medial epicondyle

Medial condyle of femur

Intercondylar eminence

Medial condyle of tibia

Soleal line

Nutrient foramen

Interosseous border

Tibia

Popliteal plane (surface)

Supracondylar line

Intercondylar line

Intercondylar fossa

Lateral epicondyle

Lateral condyle of femur

Lateral condyle of tibia

Apex of fibula

Head of fibula

Interosseous membrane

Medial crest

Fibula

Medial malleolus

Groove for tibialis posterior m.

Head of talus

Navicular bone

Metatarsal bones

Sesamoid bones

Lateral malleolus

Tuberosity

Groove for flexor
hallucis longus m.

Sustentaculum tali

Ant. tubercle

Cuboid bone

Lateral

Intermediate

Medial

Phalanges

Calcaneus

Cuneiform
bones

Gastrocnemius m.
—medial head

Adductor magnus m.

Semimembranosus m.

Popliteus m.

Flexor digitorum longus m.

Plantaris m.

Tibialis anterior m.

Fibularis [Peroneus] longus m.

Flexor hallucis longus m.

Plantaris m.

Gastrocnemius m.
—lateral head

Popliteus m.

Soleus m.

Tibialis posterior m.

Flexor hallucis
longus m.

Tendo calcaneus
(Achilles tendon)

Tibialis posterior m.

Flexor digitorum
longus m.

● **Flexor digitorum longus**   ● **Tibialis anterior**
● **Tibialis posterior**   ● **Fibularis [Peroneus] longus**
● **Flexor hallucis longus**   ● **Semimembranosus**

Posterior View

TABLE 5.1   ANTERIOR THIGH MUSCLES

Muscle	Proximal Attachment	Distal Attachment	Innervation	Main Actions
ILIOPSOAS				
Psoas major	Sides of T12 to L5 vertebral bodies, intervertebral discs between them & transverse processes of L1–L5	Lesser trochanter of femur	Ventral rami of lumbar nn. (**L1**, **L2** & L3)[a]	Flex pelvis & vertebral column on pelvis when leg & hip are extended and fixed: Act conjointly in flexing thigh at hip joint and in stabilizing this joint
Psoas minor	Sides of T12 & L1 vertebrae & intervertebral disc	Pectineal line, iliopectineal eminence via iliopubic arch lig.	Ventral rami of lumbar nn. (L1 & L2)	
Iliacus	Iliac crest, iliac fossa, ala of sacrum, ant. sacroiliac ligg. & capsule of hip joint	Tendon of psoas major & body of femur, inf. to lesser trochanter	Femoral n. (**L2** & **L3**)	
Tensor fasciae latae	Ant. sup. iliac spine & ant. part of ext. lip of iliac crest	Anterolateral aspect of lateral tibial condyle via iliotibial tract	Sup. gluteal n. (L4 & L5)	Abducts, flexes hip and helps to keep knee extended; medially rotates hip when it is flexed.
Sartorius	Ant. sup. iliac spine & sup. part of notch inf. to it	Sup. part of medial surface of tibia	Femoral n. (L2 & L3)	Flexes, abducts & laterally rotates thigh at hip joint & flexes leg at knee joint
QUADRICEPS FEMORIS				
Rectus femoris	Ant. inf. iliac spine & groove sup. to acetabulum	Base of patella & via patellar lig. to tibial tuberosity	Femoral n. (L2, **L3** & **L4**)	Extend leg at knee joint; rectus femoris also helps iliopsoas to flex thigh
Vastus lateralis	Greater trochanter & lateral lip of linea aspera of femur			
Vastus medialis	Intertrochanteric line & medial lip of linea aspera of femur			
Vastus intermedius	Ant. & lateral surfaces of shaft of femur			

[a]In this and subsequent tables, the numbers indicate the spinal cord segmental innervation of the nerves. For example, **L1**, **L2** and L3 indicate that the nerves supplying the psoas major muscle are derived from the first three lumbar segments of the spinal cord; the boldface (**L1**, **L2**) indicates the main segmental innervation. Damage to one or more of these spinal cord segments or to the motor nerve roots arising from them results in paralysis of the muscles involved.

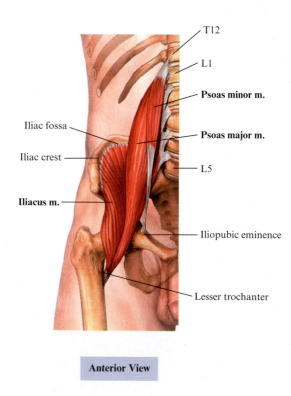

T12
L1
Psoas minor m.
Psoas major m.
Iliac fossa
Iliac crest
L5
Iliacus m.
Iliopubic eminence
Lesser trochanter

Anterior View

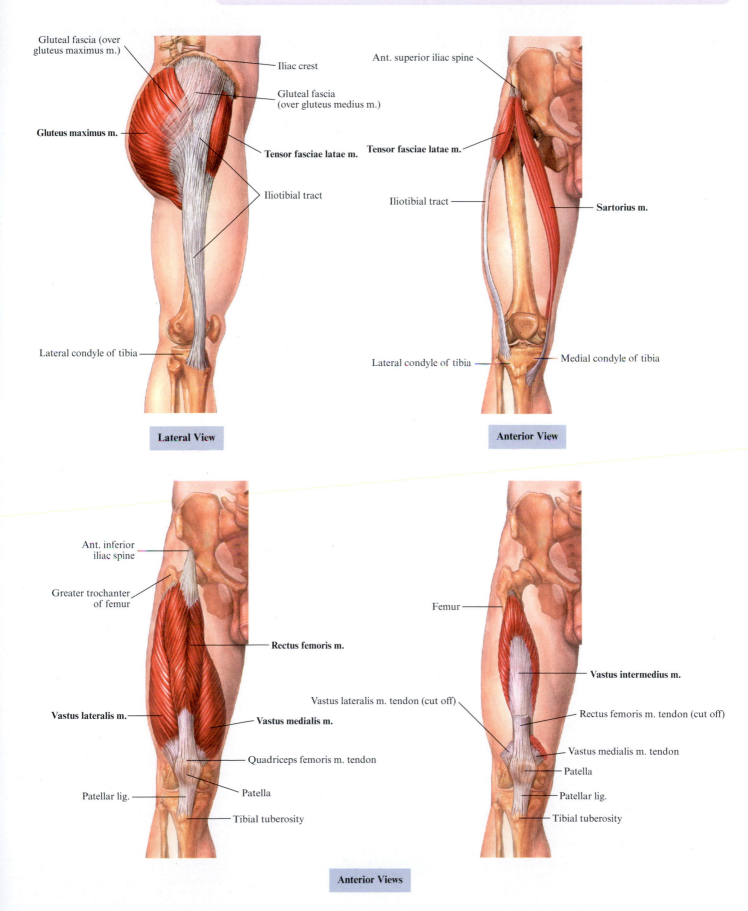

Gluteal fascia (over gluteus maximus m.)

Iliac crest

Gluteal fascia (over gluteus medius m.)

Gluteus maximus m.

Tensor fasciae latae m.

Iliotibial tract

Lateral condyle of tibia

Lateral View

Ant. superior iliac spine

Tensor fasciae latae m.

Iliotibial tract

Sartorius m.

Lateral condyle of tibia

Medial condyle of tibia

Anterior View

Ant. inferior iliac spine

Greater trochanter of femur

Rectus femoris m.

Vastus lateralis m.

Vastus medialis m.

Quadriceps femoris m. tendon

Patellar lig.

Patella

Tibial tuberosity

Femur

Vastus intermedius m.

Vastus lateralis m. tendon (cut off)

Rectus femoris m. tendon (cut off)

Vastus medialis m. tendon

Patella

Patellar lig.

Tibial tuberosity

Anterior Views

TABLE 5.2 GLUTEAL & POSTERIOR THIGH MUSCLES

Gluteal Muscle	Proximal Attachment	Distal Attachment	Innervation	Main Actions
Gluteus maximus	Ext. surface of ala of ilium, including iliac crest, dorsal surface of sacrum & coccyx and sacrotuberous lig.	Most fibers end in iliotibial tract which inserts into lateral condyle of tibia; some fibers insert on gluteal tuberosity of femur	Inf. gluteal n. (L5, **S1** & **S2**)	Extends thigh & assists in its lat. rotation; also assists in raising trunk from flexed position
Gluteus medius	Ext. surface of ilium between ant. & post. gluteal lines	Lateral surface of greater trochanter of femur	Sup. gluteal n. (**L5** & S1)	Abduct & medially rotate thigh; steady pelvis
Gluteus minimus	Ext. surface of ilium between ant. & inf. gluteal lines	Ant. surface of greater trochanter of femur		
Piriformis	Ant. surface of sacrum between S2 & S4	Superior border of greater trochanter of femur	Brr. from ventral rami of **S1** & S2	
Obturator internus	Pelvic surface of obturator membrane & surrounding bones		N. to obturator internus (L5 & **S1**)	Laterally rotate extended thigh & abduct flexed thigh
Superior gemellus	Ischial spine	Trochanteric fossa^a	Same nerve supply as obturator internus	
Inferior gemellus	Ischial tuberosity		Same nerve supply as quadratus femoris	
Quadratus femoris	Lateral border of ischial tuberosity	Quadrate tubercle and intertrochanteric crest of femur	N. to quadratus femoris (L5 & **S1**)	Laterally rotates thigh^b

^aThe gemelli muscles join the tendon of the obturator internus muscle as it attaches to the trochanteric fossa.
^bThere are six lateral rotators of the thigh: piriformis, obturator internus, gemelli (superior and inferior), quadratus femoris and obturator externus. These muscles also help to stabilize the hip joint.

Post. Thigh Muscle	Proximal Attachment	Distal Attachment	Innervation	Main Actions
Semitendinosus	Ischial tuberosity	Medial surface of sup. part of tibia	Tibial division of sciatic n. (**L5, S1** & **S2**)	Extend thigh; flex leg and rotate it medially; when thigh & leg are flexed, they can extend pelvis (and trunk)
Semimembranous		Post. part of medial condyle of tibia		
Biceps femoris Long head Short head	Ischial tuberosity Lateral lip of distal half of linea aspera & lateral supracondylar line	Lateral side of head of fibula	Tibial division of sciatic n. (L5, **S1** & **S2**) Common fibular (peroneal) division of sciatic n. (L5, **S1** & **S2**)	Flexes leg & rotates it laterally; extends thigh (e.g., when starting to walk)

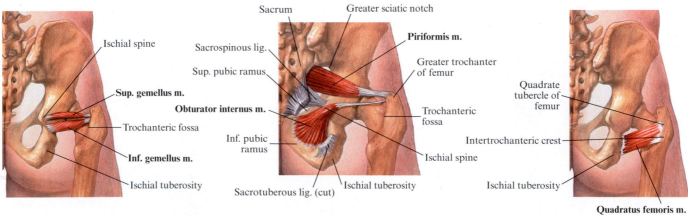

Posterior Views

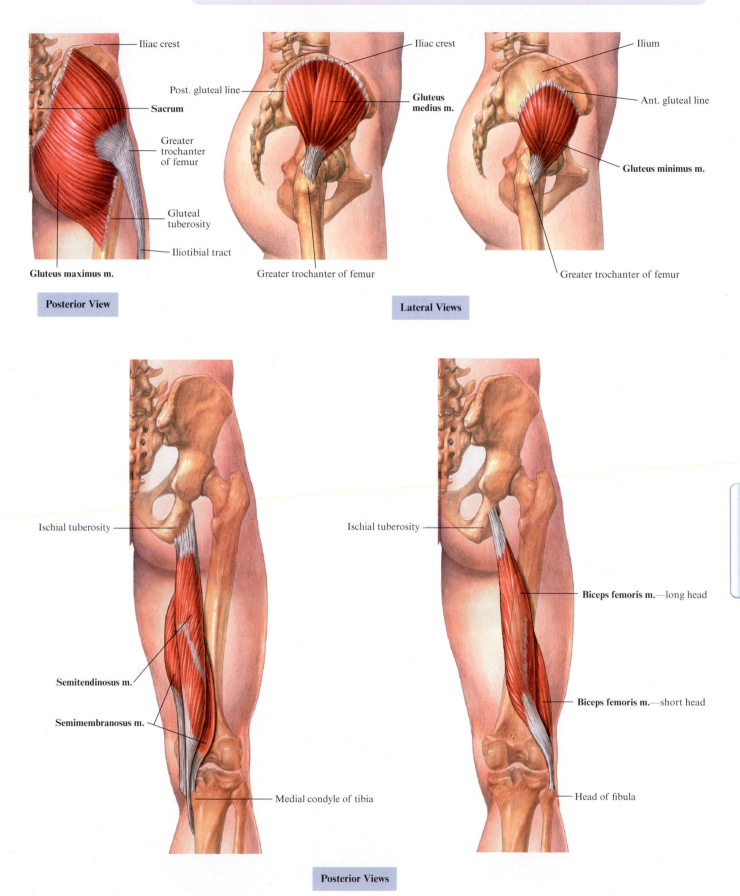

Iliac crest

Sacrum

Greater
trochanter
of femur

Gluteal
tuberosity

Iliotibial tract

Gluteus maximus m.

Posterior View

Iliac crest

Post. gluteal line

**Gluteus
medius m.**

Greater trochanter of femur

Ilium

Ant. gluteal line

Gluteus minimus m.

Greater trochanter of femur

Lateral Views

Ischial tuberosity

Semitendinosus m.

Semimembranosus m.

Medial condyle of tibia

Ischial tuberosity

Biceps femoris m.—long head

Biceps femoris m.—short head

Head of fibula

Posterior Views

TABLE 5.3   MEDIAL THIGH MUSCLES

Muscle[a]	Proximal Attachment	Distal Attachment	Innervation	Main Actions
Pectineus	Pecten pubis	Pectineal line of femur	Femoral nerve (**L2** & **L3**) & br. from obturator n. (L2, L3)	Adducts; flexes & laterally rotates thigh
Adductor longus	Body of pubis, inf. to pubic crest	Middle third of linea aspera of femur	Obturator n. ant. br. (L2, **L3** & L4)	Adducts thigh
Adductor brevis	Body & inf. ramus of pubis	Pectineal line & proximal part of linea aspera of femur	Obturator n. (L2, **L3** & L4)	Adducts thigh & may act to flex hip
Adductor magnus	Inf. ramus of pubis, ramus of ischium (adductor part) & ischial tuberosity	Gluteal tuberosity, linea aspera med. supracondylar line (adductor part) & adductor tubercle of femur (hamstring part)	*Adductor part*, obturator n. (L2, **L3** & L4) *Hamstring part*, tibial portion of sciatic n. (**L4**)	Adducts thigh; its adductor part also flexes thigh & its hamstring part extends it
Gracilis	Body & inf. ramus of pubis	Sup. part of med. surface of tibia	Obturator n. (**L2**, L3 & L4)	Adducts thigh, flexes leg & helps to rotate it medially
Obturator externus	Margins of obturator foramen & ext. surface of obturator membrane	Trochanteric fossa of femur	Obturator n. (L3 & **L4**)	Laterally rotates thigh

[a]The last five muscles are called the *adductors of the thigh*.

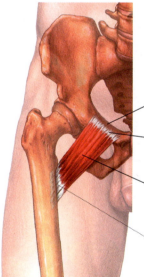

Sup. pubic ramus

Pectineal line of pubis [Pecten pubis]

Pectineus m.

Pectineal line of femur (seen through shaft of femur)

Anterior Views

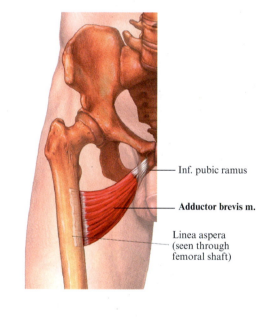

Inf. pubic ramus

Adductor brevis m.

Linea aspera (seen through femoral shaft)

Trochanteric fossa (seen through greater trochanter)

Sup. pubic ramus

Obturator externus m.

Inf. pubic ramus

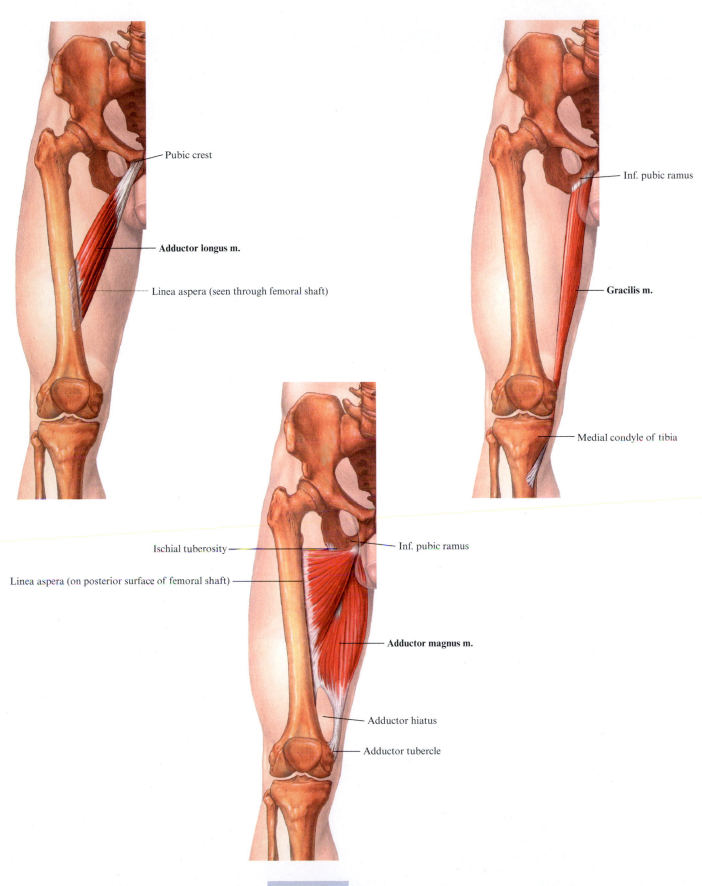

Pubic crest

Adductor longus m.

Linea aspera (seen through femoral shaft)

Inf. pubic ramus

Gracilis m.

Medial condyle of tibia

Ischial tuberosity

Inf. pubic ramus

Linea aspera (on posterior surface of femoral shaft)

Adductor magnus m.

Adductor hiatus

Adductor tubercle

Anterior Views

TABLE 5.4   ANTERIOR & LATERAL LEG MUSCLES

Anterior Muscle	Proximal Attachment	Distal Attachment	Innervation	Main Actions
Tibialis anterior	Lateral condyle & sup. half of lateral surface of tibia	Medial & inf. surfaces of medial cuneiform bone & base of 1st metatarsal bone	Deep fibular [peroneal] n. (**L4 & L5**)	Dorsiflexes & inverts foot
Extensor hallucis longus	Middle part of ant. surface of fibula & interosseous membrane	Dorsal aspect of base of distal phalanx of 1st digit (hallux)	} Deep fibular [peroneal] n. (**L5 & S1**)	Extends 1st digit & dorsiflexes foot
Extensor digitorum longus	Lateral condyle of tibia, sup. 3/4 of ant. surface of fibula & interosseous membrane	Middle & distal phalanges of lateral 4 digits via extensor expansions		Extends lateral 4 digits & dorsiflexes foot
Fibularis [Peroneus] tertius	Inferior third of ant. surface of fibula & interosseous membrane	Dorsum of base of 5th metatarsal bone		Dorsiflexes foot & aids in eversion of it

Lateral Muscle[a]	Proximal Attachment	Distal Attachment	Innervation	Main Actions
Fibularis [Peroneus] longus	Head & sup. 2/3 of lateral surface of fibula	Base of 1st metatarsal bone & medial cuneiform bone	} Superficial fibular (peroneal) n. (**L5, S1 & S2**)	Everts & plantarflexes foot
Fibularis [Peroneus] brevis	Inf. 2/3 of lateral surface of fibula	Dorsal surface of tuberosity of 5th metatarsal bone		Everts foot & weakly plantarflexes foot

[a]The fibularis [peroneus] longus and brevis were named because their proximal attachment is to the fibula. *Peroneus* is the Greek word for the Latin term *fibula* and has also been used to identify these muscles.

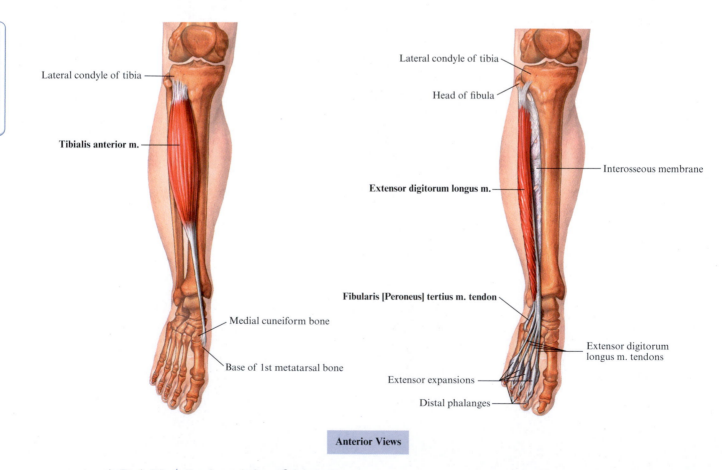

Lateral condyle of tibia

Tibialis anterior m.

Medial cuneiform bone

Base of 1st metatarsal bone

Lateral condyle of tibia

Head of fibula

Interosseous membrane

Extensor digitorum longus m.

Fibularis [Peroneus] tertius m. tendon

Extensor digitorum longus m. tendons

Extensor expansions

Distal phalanges

Anterior Views

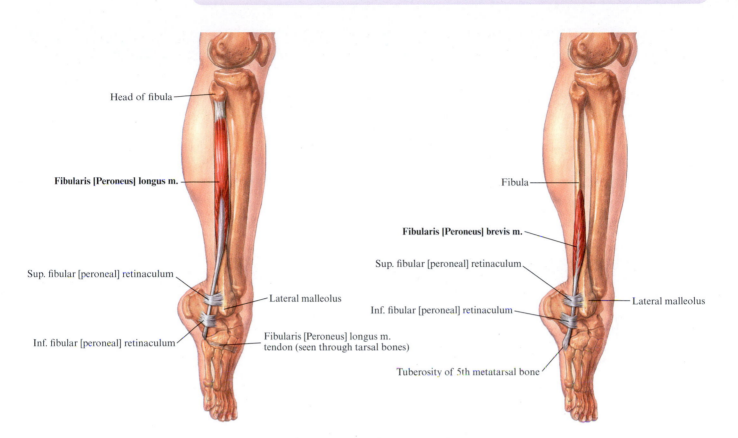

Head of fibula

Fibularis [Peroneus] longus m.

Sup. fibular [peroneal] retinaculum

Inf. fibular [peroneal] retinaculum

Lateral malleolus

Fibularis [Peroneus] longus m.
tendon (seen through tarsal bones)

Fibula

Fibularis [Peroneus] brevis m.

Sup. fibular [peroneal] retinaculum

Inf. fibular [peroneal] retinaculum

Lateral malleolus

Tuberosity of 5th metatarsal bone

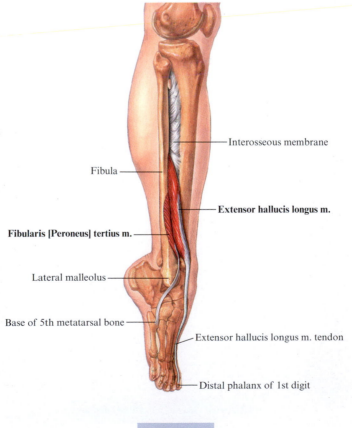

Interosseous membrane

Fibula

Extensor hallucis longus m.

Fibularis [Peroneus] tertius m.

Lateral malleolus

Base of 5th metatarsal bone

Extensor hallucis longus m. tendon

Distal phalanx of 1st digit

Lateral Views

TABLE 5.5   POSTERIOR LEG MUSCLES

Muscles	Proximal Attachment	Distal Attachment	Innervation	Main Actions
SUPERFICIAL GROUP				
Gastrocnemius	*Lateral head:* Lateral aspect of lateral condyle of femur *Medial head:* Popliteal surface of femur, sup. to medial condyle	Post. surface of tuberosity of calcaneus via tendo calcaneus	Tibial n. (L5, S1 & **S2**)	Plantarflexes foot, raises heel during walking & flexes knee joint
Soleus	Post. aspect of head of fibula, sup. 1/4th of post. surface of fibula, soleal line & medial border of tibia			Plantarflexes foot
Plantaris	Inf. end of lat. supracondylar line of femur & oblique popliteal lig.	Medial side of tendo calcaneus		Weakly assists gastronemius in plantarflexing foot & flexing knee joint

Muscles	Proximal Attachment	Distal Attachment	Innervation	Main Actions
DEEP GROUP				
Popliteus	Lateral epicondyle of femur & lateral meniscus	Post. surface of tibia, sup. to soleal line	Tibial n. (**L4, L5** & S1)	Weakly flexes knee & unlocks it
Flexor hallucis longus	Inf. 2/3 of post. surface of fibula & inf. part of interosseous membrane	Base of distal phalanx of 1st digit (hallux)	Tibial n. (**S2–S3**)	Flexes 1st digit at all joints and plantarflexes foot
Flexor digitorum longus	Medial part of post. surface of tibia, inf. to soleal line & by a broad aponeurosis to fibula	Bases of distal phalanges of lateral 4 digits		Flexes 4 digits & plantarflexes foot
Tibialis posterior	Interosseus membrane, post. surface of tibia inf. to soleal line & post. surface of fibula	Tuberosity of navicular, cuneiform & cuboid bones, & bases of 2nd, 3rd & 4th metatarsal bones	Tibial n. (L4–L5)	Plantarflexes & inverts foot

Posterior Views of Superficial Muscles

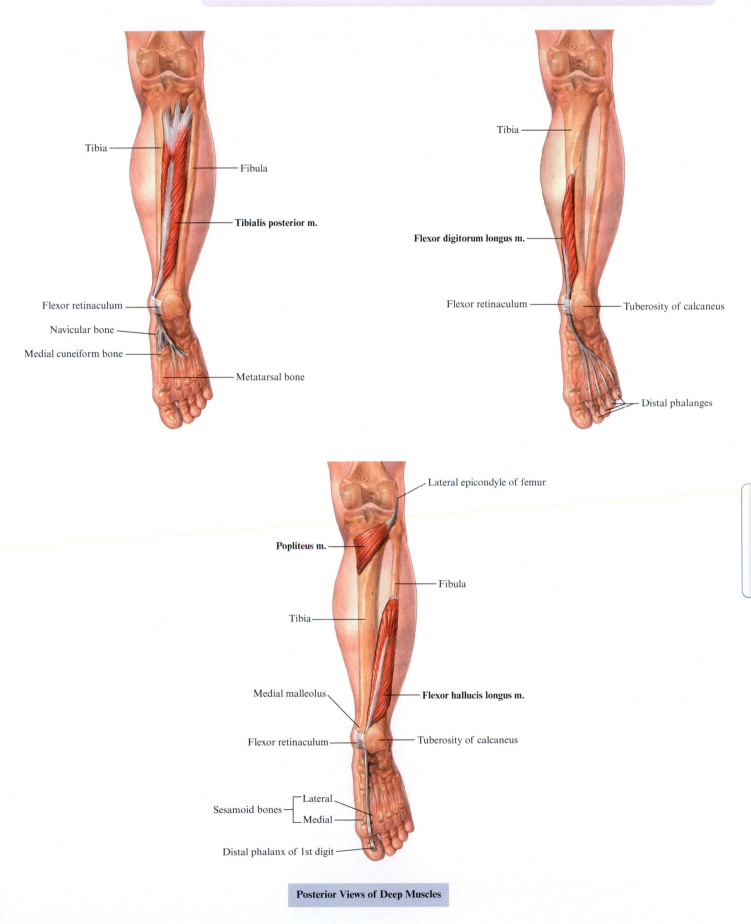

Tibia

Fibula

Tibialis posterior m.

Flexor retinaculum

Navicular bone

Medial cuneiform bone

Metatarsal bone

Tibia

Flexor digitorum longus m.

Flexor retinaculum

Tuberosity of calcaneus

Distal phalanges

Lateral epicondyle of femur

Popliteus m.

Fibula

Tibia

Medial malleolus

Flexor hallucis longus m.

Flexor retinaculum

Tuberosity of calcaneus

Sesamoid bones ⎡ Lateral
               ⎣ Medial

Distal phalanx of 1st digit

Posterior Views of Deep Muscles

TABLE 5.6   INTRINSIC FOOT MUSCLES

Muscle	Proximal Attachment	Distal Attachment	Innervation	Main Actions
FIRST LAYER[a]				
Abductor hallucis	Medial process of calcaneal tuberosity, flexor retinaculum & plantar aponeurosis	Medial side of base of proximal phalanx & medial sesamoid bone of 1st digit (hallux)	Medial plantar n. (S2 & **S3**)	Abducts & flexes 1st digit
Flexor digitorum brevis	Medial process of tuber calcanei, plantar aponeurosis & intermuscular septa	Both sides of middle phalanges of lateral 4 digits		Flexes lateral 4 digits (toes)
Abductor digiti minimi	Medial & lateral processes of calcaneal tuberosity, plantar aponeurosis & intermuscular septa	Lateral side of base of proximal phalanx of 5th digit (little toe)	Lateral plantar n. (S2 & **S3**)	Abducts & flexes 5th digit
SECOND LAYER				
Quadratus plantae	Medial surface & lateral margin of plantar surface of calcaneus	Posterolateral margin of tendon of flexor digitorum longus	Lateral plantar n. (S2 & **S3**)	Assists flexor digitorum longus in flexing lateral 4 digits
Lumbricalis	Tendons of flexor digitorum longus	Medial sides of bases of proximal phalanges of lateral 4 digits & extensor expansions of extensor digitorum longus m. tendons	*Medial one:* medial plantar n. (S2 & **S3**) *Lateral three:* lateral plantar n. (S2 & **S3**)	Flex proximal phalanges & extend middle & distal phalanges of lateral 4 digits
THIRD LAYER				
Flexor hallucis brevis	Plantar surfaces of cuboid & lateral cuneiform bones	Both sides of base of proximal phalanx of 1st digit	Medial plantar n. (S2 & **S3**)	Flexes proximal phalanx of 1st digit (hallux)
Adductor hallucis	*Oblique head:* Bases of metatarsal bones 2–4 *Transverse head:* Plantar ligg. of metatarsophalangeal joints 2–5	Tendons of both heads attached to lateral side of base of proximal phalanx & lat. sesamoid bone of 1st digit (hallux)	Deep br. of lateral plantar n. (S2 & **S3**)	Adducts 1st digit; assists in maintaining transverse arch of foot
Flexor digiti minimi brevis	Base of 5th metatarsal bone	Base of proximal phalanx of 5th digit	Superficial br. of lateral plantar n. (S2 & **S3**)	Flexes proximal phalanx of 5th digit
FOURTH LAYER				
Plantar interossei (3 muscles)	Bases & medial sides of metatarsal bones 3–5	Medial sides of bases of proximal phalanges of digits 3–5	Lateral plantar n. (S2 & **S3**)	Adduct digits (2–4) & flex metatarsophalangeal joints
Dorsal interossei (4 muscles)	Adjacent side of metatarsal bones 1–5	*1st:* medial side of proximal phalanx of 2nd digit *2nd–4th:* lateral sides of digits 2–4		Abduct digits (2–4) & flex metatarsorphalangeal joints

[a]Independent of the individual actions associated with them, the primary function of the first layer of intrinsic muscles of the foot is to sustain the longitudinal arch of the foot (i.e., resisting forces tending to spread or flatten it).

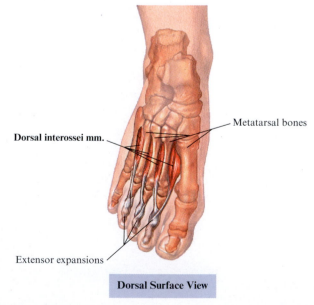

Dorsal interossei mm.

Metatarsal bones

Extensor expansions

Dorsal Surface View

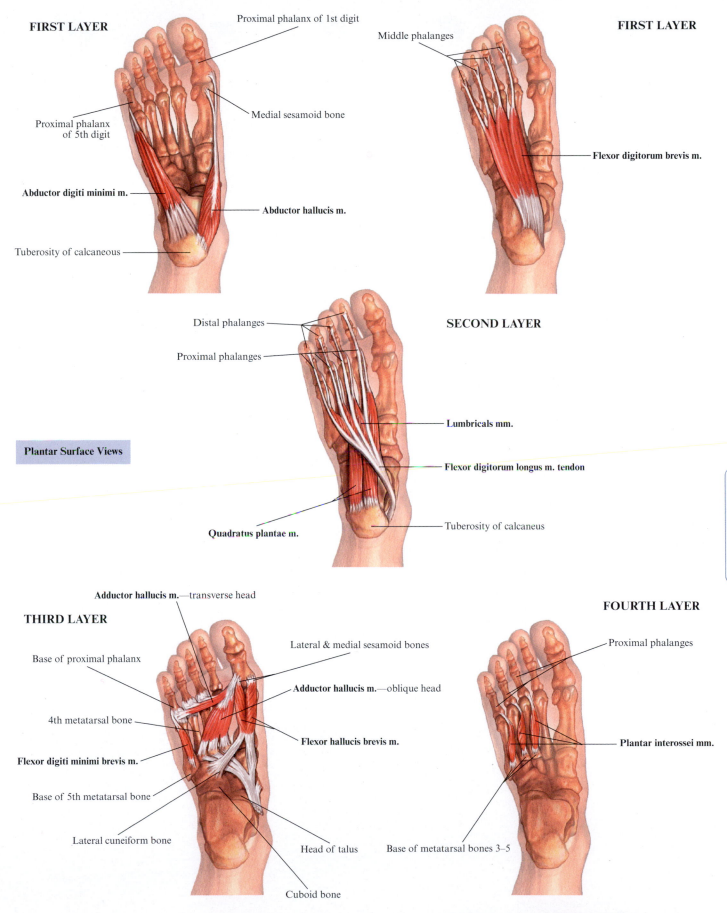

FIRST LAYER

Proximal phalanx of 1st digit

Middle phalanges

FIRST LAYER

Proximal phalanx of 5th digit

Medial sesamoid bone

Flexor digitorum brevis m.

Abductor digiti minimi m.

Abductor hallucis m.

Tuberosity of calcaneous

Distal phalanges

SECOND LAYER

Proximal phalanges

Lumbricals mm.

Plantar Surface Views

Flexor digitorum longus m. tendon

Tuberosity of calcaneus

Quadratus plantae m.

Adductor hallucis m.—transverse head

FOURTH LAYER

THIRD LAYER

Lateral & medial sesamoid bones

Proximal phalanges

Base of proximal phalanx

Adductor hallucis m.—oblique head

4th metatarsal bone

Flexor hallucis brevis m.

Plantar interossei mm.

Flexor digiti minimi brevis m.

Base of 5th metatarsal bone

Lateral cuneiform bone

Head of talus

Base of metatarsal bones 3–5

Cuboid bone

PLATE 5.13   GAIT CYCLE—STANCE PHASE

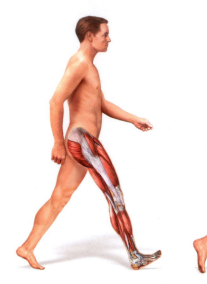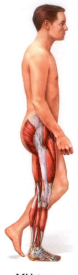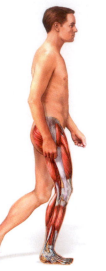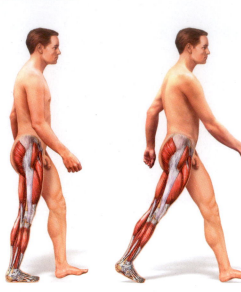

Initial contact (heel strike)   **Loading response** (foot flat)   **Midstance**   **Terminal stance** (heel off)   **Preswing** (toe off) (heel strike)

——Push Off——
Propulsion & swing limb advancement

Right Stance Phase (60%) of Gait Cycle

Double limb support (10%) Weight acceptance	Single limb support (40%) Supporting body weight	Double limb support (10%)

Phase Subdivisions	Functional Objectives	Active Muscle Groups	Primary Muscle(s)
Initial contact (heel strike)	**Lower forefoot to substrate** (controlled plantarflexion until forefoot contacts substrate)	Ankle dorsiflexors (eccentric contraction)	Tibialis anterior
	Continue deceleration (slow forward swing)	Hip extensors	Gluteus maximus
	Maintain longitudinal arch of foot	Intrinsic muscles of foot Long tendons of foot	Flexor digitorum brevis Tibialis anterior
Loading response (flat foot)	**Weight bearing**	Knee extensors	Quadriceps
	Decelerate mass (slow dorsiflexion)	Ankle plantar flexors	Triceps surae (soleus & gastrocnemius)
	Stabilize pelvis	Hip abductors	Gluteus medius & minimus, tensor of fascia lata
	Maintain longitudinal arch of foot	Intrinsic muscles of foot Long tendons of foot	Flexor digitorum brevis Tibialis posterior, long flexors of digits
Midstance	**Stabilize knee**	Knee extensors	Quadriceps
	Control dorsiflexion (sustain momentum)	Ankle plantarflexors (concentric contraction)	Triceps surae (soleus contraction)
	Stabilize pelvis	Hip abductors	Gluteus medius & minimus, tensor of fascia lata
	Maintain longitudinal arch of foot	Intrinsic muscles of foot Long tendons of foot	Flexor digitorum brevis Tibialis posterior, long flexors of digits
Terminal stance (heel off)	**Propel & accelerate mass**	Ankle plantarflexors (concentric contraction)	Triceps surae (gastrocnemius & soleus)
	Stabilize pelvis	Hip abductors	Gluteus medius & minimus, tensor fascia latae
	Maintain arches of foot, fix forefoot	Intrinsic muscles of foot Long tendons of foot	Adductor hallucis Tibialis posterior, fibularis longus

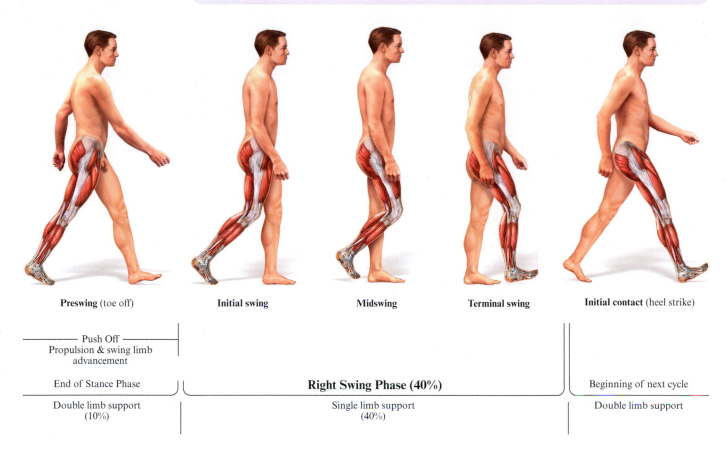

Preswing (toe off)	**Initial swing**	**Midswing**	**Terminal swing**	**Initial contact** (heel strike)

Push Off
Propulsion & swing limb advancement

End of Stance Phase **Right Swing Phase (40%)** Beginning of next cycle

Double limb support (10%)	Single limb support (40%)	Double limb support

Phase Subdivisions	Functional Objectives	Active Muscle Groups	Primary Muscle(s)
Preswing (toe off)	**Propel & accelerate mass**	Long flexors of digits	Flexor hallucis longus, flexor digitorum longus
	Maintain arches of foot, fix forefoot	Intrinsic muscles of foot	Adductor hallucis
		Long tendons of foot	Tibialis posterior, fibularis longus
	Accelerate thigh; swing	Flexors of hip (eccentric contraction)	Iliopsoas, rectus femoris
Initial swing	**Accelerate thigh**	Flexors of hip (concentric contraction)	Illiopsoas, rectus femoris, sartorius
	Clear foot	Ankle dorsiflexors	Tibialis anterior
Midswing	**Maintain flexed knee**	Knee flexors (concentric contraction)	Hamstrings, sartorius
	Clear foot	Ankle dorsiflexors	Tibialis anterior
Terminal swing (heel strike)	**Decelerate thigh & leg**	Hip extensors (eccentric contraction)	Gluteus maximus, hamstrings
	Extend knee for heel strike (control stride length), prepare for contact with substrate	Knee extensors (concentric contraction)	Quadriceps
	Position foot	Ankle dorsiflexors	Tibialis anterior
	Absorb shock at impact	Knee extensors (eccentric contraction)	Quadriceps

During normal walking on a level surface in a straight line at a constant speed, a single gait cycle begins with heel strike (initial contact) of one foot and ends with the heel strike (initial contact) of the same foot. Each cycle is divided into stance and swing phases and each phase is further subdivided into component parts.

The **stance phase** for each limb is that interval of the cycle that begins with heel strike (initial contact) and ends with toe off. During stance phase, the foot is stationary relative to the substrate and is weight bearing.

Swing phase occurs between toe off and heel strike (initial contact). The limb in swing phase is non-weight bearing and moves in the desired direction of travel.

Tables under each set of figures indicate the functional objectives of the major muscle groups and primary muscles that are active during each subdivision of stance and swing phases.

PLATE 5.15   ARTERIES OF LOWER LIMB

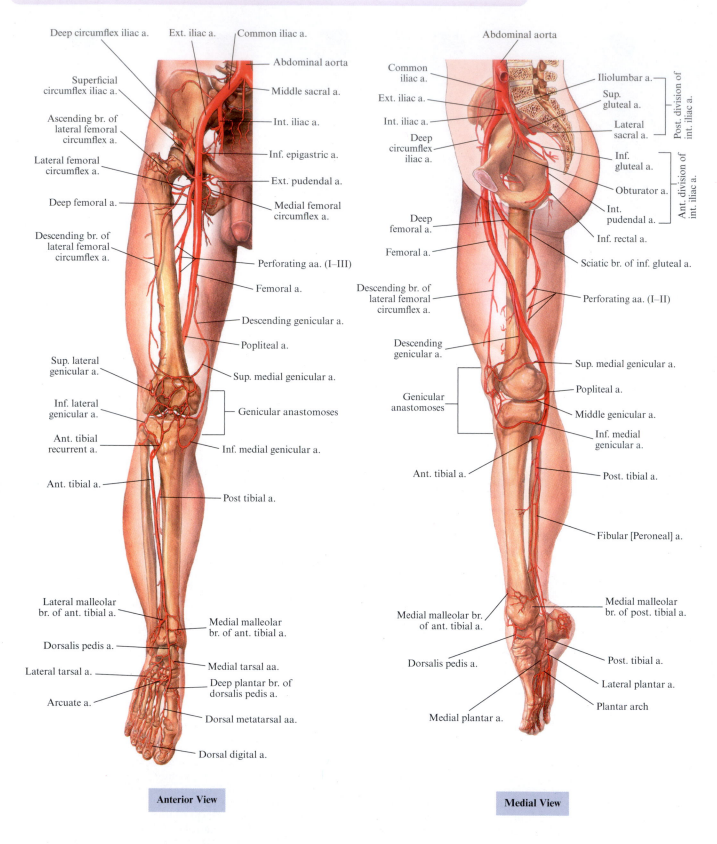

Deep circumflex iliac a.

Ext. iliac a.

Common iliac a.

Abdominal aorta

Superficial circumflex iliac a.

Middle sacral a.

Ascending br. of lateral femoral circumflex a.

Int. iliac a.

Lateral femoral circumflex a.

Inf. epigastric a.

Ext. pudendal a.

Deep femoral a.

Medial femoral circumflex a.

Descending br. of lateral femoral circumflex a.

Perforating aa. (I–III)

Femoral a.

Descending genicular a.

Popliteal a.

Sup. lateral genicular a.

Sup. medial genicular a.

Inf. lateral genicular a.

Genicular anastomoses

Ant. tibial recurrent a.

Inf. medial genicular a.

Ant. tibial a.

Post tibial a.

Lateral malleolar br. of ant. tibial a.

Medial malleolar br. of ant. tibial a.

Dorsalis pedis a.

Lateral tarsal a.

Medial tarsal aa.

Deep plantar br. of dorsalis pedis a.

Arcuate a.

Dorsal metatarsal aa.

Dorsal digital a.

Anterior View

Abdominal aorta

Common iliac a.

Iliolumbar a.

Sup. gluteal a.

Post. division of int. iliac a.

Ext. iliac a.

Int. iliac a.

Lateral sacral a.

Deep circumflex iliac a.

Inf. gluteal a.

Obturator a.

Int. pudendal a.

Ant. division of int. iliac a.

Deep femoral a.

Inf. rectal a.

Femoral a.

Sciatic br. of inf. gluteal a.

Descending br. of lateral femoral circumflex a.

Perforating aa. (I–II)

Descending genicular a.

Sup. medial genicular a.

Genicular anastomoses

Popliteal a.

Middle genicular a.

Inf. medial genicular a.

Ant. tibial a.

Post. tibial a.

Fibular [Peroneal] a.

Medial malleolar br. of post. tibial a.

Medial malleolar br. of ant. tibial a.

Dorsalis pedis a.

Post. tibial a.

Lateral plantar a.

Plantar arch

Medial plantar a.

Medial View

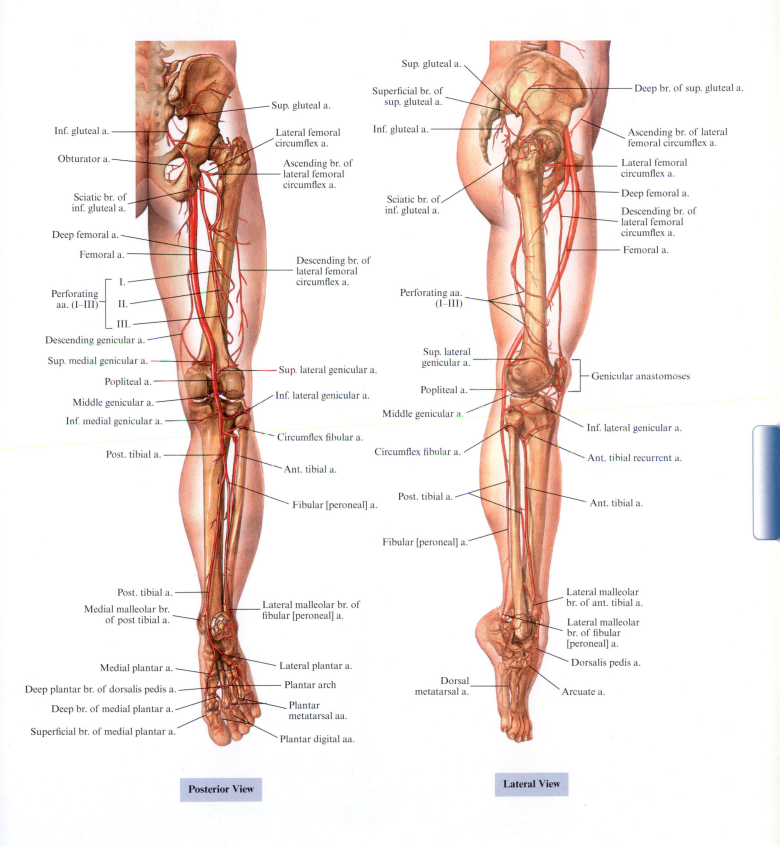

Sup. gluteal a.

Inf. gluteal a.

Obturator a.

Sciatic br. of
inf. gluteal a.

Deep femoral a.

Femoral a.

Perforating
aa. (I–III)

I.

II.

III.

Descending genicular a.

Sup. medial genicular a.

Popliteal a.

Middle genicular a.

Inf. medial genicular a.

Post. tibial a.

Sup. gluteal a.

Lateral femoral
circumflex a.

Ascending br. of
lateral femoral
circumflex a.

Descending br. of
lateral femoral
circumflex a.

Sup. lateral genicular a.

Inf. lateral genicular a.

Circumflex fibular a.

Ant. tibial a.

Fibular [peroneal] a.

Post. tibial a.

Medial malleolar br.
of post tibial a.

Medial plantar a.

Deep plantar br. of dorsalis pedis a.

Deep br. of medial plantar a.

Superficial br. of medial plantar a.

Lateral malleolar br. of
fibular [peroneal] a.

Lateral plantar a.

Plantar arch

Plantar
metatarsal aa.

Plantar digital aa.

Posterior View

Sup. gluteal a.

Superficial br. of
sup. gluteal a.

Inf. gluteal a.

Sciatic br. of
inf. gluteal a.

Deep br. of sup. gluteal a.

Ascending br. of lateral
femoral circumflex a.

Lateral femoral
circumflex a.

Deep femoral a.

Descending br. of
lateral femoral
circumflex a.

Femoral a.

Perforating aa.
(I–III)

Sup. lateral
genicular a.

Popliteal a.

Middle genicular a.

Circumflex fibular a.

Post. tibial a.

Fibular [peroneal] a.

Dorsal
metatarsal a.

Genicular anastomoses

Inf. lateral genicular a.

Ant. tibial recurrent a.

Ant. tibial a.

Lateral malleolar
br. of ant. tibial a.

Lateral malleolar
br. of fibular
[peroneal] a.

Dorsalis pedis a.

Arcuate a.

Lateral View

PLATE 5.17   SUPERFICIAL VEINS OF LOWER LIMB

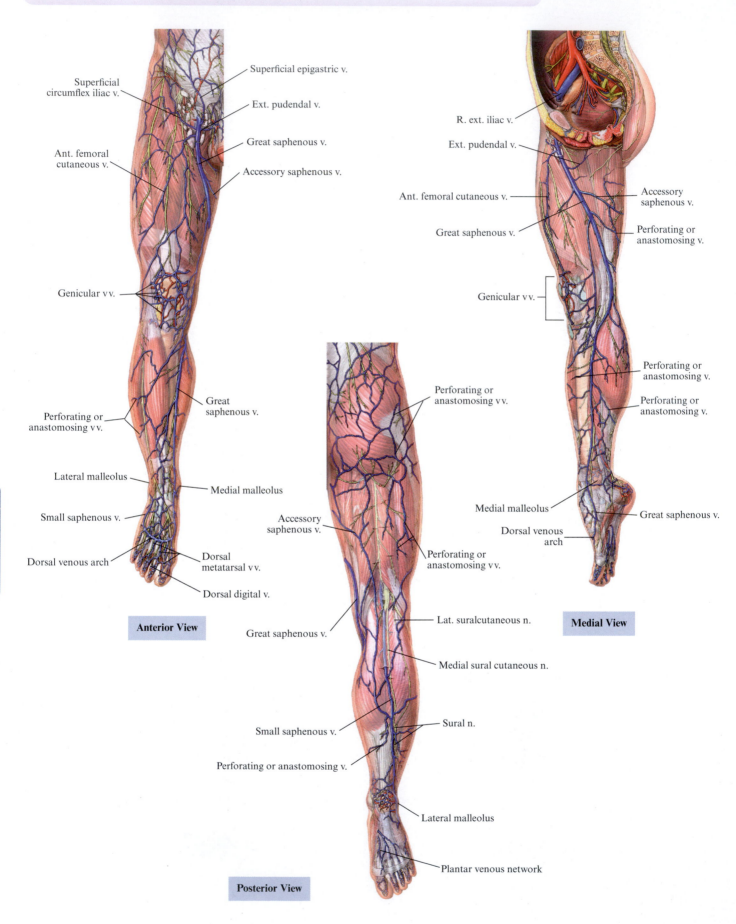

Superficial circumflex iliac v.

Superficial epigastric v.

Ext. pudendal v.

Great saphenous v.

Ant. femoral cutaneous v.

Accessory saphenous v.

Genicular vv.

Perforating or anastomosing vv.

Great saphenous v.

Lateral malleolus

Medial malleolus

Small saphenous v.

Dorsal venous arch

Dorsal metatarsal vv.

Dorsal digital v.

Anterior View

R. ext. iliac v.

Ext. pudendal v.

Ant. femoral cutaneous v.

Accessory saphenous v.

Great saphenous v.

Perforating or anastomosing v.

Genicular vv.

Perforating or anastomosing v.

Perforating or anastomosing v.

Medial malleolus

Great saphenous v.

Dorsal venous arch

Medial View

Perforating or anastomosing vv.

Accessory saphenous v.

Perforating or anastomosing vv.

Great saphenous v.

Lat. suralcutaneous n.

Medial sural cutaneous n.

Small saphenous v.

Sural n.

Perforating or anastomosing v.

Lateral malleolus

Plantar venous network

Posterior View

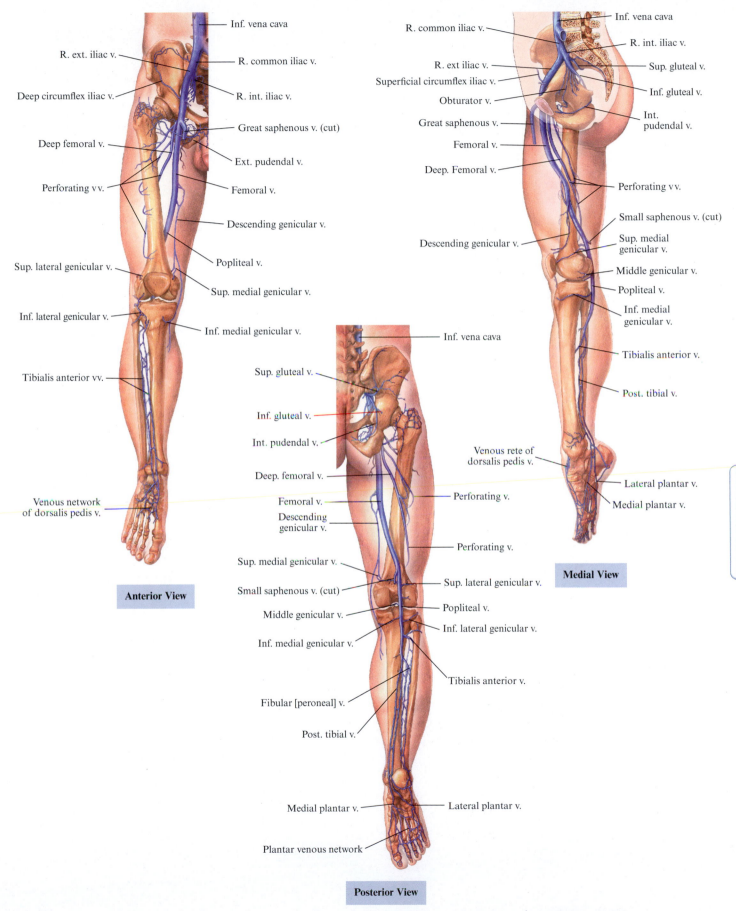

Inf. vena cava

R. ext. iliac v.

Deep circumflex iliac v.

Deep femoral v.

Perforating v v.

Sup. lateral genicular v.

Inf. lateral genicular v.

Tibialis anterior vv.

Venous network of dorsalis pedis v.

R. common iliac v.

R. int. iliac v.

Great saphenous v. (cut)

Ext. pudendal v.

Femoral v.

Descending genicular v.

Popliteal v.

Sup. medial genicular v.

Inf. medial genicular v.

Anterior View

R. common iliac v.

R. ext iliac v.

Superficial circumflex iliac v.

Obturator v.

Great saphenous v.

Femoral v.

Deep. Femoral v.

Descending genicular v.

Inf. vena cava

R. int. iliac v.

Sup. gluteal v.

Inf. gluteal v.

Int. pudendal v.

Perforating v v.

Small saphenous v. (cut)

Sup. medial genicular v.

Middle genicular v.

Popliteal v.

Inf. medial genicular v.

Tibialis anterior v.

Post. tibial v.

Venous rete of dorsalis pedis v.

Lateral plantar v.

Medial plantar v.

Medial View

Inf. vena cava

Sup. gluteal v.

Inf. gluteal v.

Int. pudendal v.

Deep. femoral v.

Femoral v.

Descending genicular v.

Sup. medial genicular v.

Small saphenous v. (cut)

Middle genicular v.

Inf. medial genicular v.

Fibular [peroneal] v.

Post. tibial v.

Perforating v.

Perforating v.

Sup. lateral genicular v.

Popliteal v.

Inf. lateral genicular v.

Tibialis anterior v.

Medial plantar v.

Lateral plantar v.

Plantar venous network

Posterior View

PLATE 5.19   DERMATOMES & CUTANEOUS NERVES OF LOWER LIMB

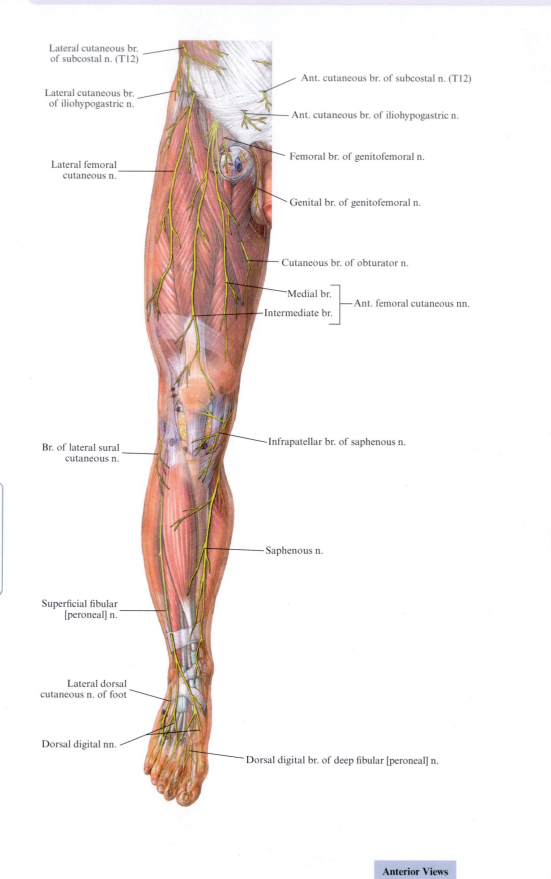

Lateral cutaneous br. of subcostal n. (T12)

Lateral cutaneous br. of iliohypogastric n.

Lateral femoral cutaneous n.

Br. of lateral sural cutaneous n.

Superficial fibular [peroneal] n.

Lateral dorsal cutaneous n. of foot

Dorsal digital nn.

Ant. cutaneous br. of subcostal n. (T12)

Ant. cutaneous br. of iliohypogastric n.

Femoral br. of genitofemoral n.

Genital br. of genitofemoral n.

Cutaneous br. of obturator n.

Medial br.
Intermediate br. } Ant. femoral cutaneous nn.

Infrapatellar br. of saphenous n.

Saphenous n.

Dorsal digital br. of deep fibular [peroneal] n.

T10
T11
T12
L1
S2
L2
S3
L3
L4
L5
S1

Anterior Views

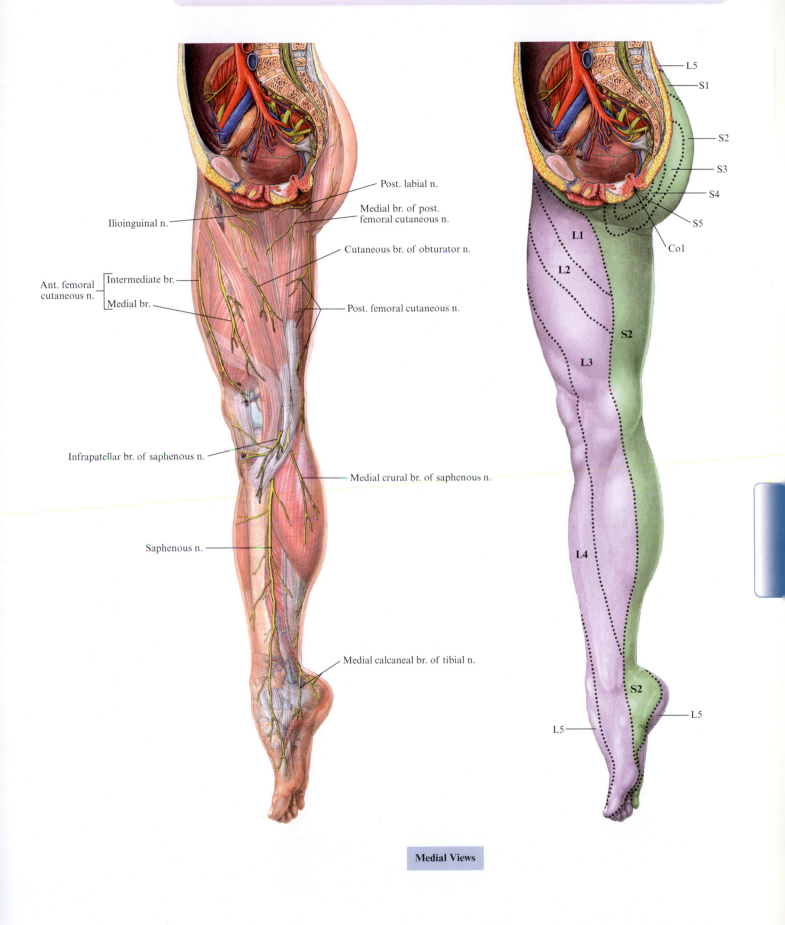

Post. labial n.

Medial br. of post.
femoral cutaneous n.

Ilioinguinal n.

Cutaneous br. of obturator n.

Ant. femoral
cutaneous n.
Intermediate br.

Medial br.

Post. femoral cutaneous n.

Infrapatellar br. of saphenous n.

Medial crural br. of saphenous n.

Saphenous n.

Medial calcaneal br. of tibial n.

L5
S1
S2
S3
S4
S5
Co1

L1
L2
S2
L3
L4
S2
L5
L5
L5

Medial Views

PLATE 5.21 DERMATOMES & CUTANEOUS NERVES OF LOWER LIMB

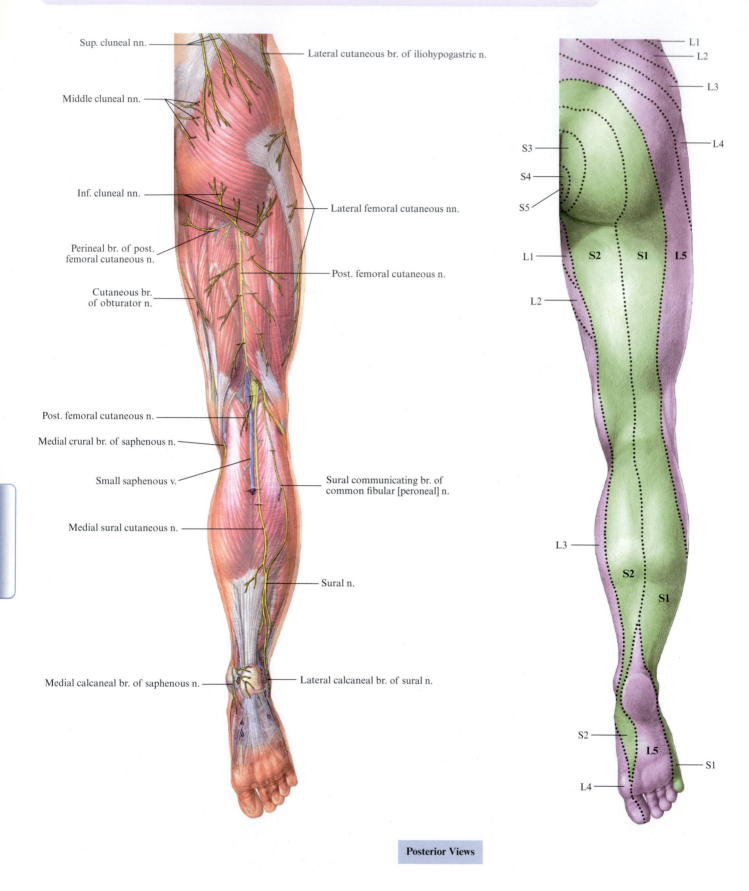

Sup. cluneal nn.

Lateral cutaneous br. of iliohypogastric n.

Middle cluneal nn.

Inf. cluneal nn.

Lateral femoral cutaneous nn.

Perineal br. of post.
femoral cutaneous n.

Cutaneous br.
of obturator n.

Post. femoral cutaneous n.

Post. femoral cutaneous n.

Medial crural br. of saphenous n.

Small saphenous v.

Sural communicating br. of
common fibular [peroneal] n.

Medial sural cutaneous n.

Sural n.

Medial calcaneal br. of saphenous n.

Lateral calcaneal br. of sural n.

L1
L2
L3
L4

S3
S4
S5

L1
L2
L3

S2 S1 L5

S2
S1

S2
L5
L4
S1

Posterior Views

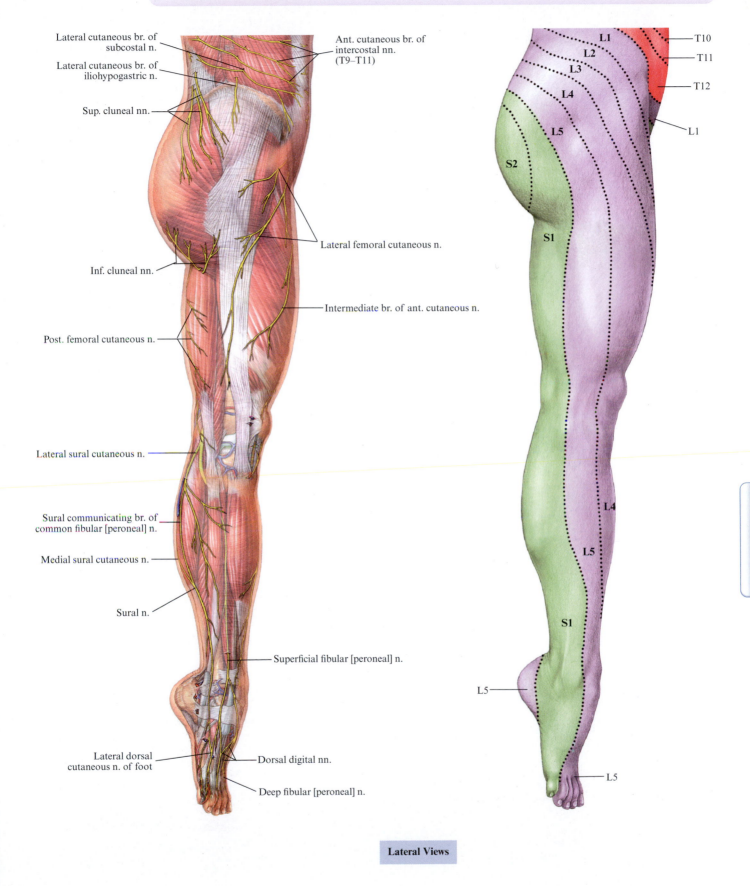

Lateral cutaneous br. of subcostal n.

Lateral cutaneous br. of iliohypogastric n.

Sup. cluneal nn.

Inf. cluneal nn.

Post. femoral cutaneous n.

Lateral sural cutaneous n.

Sural communicating br. of common fibular [peroneal] n.

Medial sural cutaneous n.

Sural n.

Lateral dorsal cutaneous n. of foot

Ant. cutaneous br. of intercostal nn. (T9–T11)

Lateral femoral cutaneous n.

Intermediate br. of ant. cutaneous n.

Superficial fibular [peroneal] n.

Dorsal digital nn.

Deep fibular [peroneal] n.

T10
T11
T12
L1
L2
L3
L4
L5
S2
S1
L5
S1
L5
L5

Lateral Views

PLATE 5.23   SEGMENTAL INNERVATION & JOINT ACTIONS

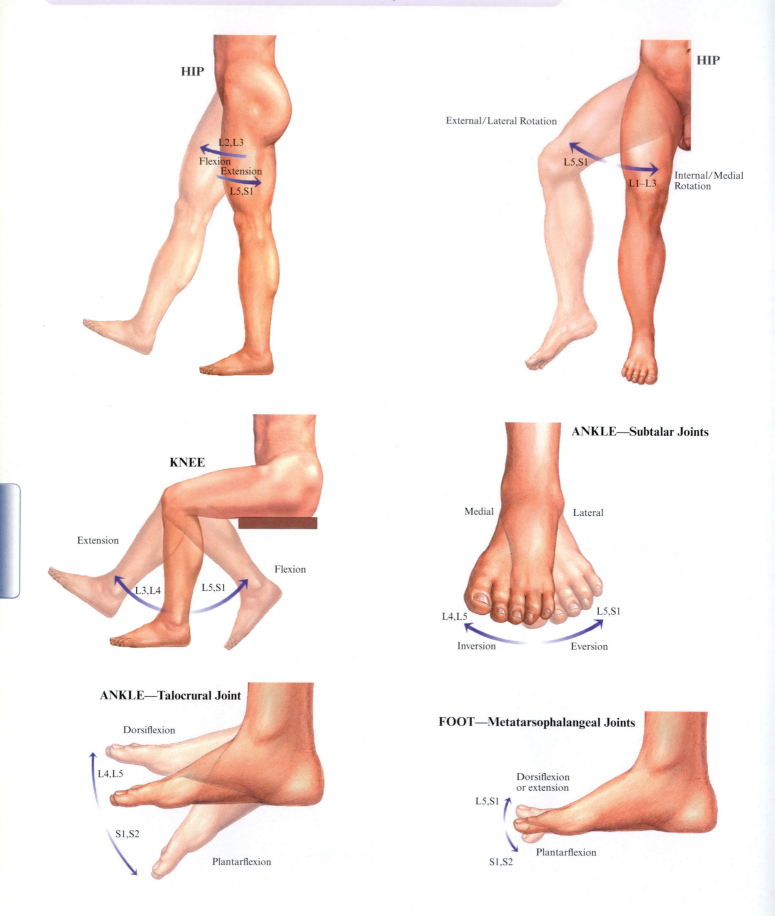

HIP

L2,L3
Flexion
Extension
L5,S1

HIP

External/Lateral Rotation

L5,S1
L1–L3
Internal/Medial Rotation

KNEE

Extension
Flexion
L3,L4   L5,S1

ANKLE—Subtalar Joints

Medial   Lateral

L4,L5   L5,S1
Inversion   Eversion

ANKLE—Talocrural Joint

Dorsiflexion
L4,L5
S1,S2
Plantarflexion

FOOT—Metatarsophalangeal Joints

Dorsiflexion or extension
L5,S1
S1,S2   Plantarflexion

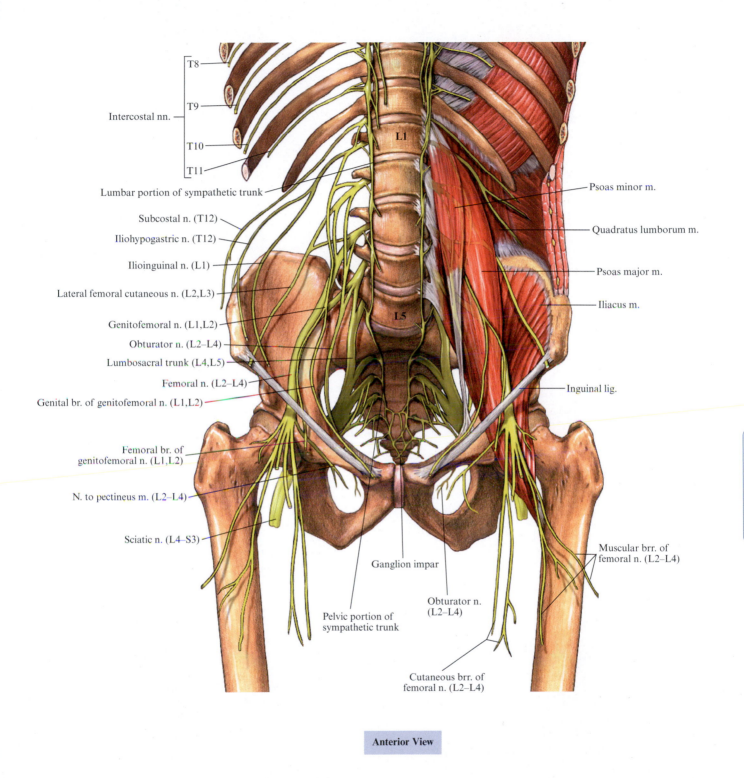

Intercostal nn. {
T8
T9
T10
T11
}

Lumbar portion of sympathetic trunk

Subcostal n. (T12)

Iliohypogastric n. (T12)

Ilioinguinal n. (L1)

Lateral femoral cutaneous n. (L2,L3)

Genitofemoral n. (L1,L2)

Obturator n. (L2–L4)

Lumbosacral trunk (L4,L5)

Femoral n. (L2–L4)

Genital br. of genitofemoral n. (L1,L2)

Femoral br. of genitofemoral n. (L1,L2)

N. to pectineus m. (L2–L4)

Sciatic n. (L4–S3)

Pelvic portion of sympathetic trunk

Ganglion impar

Psoas minor m.

Quadratus lumborum m.

Psoas major m.

Iliacus m.

Inguinal lig.

Muscular brr. of femoral n. (L2–L4)

Obturator n. (L2–L4)

Cutaneous brr. of femoral n. (L2–L4)

L1

L5

Anterior View

PLATE 5.25   DEEP NERVES OF LOWER LIMB

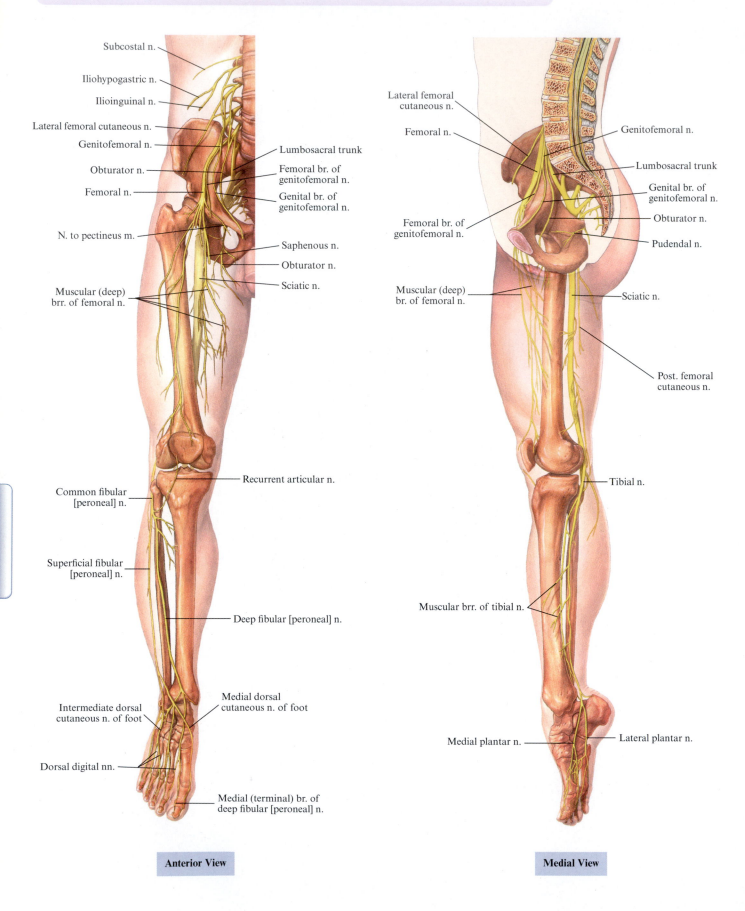

Subcostal n.

Iliohypogastric n.

Ilioinguinal n.

Lateral femoral cutaneous n.

Genitofemoral n.

Obturator n.

Femoral n.

N. to pectineus m.

Muscular (deep) brr. of femoral n.

Lumbosacral trunk

Femoral br. of genitofemoral n.

Genital br. of genitofemoral n.

Saphenous n.

Obturator n.

Sciatic n.

Common fibular [peroneal] n.

Recurrent articular n.

Superficial fibular [peroneal] n.

Deep fibular [peroneal] n.

Intermediate dorsal cutaneous n. of foot

Medial dorsal cutaneous n. of foot

Dorsal digital nn.

Medial (terminal) br. of deep fibular [peroneal] n.

Anterior View

Lateral femoral cutaneous n.

Femoral n.

Genitofemoral n.

Lumbosacral trunk

Genital br. of genitofemoral n.

Femoral br. of genitofemoral n.

Obturator n.

Pudendal n.

Muscular (deep) br. of femoral n.

Sciatic n.

Post. femoral cutaneous n.

Tibial n.

Muscular brr. of tibial n.

Medial plantar n.

Lateral plantar n.

Medial View

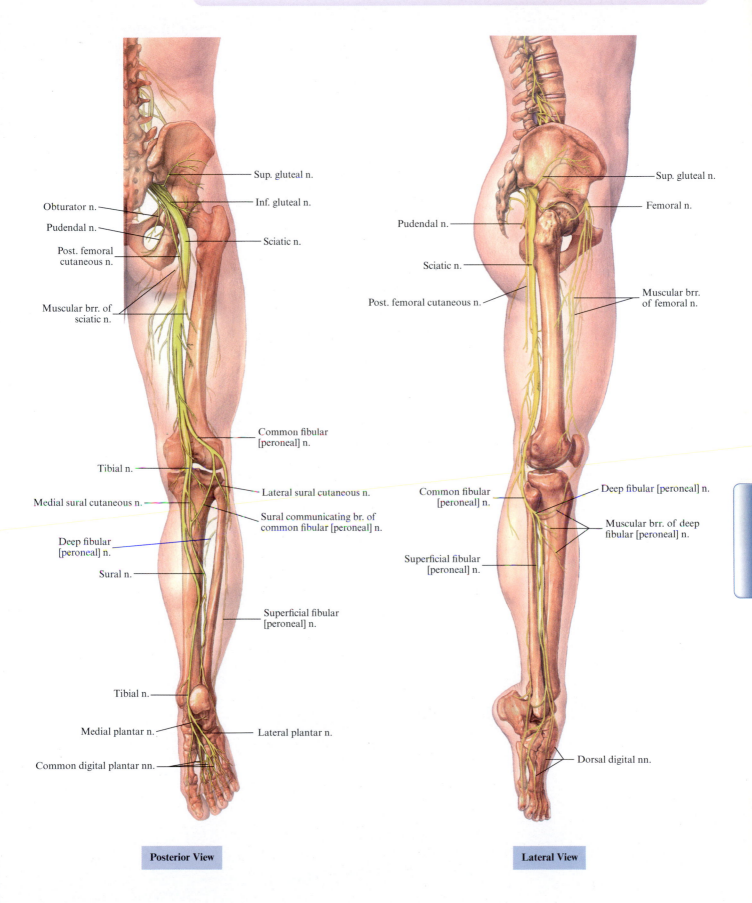

Sup. gluteal n.

Obturator n.

Inf. gluteal n.

Pudendal n.

Sciatic n.

Post. femoral
cutaneous n.

Muscular brr. of
sciatic n.

Common fibular
[peroneal] n.

Tibial n.

Lateral sural cutaneous n.

Medial sural cutaneous n.

Sural communicating br. of
common fibular [peroneal] n.

Deep fibular
[peroneal] n.

Sural n.

Superficial fibular
[peroneal] n.

Tibial n.

Medial plantar n.

Lateral plantar n.

Common digital plantar nn.

Sup. gluteal n.

Femoral n.

Pudendal n.

Sciatic n.

Muscular brr.
of femoral n.

Post. femoral cutaneous n.

Common fibular
[peroneal] n.

Deep fibular [peroneal] n.

Muscular brr. of deep
fibular [peroneal] n.

Superficial fibular
[peroneal] n.

Dorsal digital nn.

Posterior View

Lateral View

PLATE 5.27   LUMBAR PLEXUS

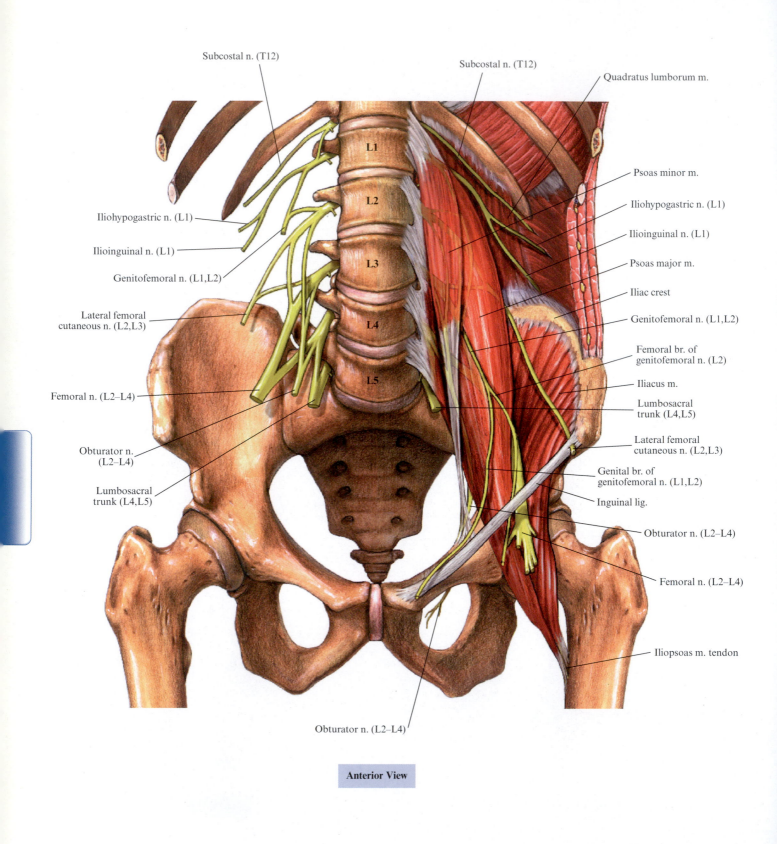

Subcostal n. (T12)

Subcostal n. (T12)

Quadratus lumborum m.

Iliohypogastric n. (L1)

Ilioinguinal n. (L1)

Genitofemoral n. (L1,L2)

Lateral femoral
cutaneous n. (L2,L3)

Femoral n. (L2–L4)

Obturator n.
(L2–L4)

Lumbosacral
trunk (L4,L5)

L1

L2

L3

L4

L5

Psoas minor m.

Iliohypogastric n. (L1)

Ilioinguinal n. (L1)

Psoas major m.

Iliac crest

Genitofemoral n. (L1,L2)

Femoral br. of
genitofemoral n. (L2)

Iliacus m.

Lumbosacral
trunk (L4,L5)

Lateral femoral
cutaneous n. (L2,L3)

Genital br. of
genitofemoral n. (L1,L2)

Inguinal lig.

Obturator n. (L2–L4)

Femoral n. (L2–L4)

Iliopsoas m. tendon

Obturator n. (L2–L4)

Anterior View

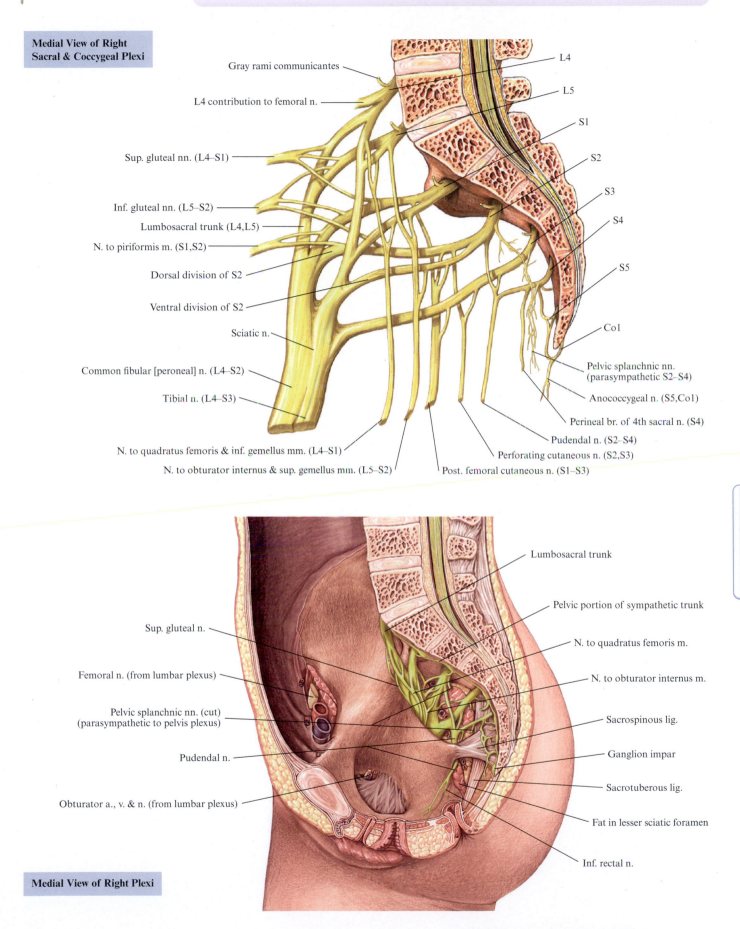

Medial View of Right Sacral & Coccygeal Plexi

Gray rami communicantes

L4 contribution to femoral n.

Sup. gluteal nn. (L4–S1)

Inf. gluteal nn. (L5–S2)

Lumbosacral trunk (L4,L5)

N. to piriformis m. (S1,S2)

Dorsal division of S2

Ventral division of S2

Sciatic n.

Common fibular [peroneal] n. (L4–S2)

Tibial n. (L4–S3)

N. to quadratus femoris & inf. gemellus mm. (L4–S1)

N. to obturator internus & sup. gemellus mm. (L5–S2)

L4

L5

S1

S2

S3

S4

S5

Co1

Pelvic splanchnic nn. (parasympathetic S2–S4)

Anococcygeal n. (S5,Co1)

Perineal br. of 4th sacral n. (S4)

Pudendal n. (S2–S4)

Perforating cutaneous n. (S2,S3)

Post. femoral cutaneous n. (S1–S3)

Medial View of Right Plexi

Sup. gluteal n.

Femoral n. (from lumbar plexus)

Pelvic splanchnic nn. (cut) (parasympathetic to pelvis plexus)

Pudendal n.

Obturator a., v. & n. (from lumbar plexus)

Lumbosacral trunk

Pelvic portion of sympathetic trunk

N. to quadratus femoris m.

N. to obturator internus m.

Sacrospinous lig.

Ganglion impar

Sacrotuberous lig.

Fat in lesser sciatic foramen

Inf. rectal n.

PLATE 5.29   SUPERFICIAL LYMPHATICS

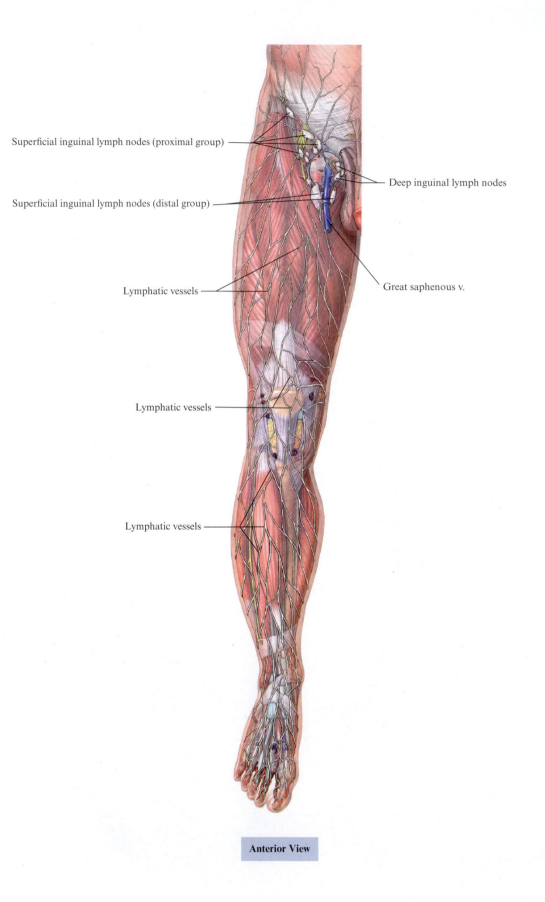

Superficial inguinal lymph nodes (proximal group)

Superficial inguinal lymph nodes (distal group)

Deep inguinal lymph nodes

Lymphatic vessels

Great saphenous v.

Lymphatic vessels

Lymphatic vessels

Anterior View

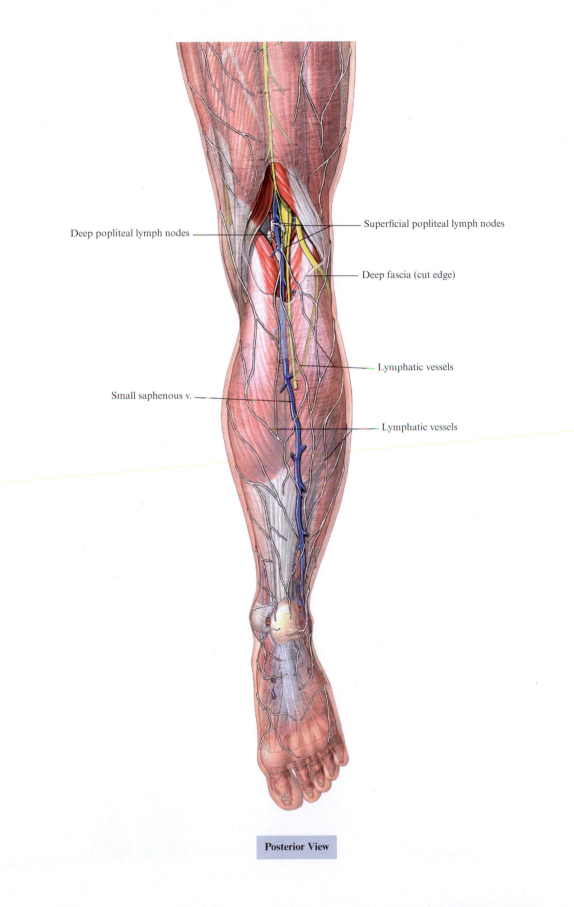

Deep popliteal lymph nodes

Superficial popliteal lymph nodes

Deep fascia (cut edge)

Lymphatic vessels

Small saphenous v.

Lymphatic vessels

Posterior View

PLATE 5.31 ANTERIOR THIGH

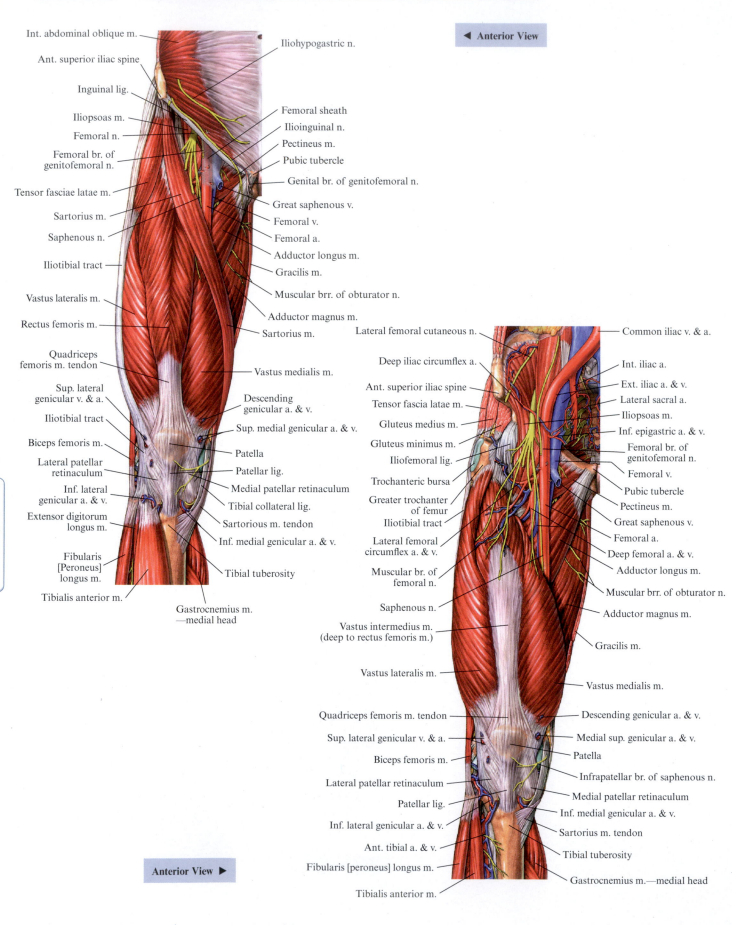

◄ **Anterior View**

Int. abdominal oblique m.
Ant. superior iliac spine
Inguinal lig.
Iliopsoas m.
Femoral n.
Femoral br. of genitofemoral n.
Tensor fasciae latae m.
Sartorius m.
Saphenous n.
Iliotibial tract
Vastus lateralis m.
Rectus femoris m.
Quadriceps femoris m. tendon
Sup. lateral genicular v. & a.
Iliotibial tract
Biceps femoris m.
Lateral patellar retinaculum
Inf. lateral genicular a. & v.
Extensor digitorum longus m.
Fibularis [Peroneus] longus m.
Tibialis anterior m.

Iliohypogastric n.
Femoral sheath
Ilioinguinal n.
Pectineus m.
Pubic tubercle
Genital br. of genitofemoral n.
Great saphenous v.
Femoral v.
Femoral a.
Adductor longus m.
Gracilis m.
Muscular brr. of obturator n.
Adductor magnus m.
Sartorius m.
Vastus medialis m.
Descending genicular a. & v.
Sup. medial genicular a. & v.
Patella
Patellar lig.
Medial patellar retinaculum
Tibial collateral lig.
Sartorious m. tendon
Inf. medial genicular a. & v.
Tibial tuberosity

Gastrocnemius m. —medial head

Lateral femoral cutaneous n.
Deep iliac circumflex a.
Ant. superior iliac spine
Tensor fascia latae m.
Gluteus medius m.
Gluteus minimus m.
Iliofemoral lig.
Trochanteric bursa
Greater trochanter of femur
Iliotibial tract
Lateral femoral circumflex a. & v.
Muscular br. of femoral n.
Saphenous n.
Vastus intermedius m. (deep to rectus femoris m.)
Vastus lateralis m.
Quadriceps femoris m. tendon
Sup. lateral genicular v. & a.
Biceps femoris m.
Lateral patellar retinaculum
Patellar lig.
Inf. lateral genicular a. & v.
Ant. tibial a. & v.
Fibularis [peroneus] longus m.
Tibialis anterior m.

Common iliac v. & a.
Int. iliac a.
Ext. iliac a. & v.
Lateral sacral a.
Iliopsoas m.
Inf. epigastric a. & v.
Femoral br. of genitofemoral n.
Femoral v.
Pubic tubercle
Pectineus m.
Great saphenous v.
Femoral a.
Deep femoral a. & v.
Adductor longus m.
Muscular brr. of obturator n.
Adductor magnus m.
Gracilis m.
Vastus medialis m.
Descending genicular a. & v.
Medial sup. genicular a. & v.
Patella
Infrapatellar br. of saphenous n.
Medial patellar retinaculum
Inf. medial genicular a. & v.
Sartorius m. tendon
Tibial tuberosity
Gastrocnemius m.—medial head

Anterior View ►

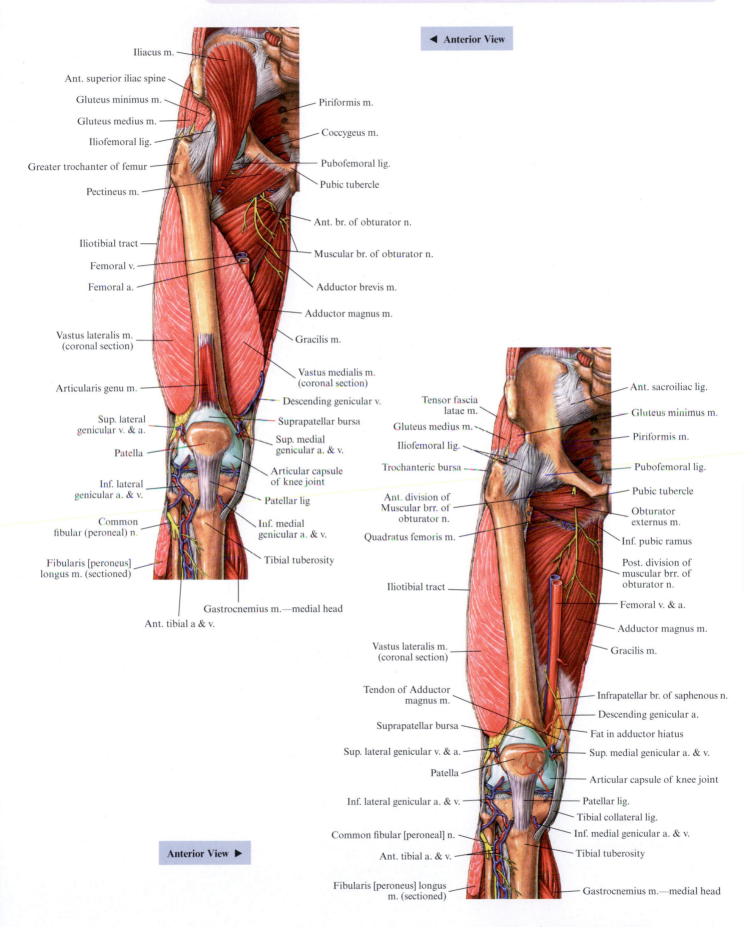

◄ **Anterior View**

Iliacus m.

Ant. superior iliac spine

Gluteus minimus m.

Gluteus medius m.

Iliofemoral lig.

Greater trochanter of femur

Pectineus m.

Iliotibial tract

Femoral v.

Femoral a.

Vastus lateralis m. (coronal section)

Articularis genu m.

Sup. lateral genicular v. & a.

Patella

Inf. lateral genicular a. & v.

Common fibular (peroneal) n.

Fibularis [peroneus] longus m. (sectioned)

Ant. tibial a & v.

Piriformis m.

Coccygeus m.

Pubofemoral lig.

Pubic tubercle

Ant. br. of obturator n.

Muscular br. of obturator n.

Adductor brevis m.

Adductor magnus m.

Gracilis m.

Vastus medialis m. (coronal section)

Descending genicular v.

Suprapatellar bursa

Sup. medial genicular a. & v.

Articular capsule of knee joint

Patellar lig

Inf. medial genicular a. & v.

Tibial tuberosity

Gastrocnemius m.—medial head

Anterior View ▶

Tensor fascia latae m.

Gluteus medius m.

Iliofemoral lig.

Trochanteric bursa

Ant. division of Muscular brr. of obturator n.

Quadratus femoris m.

Iliotibial tract

Vastus lateralis m. (coronal section)

Tendon of Adductor magnus m.

Suprapatellar bursa

Sup. lateral genicular v. & a.

Patella

Inf. lateral genicular a. & v.

Common fibular [peroneal] n.

Ant. tibial a. & v.

Fibularis [peroneus] longus m. (sectioned)

Ant. sacroiliac lig.

Gluteus minimus m.

Piriformis m.

Pubofemoral lig.

Pubic tubercle

Obturator externus m.

Inf. pubic ramus

Post. division of muscular brr. of obturator n.

Femoral v. & a.

Adductor magnus m.

Gracilis m.

Infrapatellar br. of saphenous n.

Descending genicular a.

Fat in adductor hiatus

Sup. medial genicular a. & v.

Articular capsule of knee joint

Patellar lig.

Tibial collateral lig.

Inf. medial genicular a. & v.

Tibial tuberosity

Gastrocnemius m.—medial head

PLATE 5.33   FEMORAL TRIANGLE

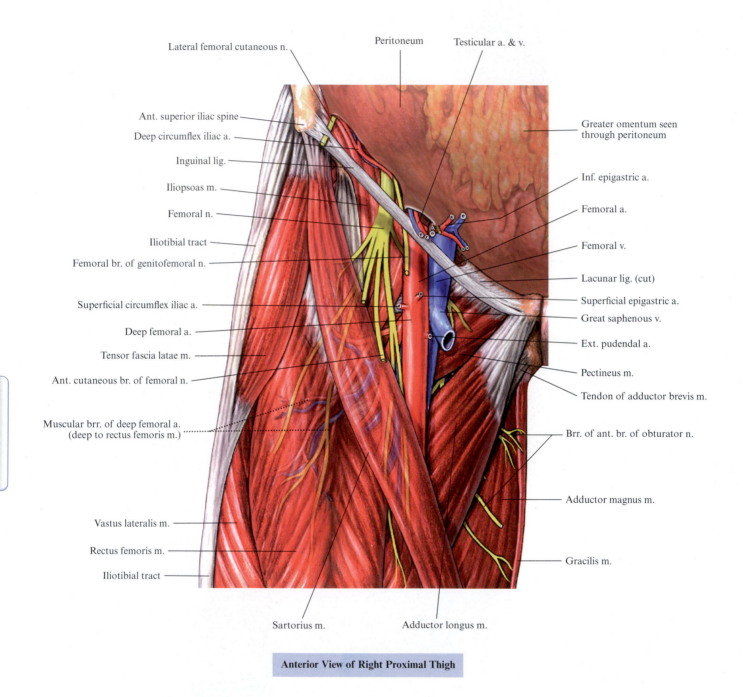

Lateral femoral cutaneous n.

Peritoneum

Testicular a. & v.

Ant. superior iliac spine

Deep circumflex iliac a.

Inguinal lig.

Iliopsoas m.

Femoral n.

Iliotibial tract

Femoral br. of genitofemoral n.

Superficial circumflex iliac a.

Deep femoral a.

Tensor fascia latae m.

Ant. cutaneous br. of femoral n.

Muscular brr. of deep femoral a.
(deep to rectus femoris m.)

Vastus lateralis m.

Rectus femoris m.

Iliotibial tract

Greater omentum seen
through peritoneum

Inf. epigastric a.

Femoral a.

Femoral v.

Lacunar lig. (cut)

Superficial epigastric a.

Great saphenous v.

Ext. pudendal a.

Pectineus m.

Tendon of adductor brevis m.

Brr. of ant. br. of obturator n.

Adductor magnus m.

Gracilis m.

Sartorius m.

Adductor longus m.

Anterior View of Right Proximal Thigh

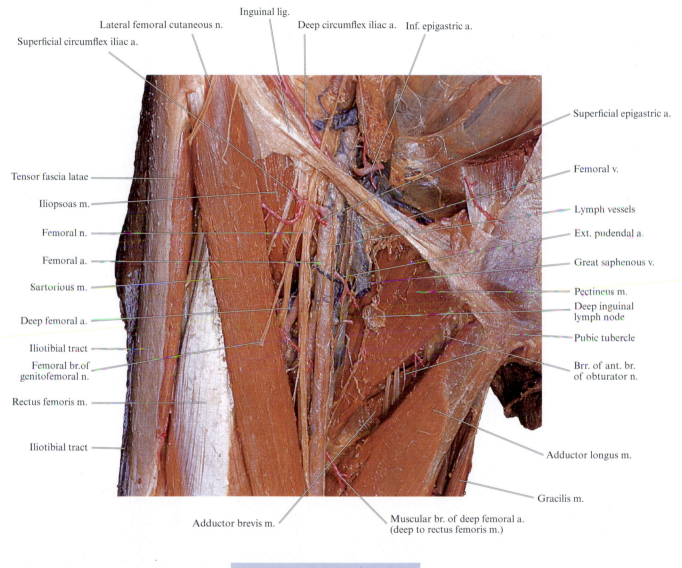

Superficial circumflex iliac a.

Lateral femoral cutaneous n.

Inguinal lig.

Deep circumflex iliac a.

Inf. epigastric a.

Superficial epigastric a.

Tensor fascia latae

Femoral v.

Iliopsoas m.

Lymph vessels

Femoral n.

Ext. pudendal a.

Femoral a.

Great saphenous v.

Sartorious m.

Pectineus m.

Deep femoral a.

Deep inguinal lymph node

Iliotibial tract

Pubic tubercle

Femoral br. of genitofemoral n.

Brr. of ant. br. of obturator n.

Rectus femoris m.

Iliotibial tract

Adductor longus m.

Gracilis m.

Adductor brevis m.

Muscular br. of deep femoral a. (deep to rectus femoris m.)

Anterior View of Right Proximal Thigh

PLATE 5.35   POSTERIOR THIGH

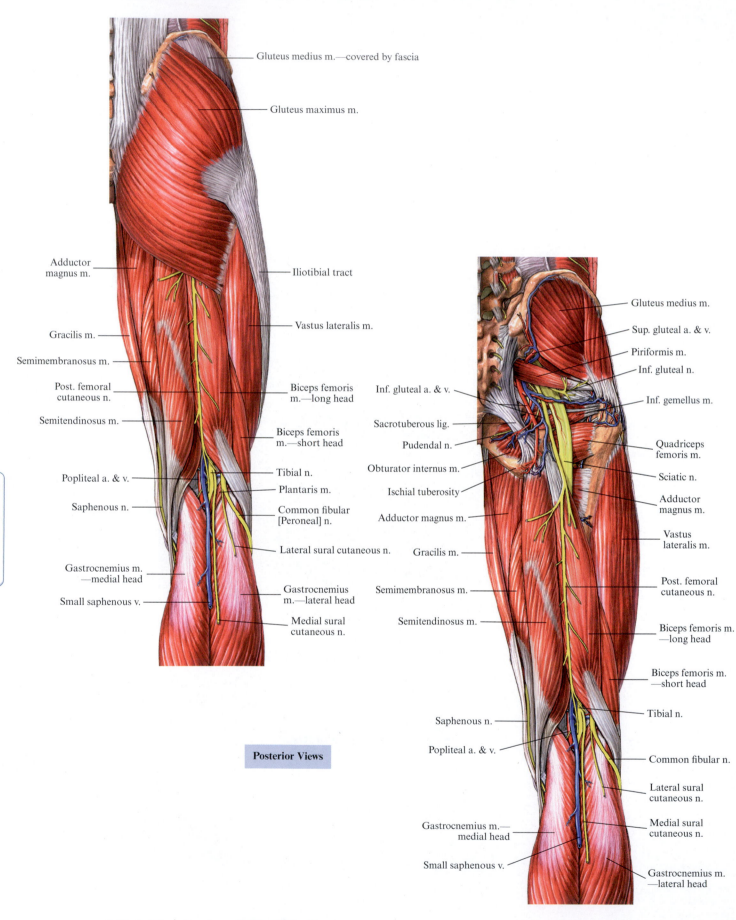

Gluteus medius m.—covered by fascia

Gluteus maximus m.

Adductor magnus m.

Iliotibial tract

Gracilis m.

Vastus lateralis m.

Semimembranosus m.

Post. femoral cutaneous n.

Biceps femoris m.—long head

Semitendinosus m.

Biceps femoris m.—short head

Popliteal a. & v.

Tibial n.

Plantaris m.

Saphenous n.

Common fibular [Peroneal] n.

Lateral sural cutaneous n.

Gastrocnemius m.—medial head

Small saphenous v.

Gastrocnemius m.—lateral head

Medial sural cutaneous n.

Inf. gluteal a. & v.

Gluteus medius m.

Sup. gluteal a. & v.

Piriformis m.

Inf. gluteal n.

Sacrotuberous lig.

Inf. gemellus m.

Pudendal n.

Obturator internus m.

Quadriceps femoris m.

Ischial tuberosity

Sciatic n.

Adductor magnus m.

Adductor magnus m.

Vastus lateralis m.

Gracilis m.

Post. femoral cutaneous n.

Semimembranosus m.

Semitendinosus m.

Biceps femoris m.—long head

Biceps femoris m.—short head

Tibial n.

Saphenous n.

Popliteal a. & v.

Common fibular n.

Lateral sural cutaneous n.

Gastrocnemius m.—medial head

Medial sural cutaneous n.

Small saphenous v.

Gastrocnemius m.—lateral head

Posterior Views

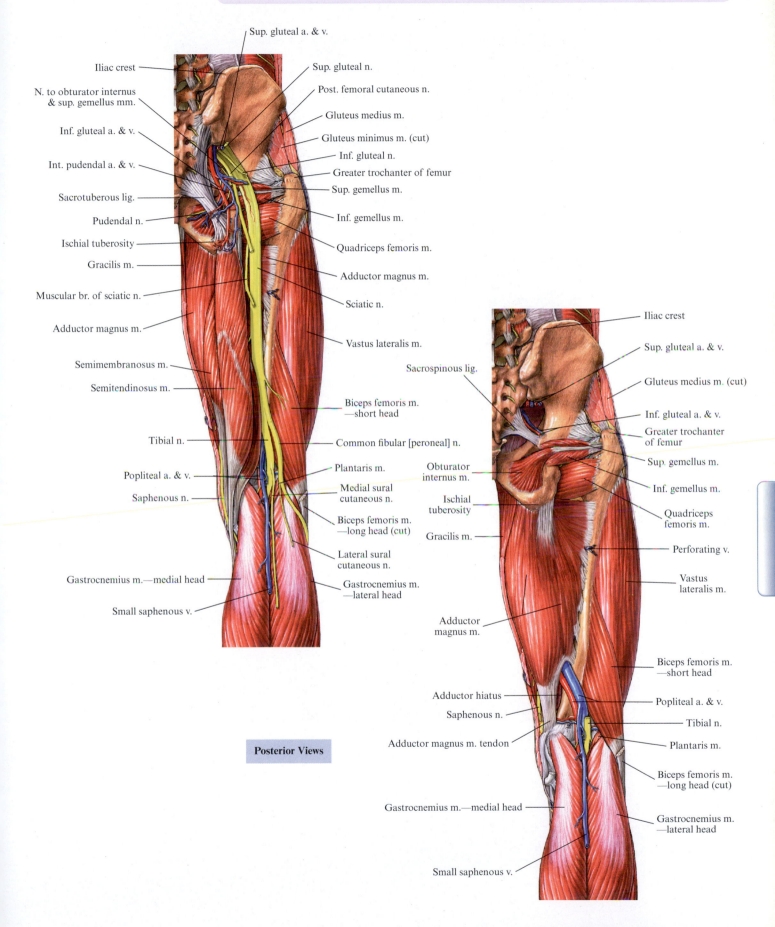

Sup. gluteal a. & v.

Iliac crest

N. to obturator internus & sup. gemellus mm.

Inf. gluteal a. & v.

Int. pudendal a. & v.

Sacrotuberous lig.

Pudendal n.

Ischial tuberosity

Gracilis m.

Muscular br. of sciatic n.

Adductor magnus m.

Semimembranosus m.

Semitendinosus m.

Tibial n.

Popliteal a. & v.

Saphenous n.

Gastrocnemius m.—medial head

Small saphenous v.

Sup. gluteal n.

Post. femoral cutaneous n.

Gluteus medius m.

Gluteus minimus m. (cut)

Inf. gluteal n.

Greater trochanter of femur

Sup. gemellus m.

Inf. gemellus m.

Quadriceps femoris m.

Adductor magnus m.

Sciatic n.

Vastus lateralis m.

Biceps femoris m. —short head

Common fibular [peroneal] n.

Plantaris m.

Medial sural cutaneous n.

Biceps femoris m. —long head (cut)

Lateral sural cutaneous n.

Gastrocnemius m. —lateral head

Posterior Views

Sacrospinous lig.

Obturator internus m.

Ischial tuberosity

Gracilis m.

Adductor magnus m.

Adductor hiatus

Saphenous n.

Adductor magnus m. tendon

Gastrocnemius m.—medial head

Small saphenous v.

Iliac crest

Sup. gluteal a. & v.

Gluteus medius m. (cut)

Inf. gluteal a. & v.

Greater trochanter of femur

Sup. gemellus m.

Inf. gemellus m.

Quadriceps femoris m.

Perforating v.

Vastus lateralis m.

Biceps femoris m. —short head

Popliteal a. & v.

Tibial n.

Plantaris m.

Biceps femoris m. —long head (cut)

Gastrocnemius m. —lateral head

PLATE 5.37   GLUTEAL REGION

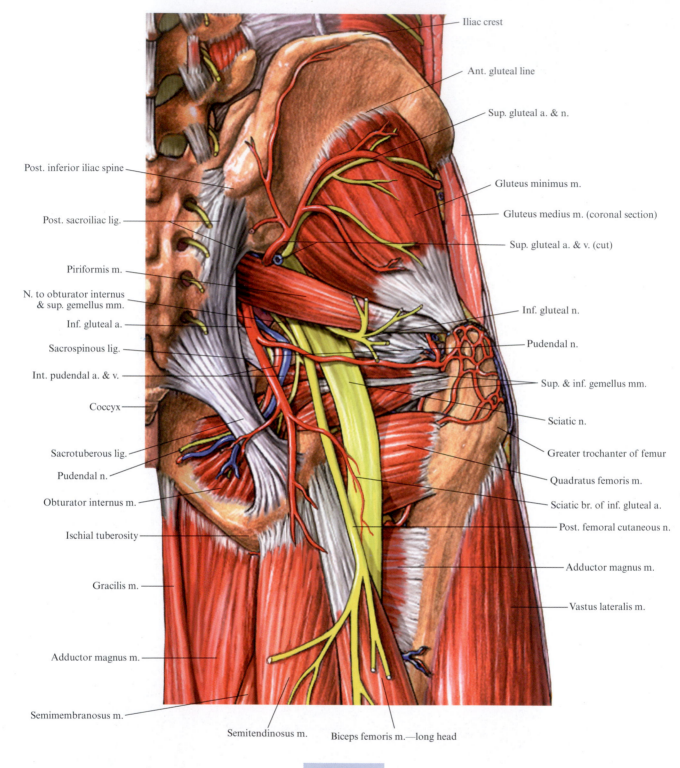

Iliac crest

Ant. gluteal line

Sup. gluteal a. & n.

Gluteus minimus m.

Gluteus medius m. (coronal section)

Sup. gluteal a. & v. (cut)

Post. inferior iliac spine

Post. sacroiliac lig.

Piriformis m.

N. to obturator internus & sup. gemellus mm.

Inf. gluteal a.

Sacrospinous lig.

Int. pudendal a. & v.

Coccyx

Sacrotuberous lig.

Pudendal n.

Obturator internus m.

Ischial tuberosity

Gracilis m.

Adductor magnus m.

Semimembranosus m.

Inf. gluteal n.

Pudendal n.

Sup. & inf. gemellus mm.

Sciatic n.

Greater trochanter of femur

Quadratus femoris m.

Sciatic br. of inf. gluteal a.

Post. femoral cutaneous n.

Adductor magnus m.

Vastus lateralis m.

Semitendinosus m.   Biceps femoris m.—long head

Posterior View

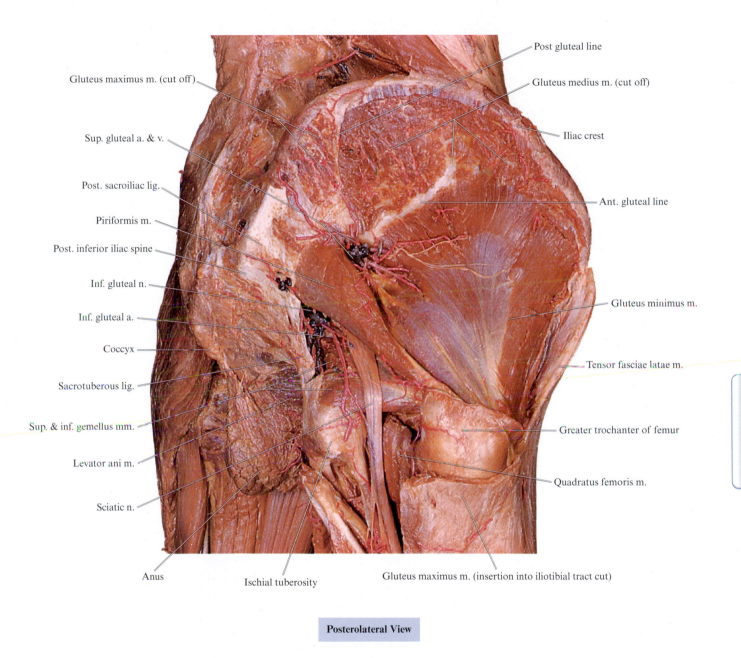

Post gluteal line

Gluteus maximus m. (cut off)

Gluteus medius m. (cut off)

Sup. gluteal a. & v.

Iliac crest

Post. sacroiliac lig.

Ant. gluteal line

Piriformis m.

Post. inferior iliac spine

Inf. gluteal n.

Gluteus minimus m.

Inf. gluteal a.

Coccyx

Tensor fasciae latae m.

Sacrotuberous lig.

Sup. & inf. gemellus mm.

Greater trochanter of femur

Levator ani m.

Quadratus femoris m.

Sciatic n.

Anus   Ischial tuberosity   Gluteus maximus m. (insertion into iliotibial tract cut)

Posterolateral View

PLATE 5.39   MEDIAL & LATERAL THIGH

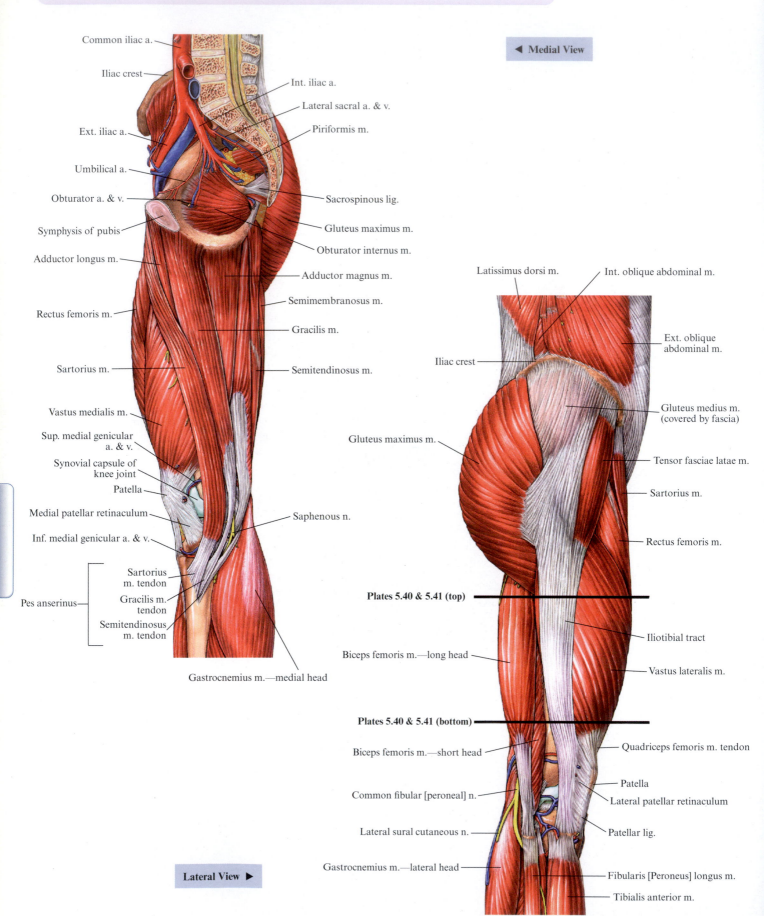

Common iliac a.
Iliac crest
Int. iliac a.
Lateral sacral a. & v.
Ext. iliac a.
Piriformis m.
Umbilical a.
Obturator a. & v.
Sacrospinous lig.
Symphysis of pubis
Gluteus maximus m.
Adductor longus m.
Obturator internus m.
Adductor magnus m.
Rectus femoris m.
Semimembranosus m.
Gracilis m.
Sartorius m.
Semitendinosus m.
Vastus medialis m.
Sup. medial genicular a. & v.
Synovial capsule of knee joint
Patella
Medial patellar retinaculum
Saphenous n.
Inf. medial genicular a. & v.
Sartorius m. tendon
Gracilis m. tendon
Pes anserinus
Semitendinosus m. tendon
Gastrocnemius m.—medial head

◄ Medial View

Latissimus dorsi m.
Int. oblique abdominal m.
Iliac crest
Ext. oblique abdominal m.
Gluteus medius m. (covered by fascia)
Gluteus maximus m.
Tensor fasciae latae m.
Sartorius m.
Rectus femoris m.
Plates 5.40 & 5.41 (top)
Iliotibial tract
Biceps femoris m.—long head
Vastus lateralis m.
Plates 5.40 & 5.41 (bottom)
Biceps femoris m.—short head
Quadriceps femoris m. tendon
Common fibular [peroneal] n.
Patella
Lateral patellar retinaculum
Lateral sural cutaneous n.
Patellar lig.
Gastrocnemius m.—lateral head
Fibularis [Peroneus] longus m.
Tibialis anterior m.

Lateral View ►

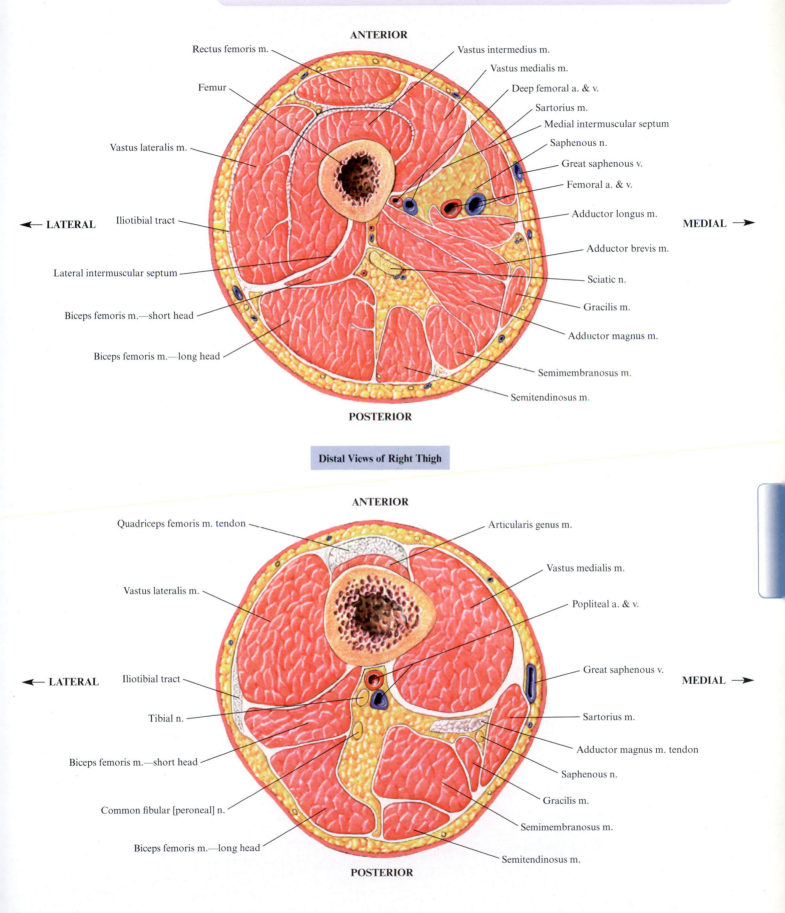

ANTERIOR

Rectus femoris m.

Femur

Vastus lateralis m.

← LATERAL

Iliotibial tract

Lateral intermuscular septum

Biceps femoris m.—short head

Biceps femoris m.—long head

Vastus intermedius m.

Vastus medialis m.

Deep femoral a. & v.

Sartorius m.

Medial intermuscular septum

Saphenous n.

Great saphenous v.

Femoral a. & v.

MEDIAL →

Adductor longus m.

Adductor brevis m.

Sciatic n.

Gracilis m.

Adductor magnus m.

Semimembranosus m.

Semitendinosus m.

POSTERIOR

Distal Views of Right Thigh

ANTERIOR

Quadriceps femoris m. tendon

Vastus lateralis m.

← LATERAL

Iliotibial tract

Tibial n.

Biceps femoris m.—short head

Common fibular [peroneal] n.

Biceps femoris m.—long head

Articularis genus m.

Vastus medialis m.

Popliteal a. & v.

Great saphenous v.

MEDIAL →

Sartorius m.

Adductor magnus m. tendon

Saphenous n.

Gracilis m.

Semimembranosus m.

Semitendinosus m.

POSTERIOR

PLATE 5.41   CROSS SECTIONS OF THIGH

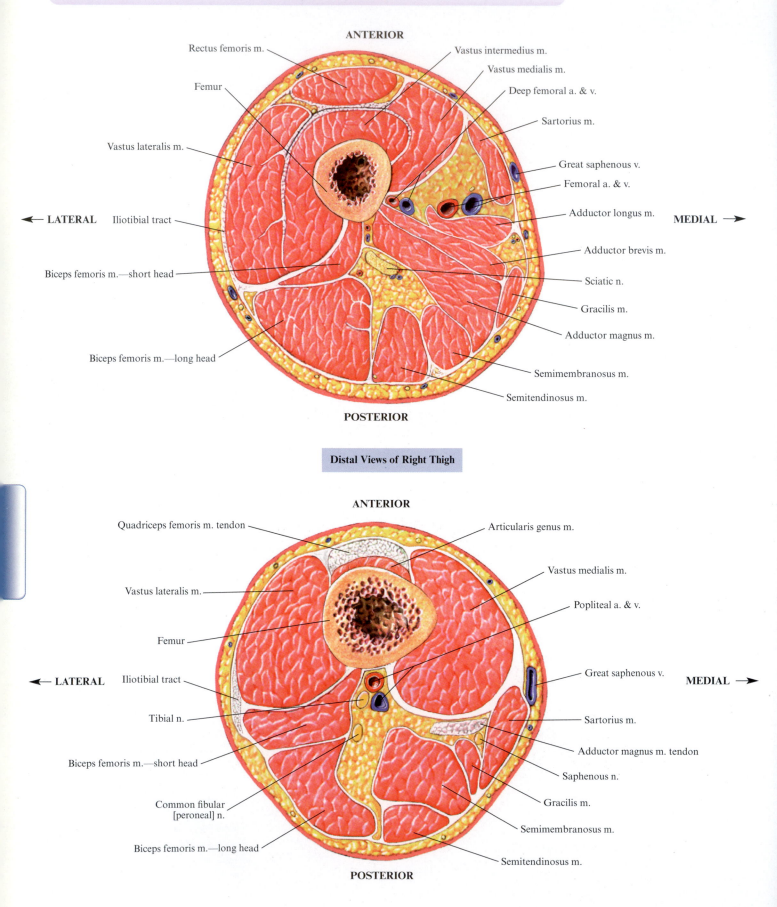

ANTERIOR

Rectus femoris m.

Femur

Vastus lateralis m.

← LATERAL   Iliotibial tract

Biceps femoris m.—short head

Biceps femoris m.—long head

Vastus intermedius m.

Vastus medialis m.

Deep femoral a. & v.

Sartorius m.

Great saphenous v.

Femoral a. & v.

Adductor longus m.   MEDIAL →

Adductor brevis m.

Sciatic n.

Gracilis m.

Adductor magnus m.

Semimembranosus m.

Semitendinosus m.

POSTERIOR

Distal Views of Right Thigh

ANTERIOR

Quadriceps femoris m. tendon

Vastus lateralis m.

Femur

← LATERAL   Iliotibial tract

Tibial n.

Biceps femoris m.—short head

Common fibular
[peroneal] n.

Biceps femoris m.—long head

Articularis genus m.

Vastus medialis m.

Popliteal a. & v.

Great saphenous v.   MEDIAL →

Sartorius m.

Adductor magnus m. tendon

Saphenous n.

Gracilis m.

Semimembranosus m.

Semitendinosus m.

POSTERIOR

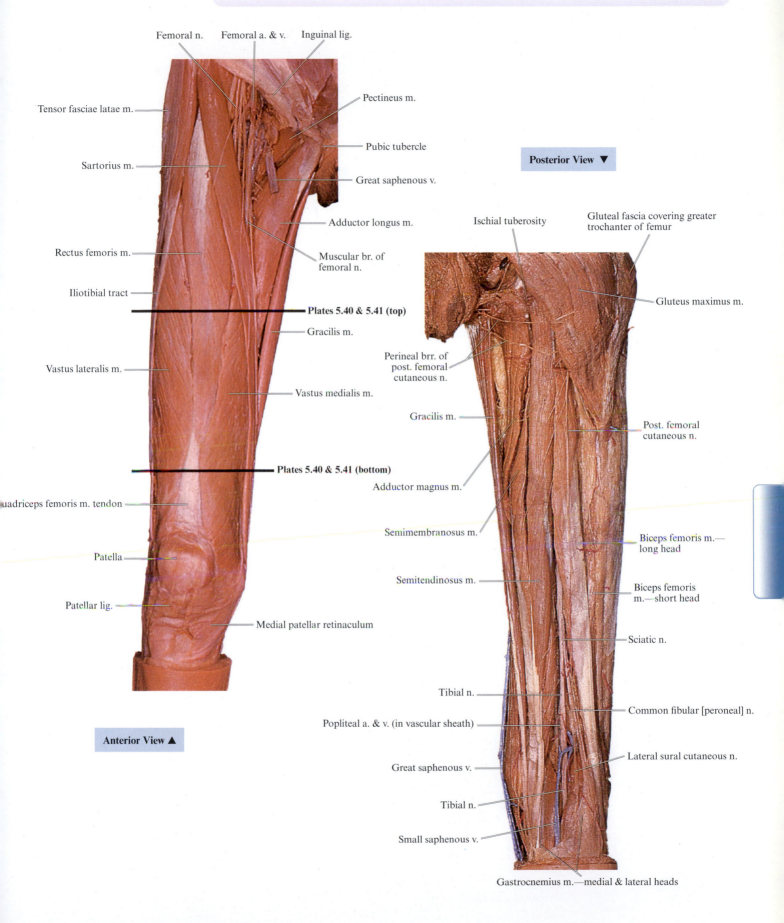

Femoral n.   Femoral a. & v.   Inguinal lig.

Tensor fasciae latae m.

Pectineus m.

Sartorius m.

Pubic tubercle

Posterior View ▼

Great saphenous v.

Adductor longus m.

Rectus femoris m.

Muscular br. of femoral n.

Iliotibial tract

Ischial tuberosity   Gluteal fascia covering greater trochanter of femur

Plates 5.40 & 5.41 (top)

Gracilis m.

Gluteus maximus m.

Vastus lateralis m.

Vastus medialis m.

Perineal brr. of post. femoral cutaneous n.

Gracilis m.

Post. femoral cutaneous n.

Plates 5.40 & 5.41 (bottom)

Adductor magnus m.

Quadriceps femoris m. tendon

Semimembranosus m.

Biceps femoris m.— long head

Patella

Semitendinosus m.

Biceps femoris m.—short head

Patellar lig.

Sciatic n.

Medial patellar retinaculum

Tibial n.

Common fibular [peroneal] n.

Popliteal a. & v. (in vascular sheath)

Anterior View ▲

Lateral sural cutaneous n.

Great saphenous v.

Tibial n.

Small saphenous v.

Gastrocnemius m.—medial & lateral heads

PLATE 5.43   HIP JOINT

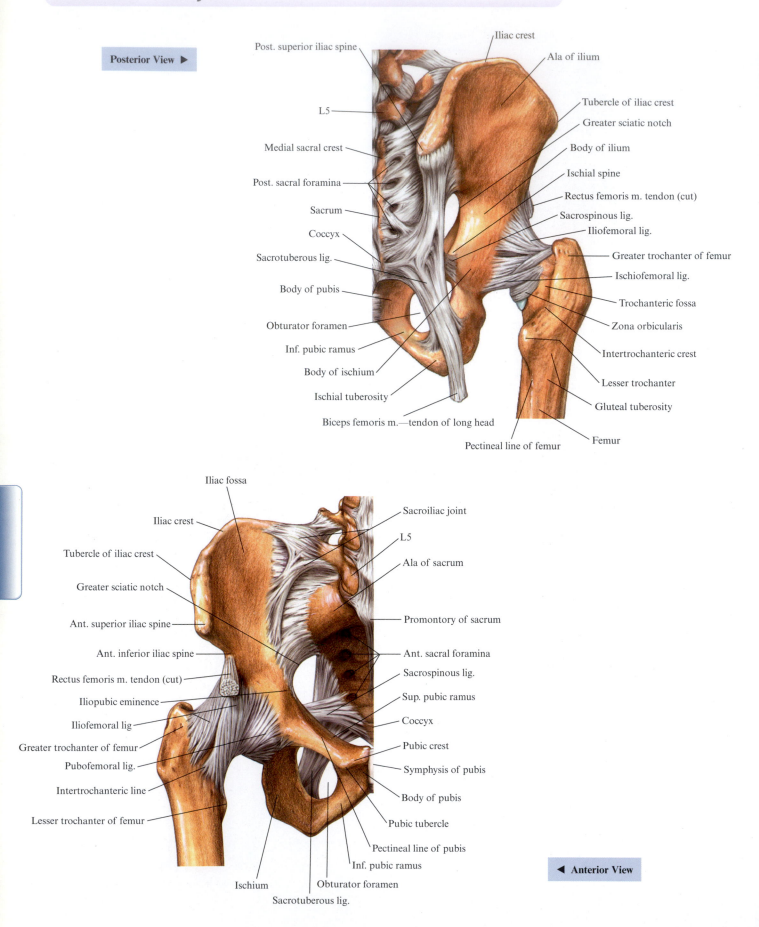

Post. superior iliac spine

Iliac crest

Ala of ilium

L5

Tubercle of iliac crest

Greater sciatic notch

Medial sacral crest

Body of ilium

Post. sacral foramina

Ischial spine

Rectus femoris m. tendon (cut)

Sacrum

Sacrospinous lig.

Coccyx

Iliofemoral lig.

Sacrotuberous lig.

Greater trochanter of femur

Body of pubis

Ischiofemoral lig.

Trochanteric fossa

Obturator foramen

Zona orbicularis

Inf. pubic ramus

Intertrochanteric crest

Body of ischium

Lesser trochanter

Ischial tuberosity

Gluteal tuberosity

Biceps femoris m.—tendon of long head

Femur

Pectineal line of femur

Iliac fossa

Iliac crest

Sacroiliac joint

L5

Tubercle of iliac crest

Ala of sacrum

Greater sciatic notch

Ant. superior iliac spine

Promontory of sacrum

Ant. inferior iliac spine

Ant. sacral foramina

Rectus femoris m. tendon (cut)

Sacrospinous lig.

Iliopubic eminence

Sup. pubic ramus

Iliofemoral lig

Coccyx

Greater trochanter of femur

Pubic crest

Pubofemoral lig.

Symphysis of pubis

Intertrochanteric line

Body of pubis

Lesser trochanter of femur

Pubic tubercle

Pectineal line of pubis

Inf. pubic ramus

Ischium

Obturator foramen

Sacrotuberous lig.

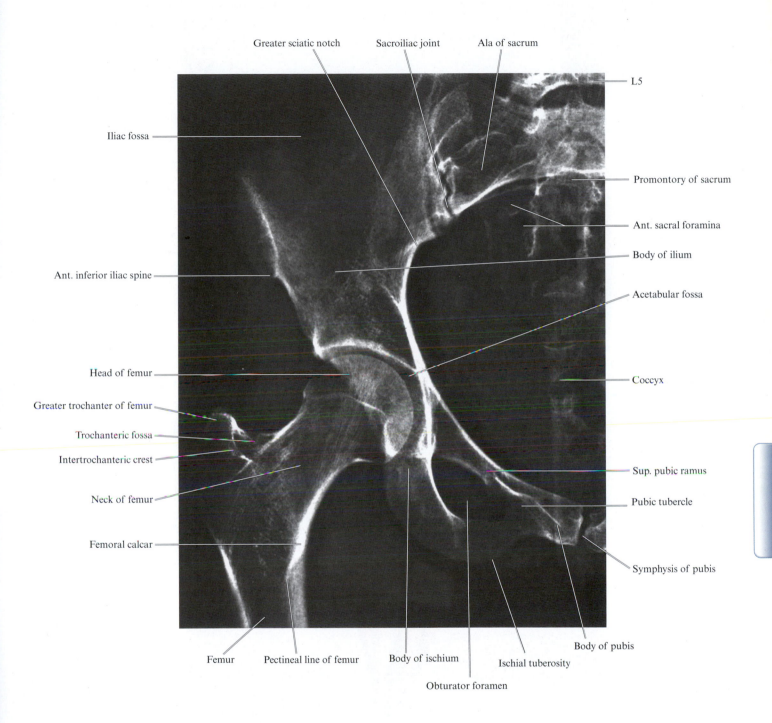

Greater sciatic notch

Sacroiliac joint

Ala of sacrum

L5

Iliac fossa

Promontory of sacrum

Ant. sacral foramina

Body of ilium

Ant. inferior iliac spine

Acetabular fossa

Head of femur

Coccyx

Greater trochanter of femur

Trochanteric fossa

Intertrochanteric crest

Sup. pubic ramus

Neck of femur

Pubic tubercle

Femoral calcar

Symphysis of pubis

Body of pubis

Femur

Pectineal line of femur

Body of ischium

Ischial tuberosity

Obturator foramen

PLATE 5.45 ANTERIOR LEG

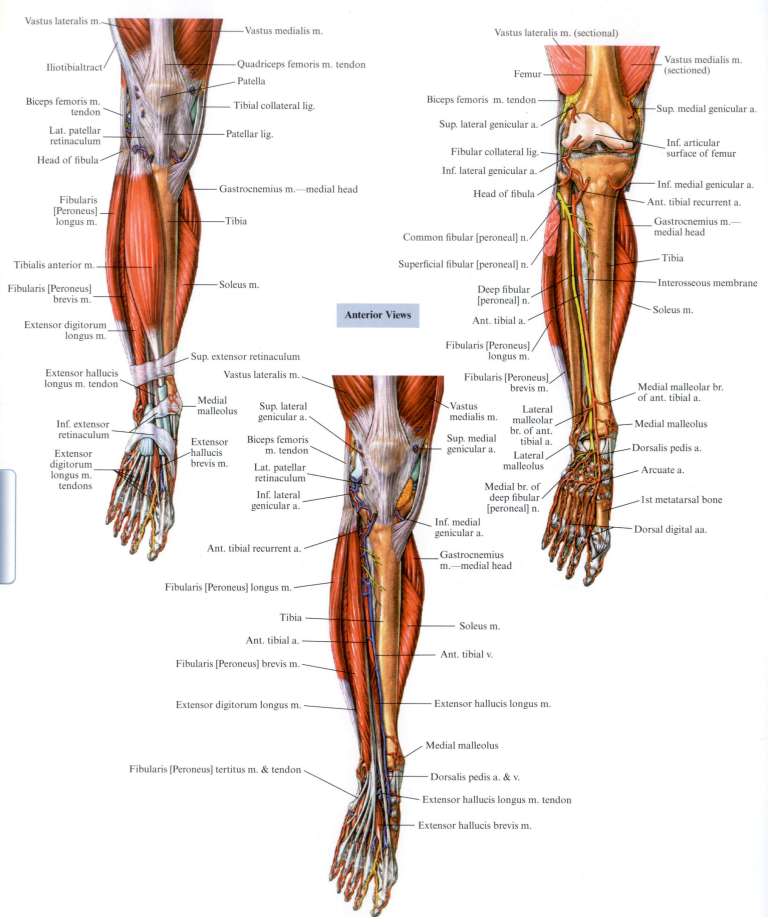

Vastus lateralis m.

Vastus medialis m.

Iliotibialtract

Quadriceps femoris m. tendon

Patella

Biceps femoris m. tendon

Tibial collateral lig.

Lat. patellar retinaculum

Patellar lig.

Head of fibula

Fibularis [Peroneus] longus m.

Gastrocnemius m.—medial head

Tibia

Tibialis anterior m.

Fibularis [Peroneus] brevis m.

Soleus m.

Extensor digitorum longus m.

Extensor hallucis longus m. tendon

Sup. extensor retinaculum

Inf. extensor retinaculum

Medial malleolus

Extensor digitorum longus m. tendons

Extensor hallucis brevis m.

Vastus lateralis m. (sectional)

Vastus medialis m. (sectioned)

Femur

Biceps femoris m. tendon

Sup. medial genicular a.

Sup. lateral genicular a.

Inf. articular surface of femur

Fibular collateral lig.

Inf. lateral genicular a.

Inf. medial genicular a.

Head of fibula

Ant. tibial recurrent a.

Common fibular [peroneal] n.

Gastrocnemius m.—medial head

Superficial fibular [peroneal] n.

Tibia

Deep fibular [peroneal] n.

Interosseous membrane

Ant. tibial a.

Soleus m.

Fibularis [Peroneus] longus m.

Fibularis [Peroneus] brevis m.

Medial malleolar br. of ant. tibial a.

Lateral malleolar br. of ant. tibial a.

Medial malleolus

Lateral malleolus

Dorsalis pedis a.

Medial br. of deep fibular [peroneal] n.

Arcuate a.

1st metatarsal bone

Dorsal digital aa.

Anterior Views

Vastus lateralis m.

Sup. lateral genicular a.

Vastus medialis m.

Biceps femoris m. tendon

Sup. medial genicular a.

Lat. patellar retinaculum

Inf. lateral genicular a.

Inf. medial genicular a.

Ant. tibial recurrent a.

Gastrocnemius m.—medial head

Fibularis [Peroneus] longus m.

Tibia

Soleus m.

Ant. tibial a.

Ant. tibial v.

Fibularis [Peroneus] brevis m.

Extensor digitorum longus m.

Extensor hallucis longus m.

Medial malleolus

Fibularis [Peroneus] tertitus m. & tendon

Dorsalis pedis a. & v.

Extensor hallucis longus m. tendon

Extensor hallucis brevis m.

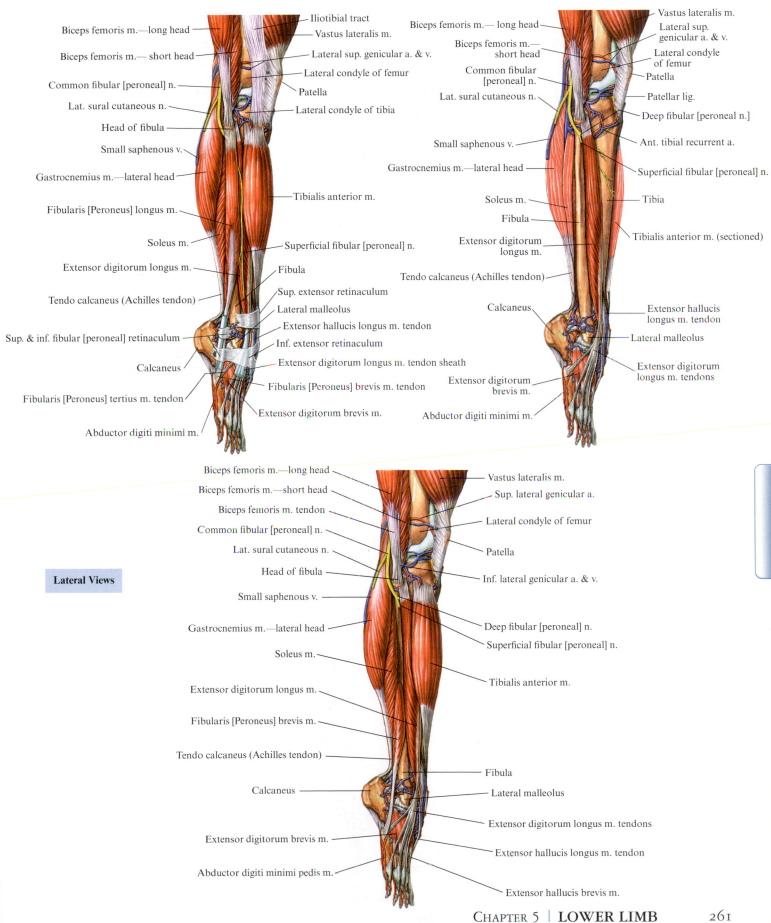

Biceps femoris m.—long head
Iliotibial tract
Vastus lateralis m.
Biceps femoris m.— short head
Lateral sup. genicular a. & v.
Common fibular [peroneal] n.
Lateral condyle of femur
Lat. sural cutaneous n.
Patella
Head of fibula
Lateral condyle of tibia
Small saphenous v.
Gastrocnemius m.—lateral head
Tibialis anterior m.
Fibularis [Peroneus] longus m.
Soleus m.
Superficial fibular [peroneal] n.
Extensor digitorum longus m.
Fibula
Tendo calcaneus (Achilles tendon)
Sup. extensor retinaculum
Lateral malleolus
Sup. & inf. fibular [peroneal] retinaculum
Extensor hallucis longus m. tendon
Inf. extensor retinaculum
Calcaneus
Extensor digitorum longus m. tendon sheath
Fibularis [Peroneus] tertius m. tendon
Fibularis [Peroneus] brevis m. tendon
Extensor digitorum brevis m.
Abductor digiti minimi m.

Biceps femoris m.— long head
Vastus lateralis m.
Biceps femoris m.— short head
Lateral sup. genicular a. & v.
Common fibular [peroneal] n.
Lateral condyle of femur
Lat. sural cutaneous n.
Patella
Patellar lig.
Deep fibular [peroneal n.]
Small saphenous v.
Ant. tibial recurrent a.
Gastrocnemius m.—lateral head
Superficial fibular [peroneal] n.
Soleus m.
Tibia
Fibula
Extensor digitorum longus m.
Tibialis anterior m. (sectioned)
Tendo calcaneus (Achilles tendon)
Calcaneus
Extensor hallucis longus m. tendon
Lateral malleolus
Extensor digitorum longus m. tendons
Extensor digitorum brevis m.
Abductor digiti minimi m.

Lateral Views

Biceps femoris m.—long head
Vastus lateralis m.
Biceps femoris m.—short head
Sup. lateral genicular a.
Biceps femoris m. tendon
Lateral condyle of femur
Common fibular [peroneal] n.
Patella
Lat. sural cutaneous n.
Head of fibula
Inf. lateral genicular a. & v.
Small saphenous v.
Gastrocnemius m.—lateral head
Deep fibular [peroneal] n.
Soleus m.
Superficial fibular [peroneal] n.
Extensor digitorum longus m.
Tibialis anterior m.
Fibularis [Peroneus] brevis m.
Tendo calcaneus (Achilles tendon)
Fibula
Calcaneus
Lateral malleolus
Extensor digitorum longus m. tendons
Extensor digitorum brevis m.
Extensor hallucis longus m. tendon
Abductor digiti minimi pedis m.
Extensor hallucis brevis m.

PLATE 5.49   MEDIAL LEG

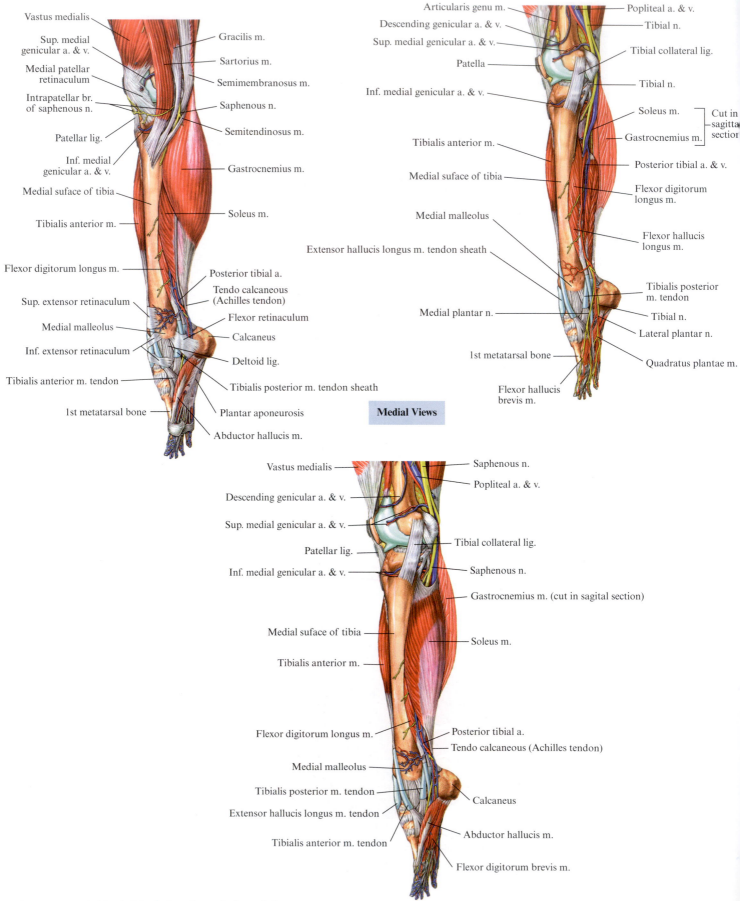

Vastus medialis

Sup. medial
genicular a. & v.

Medial patellar
retinaculum

Intrapatellar br.
of saphenous n.

Patellar lig.

Inf. medial
genicular a. & v.

Medial suface of tibia

Tibialis anterior m.

Flexor digitorum longus m.

Sup. extensor retinaculum

Medial malleolus

Inf. extensor retinaculum

Tibialis anterior m. tendon

1st metatarsal bone

Gracilis m.

Sartorius m.

Semimembranosus m.

Saphenous n.

Semitendinosus m.

Gastrocnemius m.

Soleus m.

Posterior tibial a.

Tendo calcaneous
(Achilles tendon)

Flexor retinaculum

Calcaneus

Deltoid lig.

Tibialis posterior m. tendon sheath

Plantar aponeurosis

Abductor hallucis m.

Articularis genu m.

Descending genicular a. & v.

Sup. medial genicular a. & v.

Patella

Inf. medial genicular a. & v.

Tibialis anterior m.

Medial suface of tibia

Medial malleolus

Extensor hallucis longus m. tendon sheath

Medial plantar n.

1st metatarsal bone

Flexor hallucis
brevis m.

Popliteal a. & v.

Tibial n.

Tibial collateral lig.

Tibial n.

Soleus m.   } Cut in
                  sagitta
Gastrocnemius m.   section

Posterior tibial a. & v.

Flexor digitorum
longus m.

Flexor hallucis
longus m.

Tibialis posterior
m. tendon

Tibial n.

Lateral plantar n.

Quadratus plantae m.

Medial Views

Vastus medialis

Descending genicular a. & v.

Sup. medial genicular a. & v.

Patellar lig.

Inf. medial genicular a. & v.

Medial suface of tibia

Tibialis anterior m.

Flexor digitorum longus m.

Medial malleolus

Tibialis posterior m. tendon

Extensor hallucis longus m. tendon

Tibialis anterior m. tendon

Saphenous n.

Popliteal a. & v.

Tibial collateral lig.

Saphenous n.

Gastrocnemius m. (cut in sagital section)

Soleus m.

Posterior tibial a.

Tendo calcaneous (Achilles tendon)

Calcaneus

Abductor hallucis m.

Flexor digitorum brevis m.

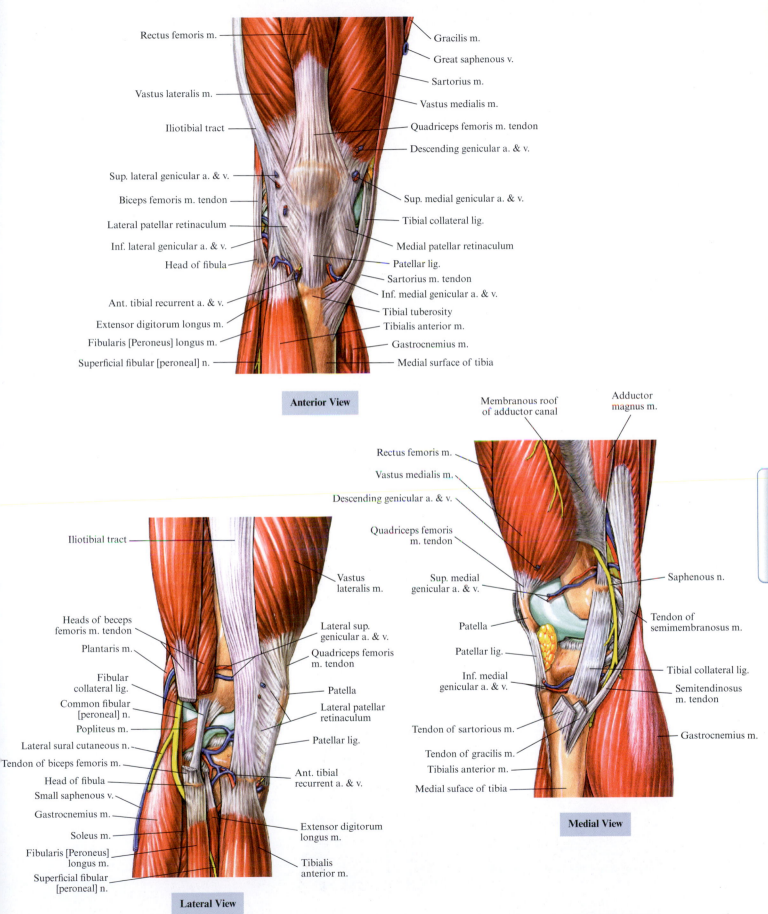

Rectus femoris m.

Gracilis m.

Great saphenous v.

Sartorius m.

Vastus lateralis m.

Vastus medialis m.

Iliotibial tract

Quadriceps femoris m. tendon

Descending genicular a. & v.

Sup. lateral genicular a. & v.

Biceps femoris m. tendon

Sup. medial genicular a. & v.

Lateral patellar retinaculum

Tibial collateral lig.

Inf. lateral genicular a. & v.

Medial patellar retinaculum

Head of fibula

Patellar lig.

Sartorius m. tendon

Inf. medial genicular a. & v.

Ant. tibial recurrent a. & v.

Tibial tuberosity

Extensor digitorum longus m.

Tibialis anterior m.

Fibularis [Peroneus] longus m.

Gastrocnemius m.

Superficial fibular [peroneal] n.

Medial surface of tibia

Anterior View

Membranous roof of adductor canal

Adductor magnus m.

Rectus femoris m.

Vastus medialis m.

Descending genicular a. & v.

Quadriceps femoris m. tendon

Saphenous n.

Sup. medial genicular a. & v.

Patella

Tendon of semimembranosus m.

Patellar lig.

Tibial collateral lig.

Inf. medial genicular a. & v.

Semitendinosus m. tendon

Tendon of sartorious m.

Gastrocnemius m.

Tendon of gracilis m.

Tibialis anterior m.

Medial suface of tibia

Medial View

Iliotibial tract

Vastus lateralis m.

Lateral sup. genicular a. & v.

Heads of beceps femoris m. tendon

Quadriceps femoris m. tendon

Plantaris m.

Fibular collateral lig.

Patella

Common fibular [peroneal] n.

Lateral patellar retinaculum

Popliteus m.

Patellar lig.

Lateral sural cutaneous n.

Tendon of biceps femoris m.

Head of fibula

Ant. tibial recurrent a. & v.

Small saphenous v.

Gastrocnemius m.

Soleus m.

Extensor digitorum longus m.

Fibularis [Peroneus] longus m.

Tibialis anterior m.

Superficial fibular [peroneal] n.

Lateral View

PLATE 5.51   POSTERIOR KNEE

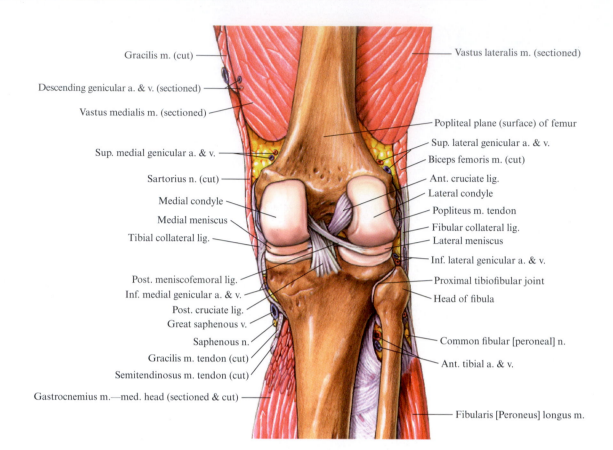

Gracilis m. (cut)

Descending genicular a. & v. (sectioned)

Vastus medialis m. (sectioned)

Sup. medial genicular a. & v.

Sartorius n. (cut)

Medial condyle

Medial meniscus

Tibial collateral lig.

Post. meniscofemoral lig.

Inf. medial genicular a. & v.

Post. cruciate lig.

Great saphenous v.

Saphenous n.

Gracilis m. tendon (cut)

Semitendinosus m. tendon (cut)

Gastrocnemius m.—med. head (sectioned & cut)

Vastus lateralis m. (sectioned)

Popliteal plane (surface) of femur

Sup. lateral genicular a. & v.

Biceps femoris m. (cut)

Ant. cruciate lig.

Lateral condyle

Popliteus m. tendon

Fibular collateral lig.

Lateral meniscus

Inf. lateral genicular a. & v.

Proximal tibiofibular joint

Head of fibula

Common fibular [peroneal] n.

Ant. tibial a. & v.

Fibularis [Peroneus] longus m.

Posterior Views

Gracilis m. (cut)

Descending genicular a. & v.

Vastus medialis m. (sectioned)

Sup. medial genicular a. & v.

Sartorius m. (cut)

Post. surface of articular
capsule of knee joint

Gastrocnemius m.—medial head (cut)

Tibial collateral lig.

Semimembranosus m. tendon

Oblique popliteal lig.

Great saphenous v.

Saphenous n.

Gracilis m. tendon (cut)

Semitendinosus m. tendon (cut)

Gastrocnemius m.—med. head (sectioned & cut)

Vastus lateralis m. (sectioned)

Popliteal plane (surface) of femur

Sup. lateral genicular a. & v.

Plantaris m. (cut)

Biceps femoris m.—short head (coronal section)

Gastrocnemius m.—lateral head (cut)

Fibular collateral lig.

Biceps femoris m.—long head tendon (cut)

Arcuate popliteal lig.

Post. lig. of head of fibula

Head of fibula

Popliteus m. (cut ends)

Common fibular [peroneal] n.

Tibialis posterior m.

Fibularis [Peroneus] longus m.

Distal View of Articular Surface of Right Femur

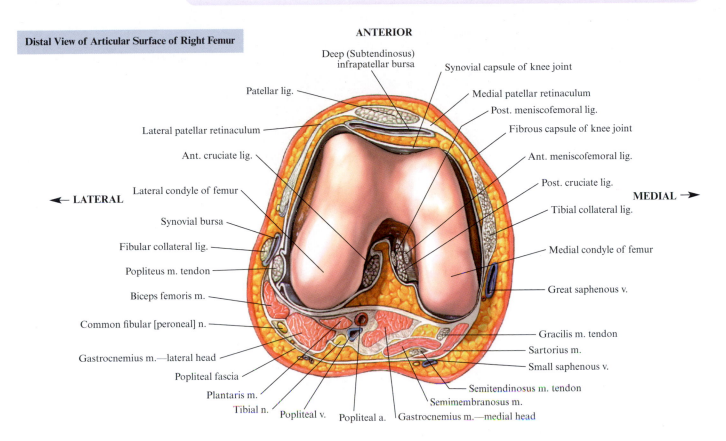

ANTERIOR

Deep (Subtendinosus) infrapatellar bursa

Patellar lig.

Synovial capsule of knee joint

Medial patellar retinaculum

Post. meniscofemoral lig.

Fibrous capsule of knee joint

Lateral patellar retinaculum

Ant. meniscofemoral lig.

Ant. cruciate lig.

Post. cruciate lig.

Lateral condyle of femur

Tibial collateral lig.

← LATERAL

MEDIAL →

Synovial bursa

Medial condyle of femur

Fibular collateral lig.

Popliteus m. tendon

Great saphenous v.

Biceps femoris m.

Common fibular [peroneal] n.

Gracilis m. tendon

Sartorius m.

Gastrocnemius m.—lateral head

Small saphenous v.

Popliteal fascia

Semitendinosus m. tendon

Plantaris m.

Semimembranosus m.

Tibial n.   Popliteal v.   Popliteal a.   Gastrocnemius m.—medial head

POSTERIOR

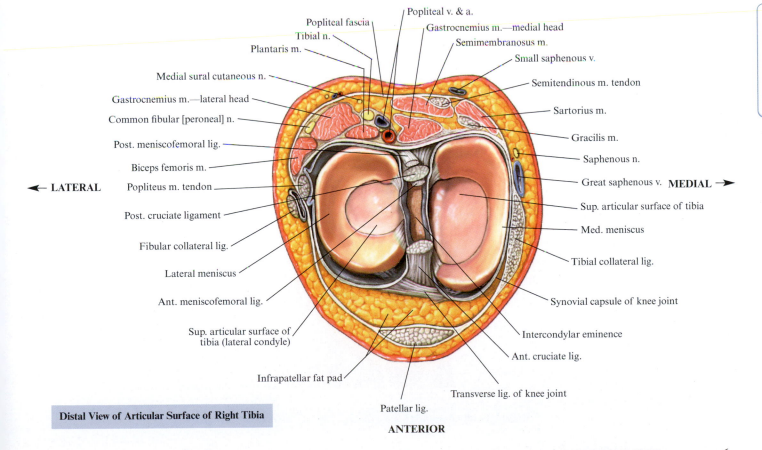

Popliteal v. & a.

Popliteal fascia

Gastrocnemius m.—medial head

Tibial n.

Semimembranosus m.

Plantaris m.

Small saphenous v.

Medial sural cutaneous n.

Semitendinous m. tendon

Gastrocnemius m.—lateral head

Sartorius m.

Common fibular [peroneal] n.

Post. meniscofemoral lig.

Gracilis m.

Biceps femoris m.

Saphenous n.

Popliteus m. tendon

Great saphenous v.   MEDIAL →

← LATERAL

Post. cruciate ligament

Sup. articular surface of tibia

Fibular collateral lig.

Med. meniscus

Lateral meniscus

Tibial collateral lig.

Ant. meniscofemoral lig.

Synovial capsule of knee joint

Sup. articular surface of tibia (lateral condyle)

Intercondylar eminence

Ant. cruciate lig.

Infrapatellar fat pad

Transverse lig. of knee joint

Patellar lig.

Distal View of Articular Surface of Right Tibia

ANTERIOR

PLATE 5.53   KNEE JOINT

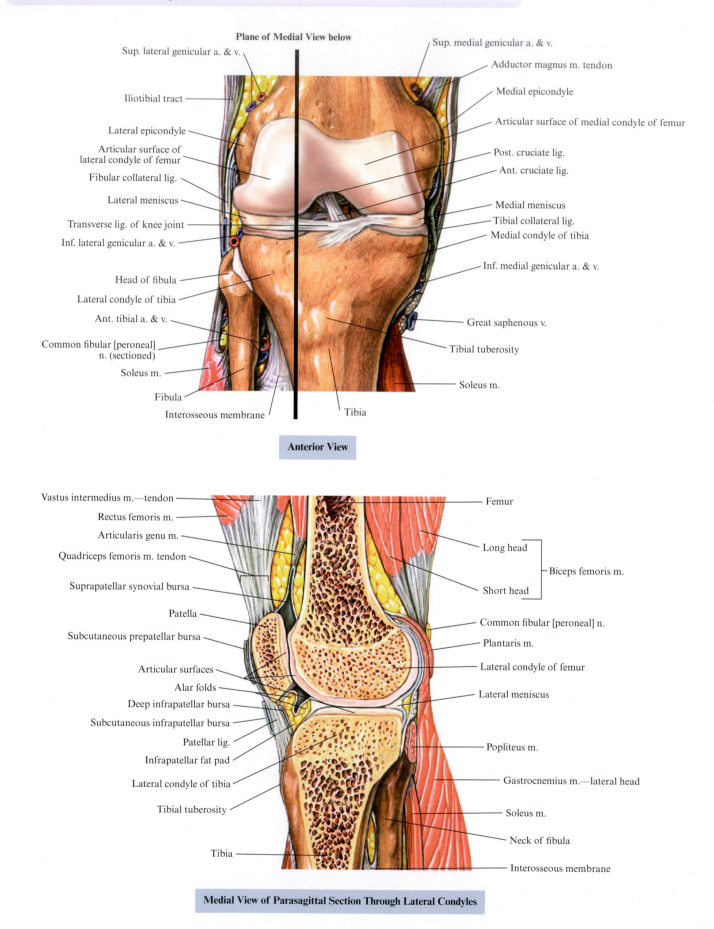

Plane of Medial View below

Sup. lateral genicular a. & v.

Iliotibial tract

Lateral epicondyle

Articular surface of
lateral condyle of femur

Fibular collateral lig.

Lateral meniscus

Transverse lig. of knee joint

Inf. lateral genicular a. & v.

Head of fibula

Lateral condyle of tibia

Ant. tibial a. & v.

Common fibular [peroneal]
n. (sectioned)

Soleus m.

Fibula

Interosseous membrane

Sup. medial genicular a. & v.

Adductor magnus m. tendon

Medial epicondyle

Articular surface of medial condyle of femur

Post. cruciate lig.

Ant. cruciate lig.

Medial meniscus

Tibial collateral lig.

Medial condyle of tibia

Inf. medial genicular a. & v.

Great saphenous v.

Tibial tuberosity

Soleus m.

Tibia

Anterior View

Vastus intermedius m.—tendon

Rectus femoris m.

Articularis genu m.

Quadriceps femoris m. tendon

Suprapatellar synovial bursa

Patella

Subcutaneous prepatellar bursa

Articular surfaces

Alar folds

Deep infrapatellar bursa

Subcutaneous infrapatellar bursa

Patellar lig.

Infrapatellar fat pad

Lateral condyle of tibia

Tibial tuberosity

Tibia

Femur

Long head

Short head

} Biceps femoris m.

Common fibular [peroneal] n.

Plantaris m.

Lateral condyle of femur

Lateral meniscus

Popliteus m.

Gastrocnemius m.—lateral head

Soleus m.

Neck of fibula

Interosseous membrane

Medial View of Parasagittal Section Through Lateral Condyles

 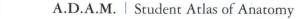

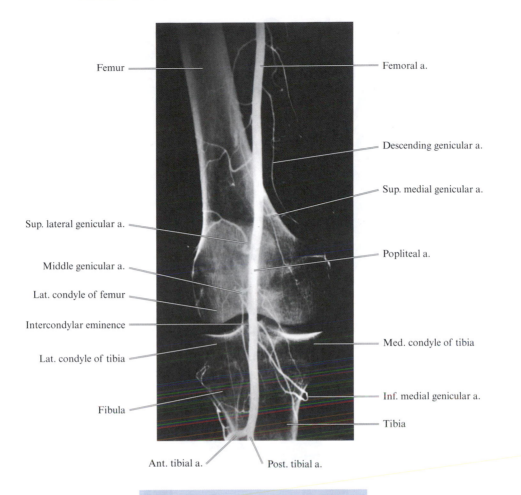

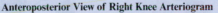

Femur — Femoral a.

Descending genicular a.

Sup. medial genicular a.

Sup. lateral genicular a. —

Middle genicular a. — — Popliteal a.

Lat. condyle of femur —

Intercondylar eminence —

Lat. condyle of tibia — — Med. condyle of tibia

Fibula — — Inf. medial genicular a.

— Tibia

Ant. tibial a. — — Post. tibial a.

Anteroposterior View of Right Knee Arteriogram

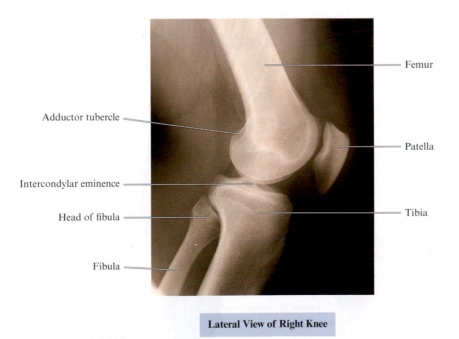

Femur

Adductor tubercle —

— Patella

Intercondylar eminence —

Head of fibula —

— Tibia

Fibula —

Lateral View of Right Knee

PLATE 5.57   DORSUM OF FOOT

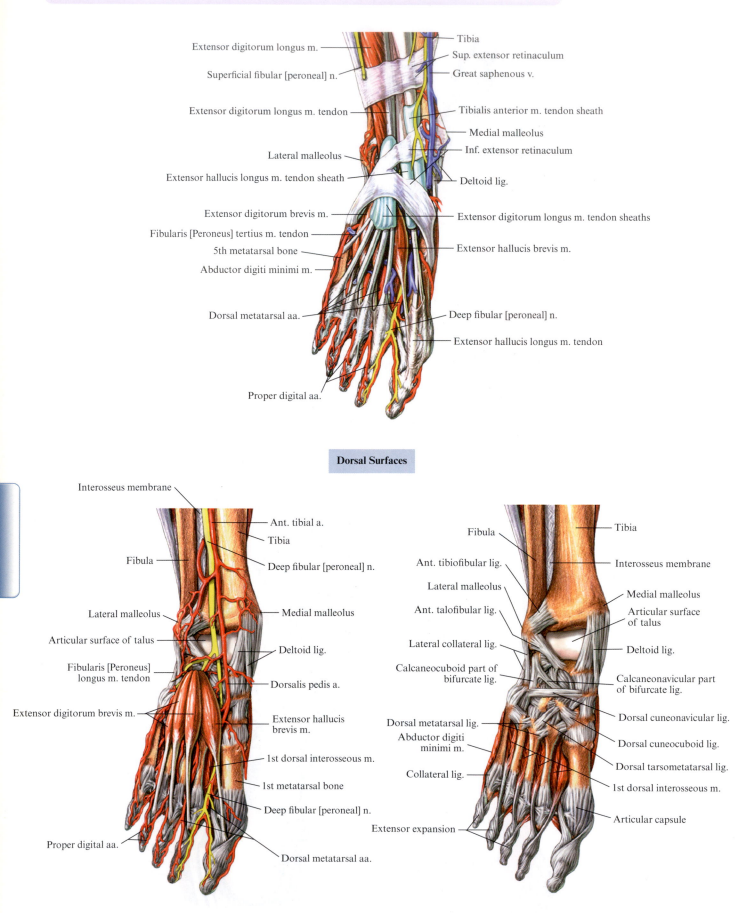

Extensor digitorum longus m. — Tibia
— Sup. extensor retinaculum
Superficial fibular [peroneal] n. — Great saphenous v.

Extensor digitorum longus m. tendon — Tibialis anterior m. tendon sheath
— Medial malleolus
Lateral malleolus — Inf. extensor retinaculum
Extensor hallucis longus m. tendon sheath — Deltoid lig.

Extensor digitorum brevis m. — Extensor digitorum longus m. tendon sheaths
Fibularis [Peroneus] tertius m. tendon —
5th metatarsal bone — Extensor hallucis brevis m.
Abductor digiti minimi m. —

Dorsal metatarsal aa. — Deep fibular [peroneal] n.
— Extensor hallucis longus m. tendon

Proper digital aa. —

Dorsal Surfaces

Interosseus membrane —
— Ant. tibial a.
— Tibia
Fibula — — Deep fibular [peroneal] n.

Lateral malleolus — — Medial malleolus
Articular surface of talus —
Fibularis [Peroneus] longus m. tendon — — Deltoid lig.
— Dorsalis pedis a.
Extensor digitorum brevis m. —
— Extensor hallucis brevis m.
— 1st dorsal interosseous m.
— 1st metatarsal bone
Proper digital aa. — — Deep fibular [peroneal] n.
— Dorsal metatarsal aa.

Fibula — — Tibia
Ant. tibiofibular lig. — — Interosseus membrane
Lateral malleolus — — Medial malleolus
Ant. talofibular lig. — — Articular surface of talus
Lateral collateral lig. — — Deltoid lig.
Calcaneocuboid part of bifurcate lig. — — Calcaneonavicular part of bifurcate lig.
— Dorsal cuneonavicular lig.
Dorsal metatarsal lig. — — Dorsal cuneocuboid lig.
Abductor digiti minimi m. — — Dorsal tarsometatarsal lig.
Collateral lig. — — 1st dorsal interosseous m.
— Articular capsule
Extensor expansion —

Medial View

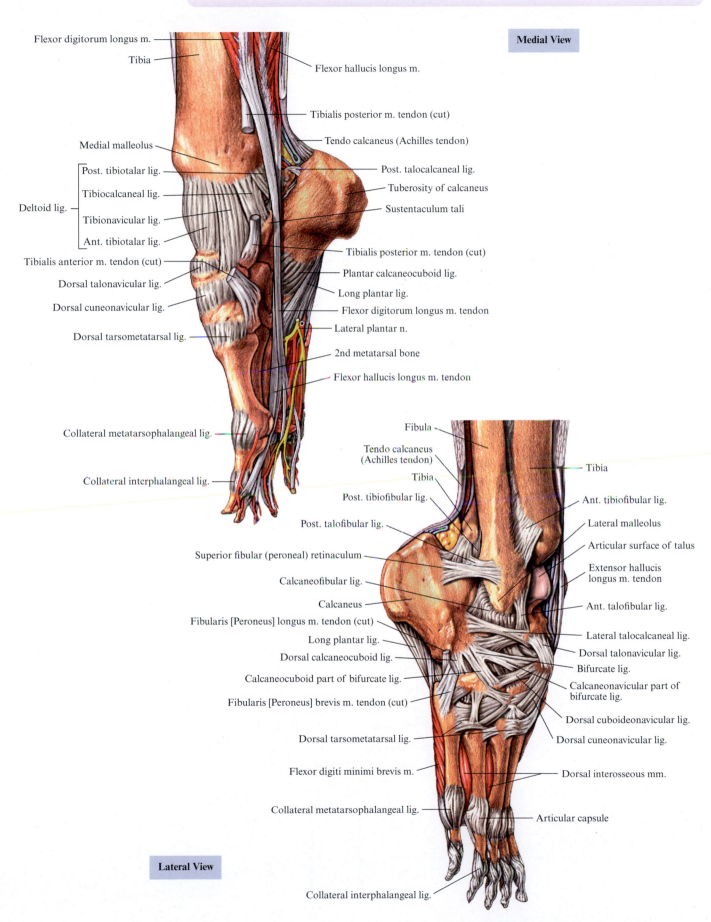

Flexor digitorum longus m.

Tibia

Flexor hallucis longus m.

Tibialis posterior m. tendon (cut)

Tendo calcaneus (Achilles tendon)

Medial malleolus

Post. talocalcaneal lig.

Post. tibiotalar lig.

Tibiocalcaneal lig.

Tuberosity of calcaneus

Deltoid lig.

Sustentaculum tali

Tibionavicular lig.

Ant. tibiotalar lig.

Tibialis posterior m. tendon (cut)

Tibialis anterior m. tendon (cut)

Plantar calcaneocuboid lig.

Dorsal talonavicular lig.

Long plantar lig.

Dorsal cuneonavicular lig.

Flexor digitorum longus m. tendon

Lateral plantar n.

Dorsal tarsometatarsal lig.

2nd metatarsal bone

Flexor hallucis longus m. tendon

Collateral metatarsophalangeal lig.

Collateral interphalangeal lig.

Fibula

Tendo calcaneus
(Achilles tendon)

Tibia

Tibia

Post. tibiofibular lig.

Ant. tibiofibular lig.

Post. talofibular lig.

Lateral malleolus

Superior fibular (peroneal) retinaculum

Articular surface of talus

Calcaneofibular lig.

Extensor hallucis
longus m. tendon

Calcaneus

Ant. talofibular lig.

Fibularis [Peroneus] longus m. tendon (cut)

Lateral talocalcaneal lig.

Long plantar lig.

Dorsal talonavicular lig.

Dorsal calcaneocuboid lig.

Bifurcate lig.

Calcaneocuboid part of bifurcate lig.

Calcaneonavicular part of
bifurcate lig.

Fibularis [Peroneus] brevis m. tendon (cut)

Dorsal cuboideonavicular lig.

Dorsal tarsometatarsal lig.

Dorsal cuneonavicular lig.

Flexor digiti minimi brevis m.

Dorsal interosseous mm.

Collateral metatarsophalangeal lig.

Articular capsule

Lateral View

Collateral interphalangeal lig.

PLATE 5.59   FOOT—SKELETON

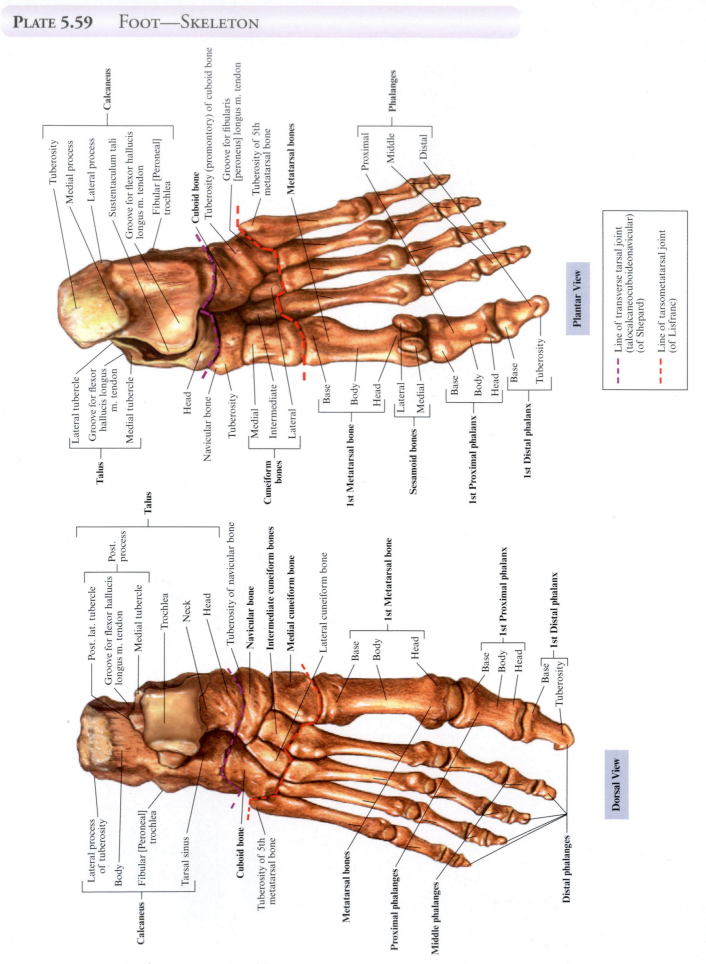

Plantar View

Tuberosity
Medial process
Lateral process
Sustentaculum tali
Groove for flexor hallucis longus m. tendon
Fibular [Peroneal] trochlea
Calcaneus

Cuboid bone
Tuberosity (promontory) of cuboid bone
Groove for fibularis [peroneus] longus m. tendon
Tuberosity of 5th metatarsal bone
Metatarsal bones

Proximal
Middle
Distal
Phalanges

Lateral tubercle
Groove for flexor hallucis longus m. tendon
Medial tubercle
Talus

Head
Navicular bone
Tuberosity

Medial
Intermediate
Lateral
Cuneiform bones

Base
Body
Head

Lateral
Medial
Sesamoid bones

Base
Body
Head
1st Proximal phalanx

Base
Tuberosity
1st Distal phalanx

1st Metatarsal bone

Line of transverse tarsal joint (talocalcaneocuboideonavicular) (of Shepard)
Line of tarsometatarsal joint (of Lisfranc)

Dorsal View

Talus
Post. process

Post. lat. tubercle
Groove for flexor hallucis longus m. tendon
Medial tubercle
Trochlea
Neck
Head
Tuberosity of navicular bone
Navicular bone
Intermediate cuneiform bones
Medial cuneiform bone
Lateral cuneiform bone
1st Metatarsal bone

Base
Body
Head
1st Proximal phalanx

Base
Body
Head

Base
Tuberosity
1st Distal phalanx

Lateral process of tuberosity
Body
Fibular [Peroneal] trochlea
Tarsal sinus
Calcaneus

Cuboid bone
Tuberosity of 5th metatarsal bone

Metatarsal bones

Proximal phalanges

Middle phalanges

Distal phalanges

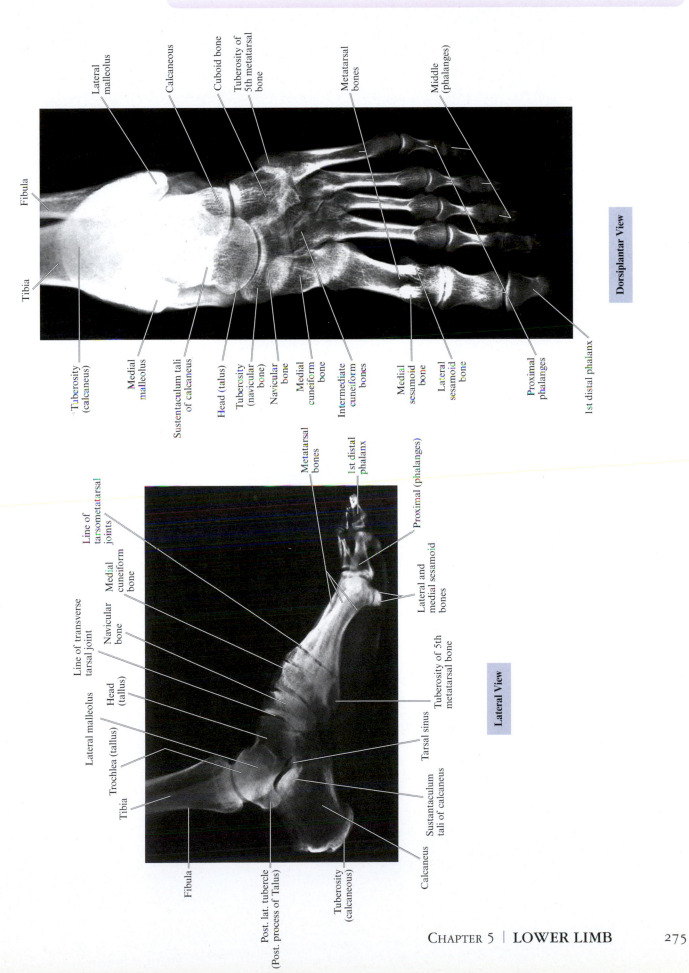

Dorsiplantar View

Lateral malleolus

Calcaneous

Cuboid bone

Tuberosity of 5th metatarsal bone

Metatarsal bones

Middle (phalanges)

Fibula

Tibia

Tuberosity (calcaneus)

Medial malleolus

Sustentaculum tali of calcaneus

Head (talus)

Tuberosity (navicular bone)

Navicular bone

Medial cuneiform bone

Intermediate cuneiform bones

Medial sesamoid bone

Lateral sesamoid bone

Proximal phalanges

1st distal phalanx

Lateral View

Metatarsal bones

1st distal phalanx

Proximal (phalanges)

Line of tarsometatarsal joints

Medial cuneiform bone

Navicular bone

Line of transverse tarsal joint

Head (tallus)

Lateral malleolus

Trochlea (tallus)

Tibia

Fibula

Post. lat. tubercle (Post. process of Talus)

Tuberosity (calcaneous)

Calcaneus

Sustantaculum tali of calcaneus

Tarsal sinus

Tuberosity of 5th metatarsal bone

Lateral and medial sesamoid bones

6 UPPER LIMB

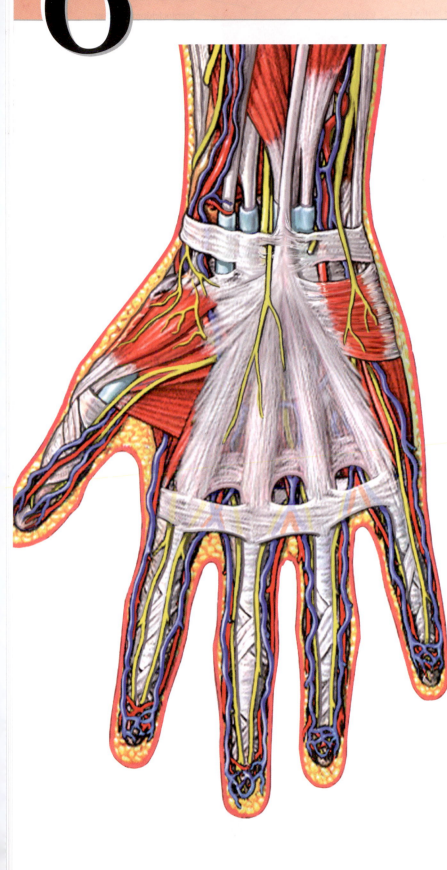

TABLE 6.2   SCAPULAR & POSTERIOR ARM MUSCLES

Scapular Muscles

Muscle	Proximal/Medial Attachment	Distal/Lateral Attachment	Innervation[a]	Main Actions
Deltoid	Lateral third of clavicle, acromion & spine of scapula	Deltoid tuberosity of humerus	Axillary n. (**C5** & C6)	*Anterior part:* flexes & medially rotates arm *Middle part:* abducts arm *Posterior part:* extends & laterally rotates arm
Supraspinatus[a]	Supraspinous fossa of scapula	Sup. facet on greater tubercle of humerus	Suprascapular n. (C4, **C5** & C6)	Helps deltoid to abduct arm[a]
Infraspinatus[a]	Infraspinous fossa of scapula	Middle facet on greater tubercle of humerus	Suprascapular n. (C4, **C5** & C6)	Laterally rotates arm; helps to hold humeral head in glenoid cavity of scapula
Teres minor[a]	Sup. part of lateral border of scapula	Inf. facet on greater tubercle of humerus	Axillary n. (**C5** & C6)	
Teres major	Dorsal surface of inf. angle of scapula	Medial lip of intertubular groove of humerus	Lower subscapular n. (**C6** & C7)	Adducts & medially rotates arm
Subscapularis[a]	Subscapular fossa	Lesser tubercle of humerus	Upper & lower subscapular nn. (C5, **C6** & C7)	Medially rotates arm & adducts it; helps to hold humeral head in glenoid cavity

[a]Collectively, the supraspinatus, infraspinatus, teres minor, and subscapularis muscles are referred to as the **rotator cuff muscles**. Their prime function during all movements of the shoulder joint is to hold the head of the humerus in the glenoid cavity of the scapula.

Posterior Arm Muscles

Muscle	Proximal Attachment	Distal Attachment	Innervation	Main Actions
Triceps brachii	*Long head:* infraglenoid tubercle of scapula *Lateral head:* post. surface of humerus, sup. to radial n. groove *Medial head:* post. surface of humerus, inf. to radial n. groove	Proximal end of olecranon ulna & fascia of forearm	Radial n. (**C6, C7,** & C8)	Extends the forearm; it is *chief extensor of forearm,* long head steadies head of abducted humerus
Anconeus	Lateral epicondyle of humerus	Lateral surface of olecranon & sup. part of post. surface of ulna	Radial n. (C7, C8 & T1)	Assists triceps in extending forearm; stabilizes elbow joint; abducts ulna during pronation

Sup. angle of scapula

Lesser tubercle of humerus

Subscapularis m.

Coracoid process of scapula

Coracobrachialis m.

Crest of lesser tubercle

Subscapular fossa

Anterior Views

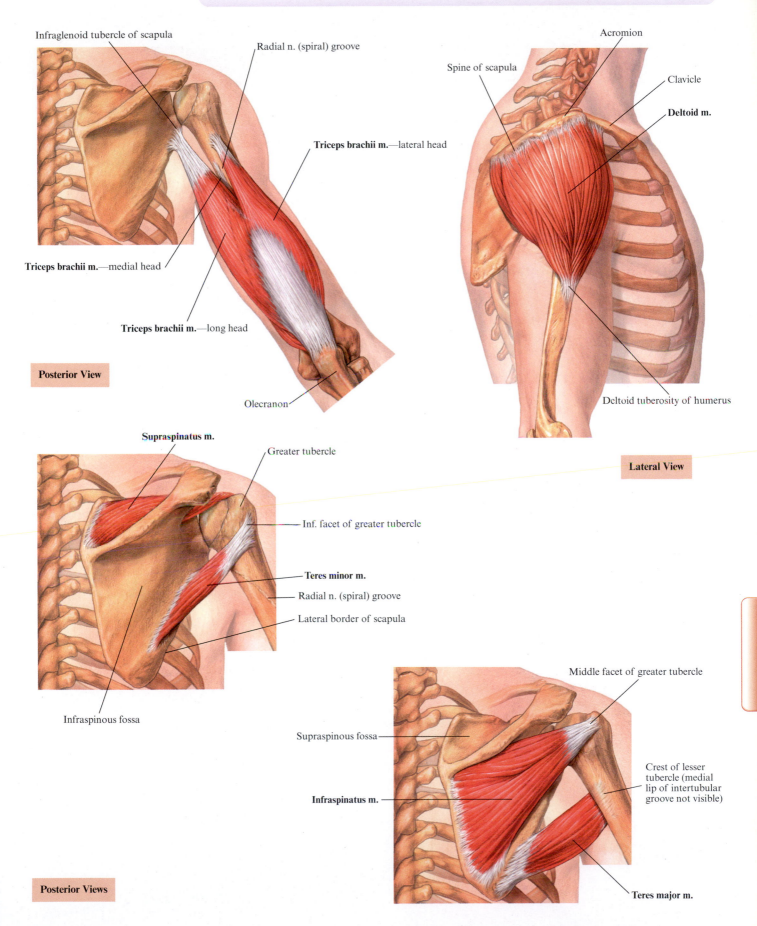

Infraglenoid tubercle of scapula

Radial n. (spiral) groove

Acromion

Spine of scapula

Clavicle

Deltoid m.

Triceps brachii m.—lateral head

Triceps brachii m.—medial head

Triceps brachii m.—long head

Posterior View

Olecranon

Deltoid tuberosity of humerus

Lateral View

Supraspinatus m.

Greater tubercle

Inf. facet of greater tubercle

Teres minor m.

Radial n. (spiral) groove

Lateral border of scapula

Infraspinous fossa

Middle facet of greater tubercle

Supraspinous fossa

Crest of lesser tubercle (medial lip of intertubular groove not visible)

Infraspinatus m.

Posterior Views

Teres major m.

TABLE **6.3**   ANTERIOR ARM & FOREARM MUSCLES

Muscles of Anterior Arm

Muscle	Proximal Attachment	Distal Attachment	Innervation[a]	Main Actions
Biceps brachii	*Short head:* Tip of coracoid process of scapula *Long head:* Supraglenoid tubercle of scapula	Tuberosity of radius & fascia of forearm via bicipital aponeurosis	Musculocutaneous n. (C5 & **C6**)	Supinates forearm and, when it is supine, flexes forearm
Brachialis	Distal half of ant. surface of humerus	Coronoid process & tuberosity of ulna		Flexes forearm in all positions
Coracobrachialis	Tip of coracoid process of scapula	Middle third of medial surface of humerus	Musculocutaneous n. (C5, **C6** & C7)	Helps to flex & adduct arm

Superficial and Intermediate Layers of Muscles on Anterior Surface of Forearm[a]

Muscle	Proximal Attachment	Distal Attachment	Innervation[a]	Main Actions
Pronator teres	Medial epicondyle of humerus & coronoid process of ulna	Middle of lateral surface of radius	Median n. (C6 & **C7**)	Pronates forearm & flexes it
Flexor carpi radialis	Medial epicondyle of humerus	Base of 2nd metacarpal bone		Flexes hand & abducts it radially
Palmaris longus	Medial epicondyle of humerus	Distal half of flexor retinaculum & palmar aponeurosis	Median n. (C7 & C8)	Flexes hand & tightens palmar aponeurosis
Flexor carpi ulnaris[b]	*Humeral head:* medial epicondyle of humerus *Ulnar head:* olecranon & post. border of ulna	Pisiform bone (hook of hamate bone & 5th metacarpal bone)	Ulnar n. (C7 & **C8**)	Flexes hand & adducts it ulnarly
Flexor digitorum superficialis[c]	*Humeroulnar head:* medial epicondyle of humerus, ulnar collateral lig. & coronoid process of ulna *Radial head:* sup. half of ant. border of radius	Bodies of the middle phalanges of medial four digits	Median n. (C7, **C8** & T1)	Flexes middle of phalanges of medial four digits; acting more strongly, it flexes proximal phalanges & hand

[a]The superficial muscles of the *flexor-pronator group* are attached, in whole or in part, to the anterior surface of the medial epicondyle by a *common flexor tendon.*
[b]In contrast to the other superficial flexor muscles, the flexor carpi ulnaris is supplied by the ulnar nerve.
[c]This muscle comprises the *intermediate muscle layer* in the anterior part of the forearm. In some clinical texts, this muscle is referred to by its old name, "flexor digitorum sublimis."

Deep Layer of Muscles on Anterior Surface of Forearm

Muscle	Proximal Attachment	Distal Attachment	Innervation	Main Actions
Pronator quadratus	Distal fourth of ant. surface of ulna	Distal fourth of ant. surface of radius	Ant. interosseous n. from median (**C8** & T1)	Pronates forearm; deep fibers bind radius & ulna together

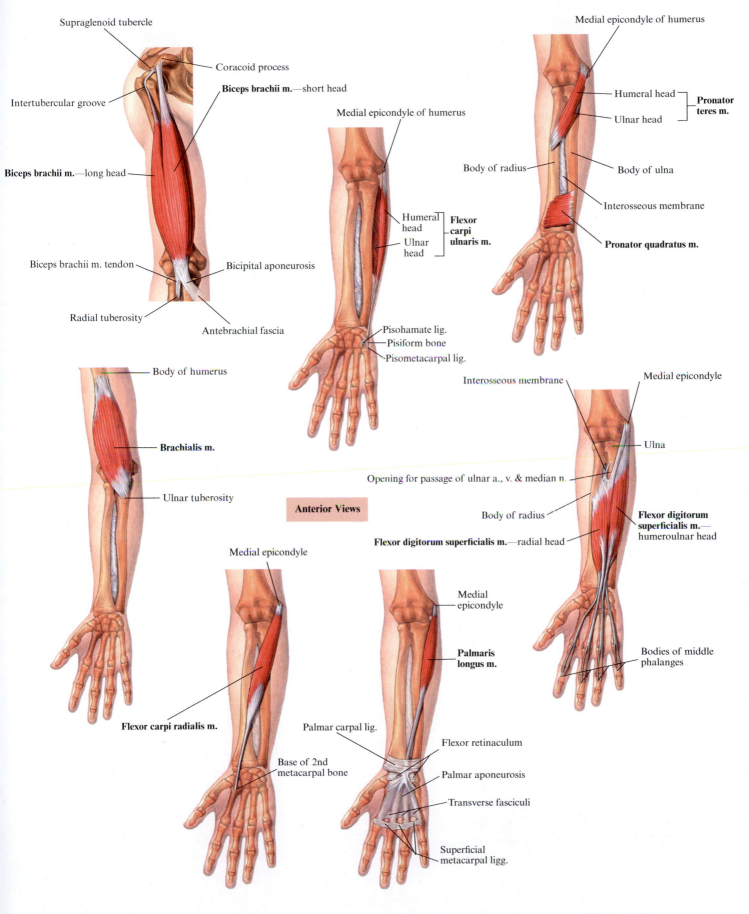

Supraglenoid tubercle

Coracoid process

Biceps brachii m.—short head

Intertubercular groove

Medial epicondyle of humerus

Medial epicondyle of humerus

Biceps brachii m.—long head

Humeral head
Ulnar head

Pronator teres m.

Body of radius

Body of ulna

Interosseous membrane

Biceps brachii m. tendon

Bicipital aponeurosis

Humeral head
Ulnar head

Flexor carpi ulnaris m.

Pronator quadratus m.

Radial tuberosity

Antebrachial fascia

Body of humerus

Pisohamate lig.
Pisiform bone
Pisometacarpal lig.

Interosseous membrane

Medial epicondyle

Brachialis m.

Ulna

Opening for passage of ulnar a., v. & median n.

Ulnar tuberosity

Anterior Views

Body of radius

Flexor digitorum superficialis m.—radial head

Flexor digitorum superficialis m.— humeroulnar head

Medial epicondyle

Medial epicondyle

Bodies of middle phalanges

Palmaris longus m.

Flexor carpi radialis m.

Palmar carpal lig.

Flexor retinaculum

Base of 2nd metacarpal bone

Palmar aponeurosis

Transverse fasciculi

Superficial metacarpal ligg.

TABLE 6.4 FOREARM MUSCLES

Deep Layer of Muscles on Anterior Surface of Forearm

Muscle	Proximal Attachment	Distal Attachment	Innervation	Main Actions
Flexor digitorum profundus	Proximal three-fourths of medial & ant. surfaces of ulna & interosseous membrane	Bases of distal phalanges of medial four digits	*Medial part:* Ulnar n. (**C8** & T1) *Lateral part:* Median n. (**C8** & T1)	Flexes distal phalanges of medial four digits (fingers)
Flexor pollicis longus	Ant. surface of the distal radius & adjacent interosseous membrane	Base of distal phalanx of thumb	Ant. interosseous n. from Median n. (**C8** & T1)	Flexes phalanges of first digit (thumb)

Superficial Muscles on Posterior or Extensor Surface of Forearm

Muscle	Proximal Attachment	Distal Attachment	Innervation	Main Actions
Brachioradialis	Proximal two-thirds of lateral supracondylar ridge of humerus, lat. intermuscular septum	Lateral surface of distal end of radius	Radial n. (C5, **C6** & C7)	Flexes forearm
Extensor carpi radialis longus	Lateral supracondylar ridge of humerus, lat. intermuscular septum	Base of 2nd metacarpal bone	Radial n. (**C6** & C7)	Extend & abduct hand at wrist joint
Extensor carpi radialis brevis	Lateral epicondyle of humerus	Base of 3rd metacarpal bone	Deep br. of radial n. (**C7** & C8)	
Extensor digitorum	Lateral epicondyle of humerus	Extensor expansions of medial four digits	Post. interosseous n. (**C7** & C8), a br. of the radial n.	Extends medial four digits at metacarpophalangeal joints; extends hand at wrist joint
Extensor carpi ulnaris	Lateral epicondyle of humerus & post. border of ulna	Base of 5th metacarpal bone		Extends & adducts hand at wrist joint

Body of radius

Flexor pollicis longus m.

Trapezium bone

Base of distal phalanx of thumb

Interosseous membrane

Anterior View

Lateral epicondyle

Extensor carpi ulnaris m.

Base of 5th metacarpal bone

Posterior View

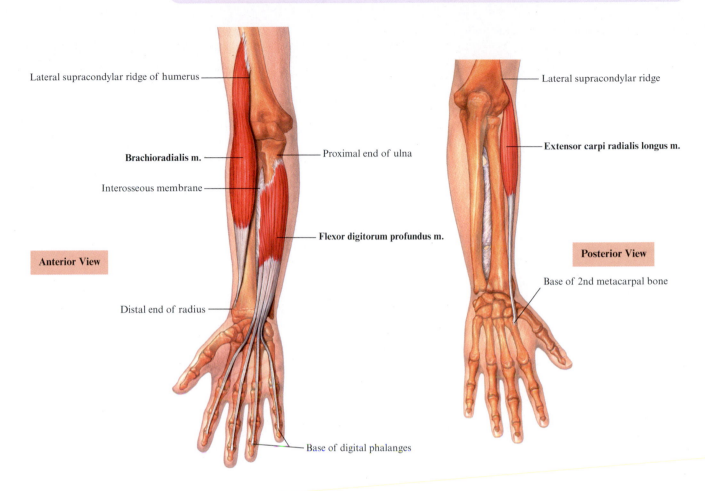

Lateral supracondylar ridge of humerus

Brachioradialis m.

Interosseous membrane

Anterior View

Distal end of radius

Proximal end of ulna

Flexor digitorum profundus m.

Base of digital phalanges

Lateral supracondylar ridge

Extensor carpi radialis longus m.

Posterior View

Base of 2nd metacarpal bone

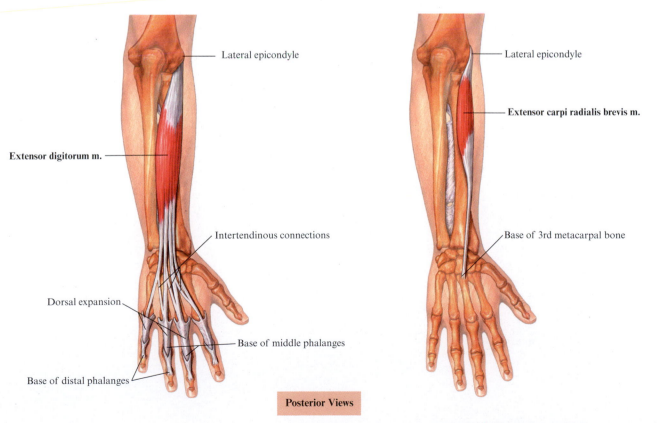

Lateral epicondyle

Extensor digitorum m.

Intertendinous connections

Dorsal expansion

Base of middle phalanges

Base of distal phalanges

Posterior Views

Lateral epicondyle

Extensor carpi radialis brevis m.

Base of 3rd metacarpal bone

TABLE **6.5** POSTERIOR FOREARM MUSCLES

Deep Muscles on Posterior or Extensor Surface of Forearm

Muscle	Proximal Attachment	Distal Attachment	Innervation	Main Actions
Supinator	Lateral epicondyle of humerus, radial collateral & anular ligaments, supinator fossa & crest of ulna	Lateral, post. & ant. surfaces of proximal third of radius	Deep br. of radial n. (C5 & **C6**)	Supinates forearm, *i.e.,* rotates radius to turn palm anteriorly
Abductor pollicis longus	Post. surfaces of ulna & radius & interosseous membrane	Base of 1st metacarpalbone	Post. interosseous n. (C7 & **C8**)	Abducts thumb & extends it at carpometacarpal joint
Extensor pollicis brevis	Post. surface of radius & interosseous membrane	Base of proximal phalanx of thumb		Extends proximal phalanx of thumb at carpometacarpal joint
Extensor pollicis longus	Post. surface of middle third of ulnar & interosseous membrane	Base of distal phalanx of thumb		Extends distal phalanx of thumb at metacarpophalangeal & interphalangeal joints
Extensor indicis	Post. surface of ulna & interosseous membrane	Extensor expansion of second digit (index finger)		Extends digit 2 & helps to extend wrist
Extensor digit minimi	Lateral epicondyle of humerus	Extensor expansion of 5th digit	Post. interosseous n. (**C7** & C8), a br. of the radial n.	Extends digit 5 at metacarpophalangeal & interphalangeal joints

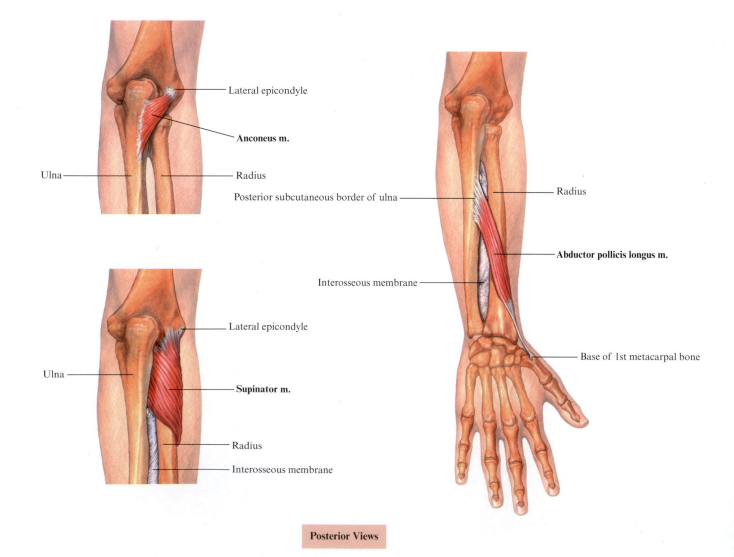

Posterior Views

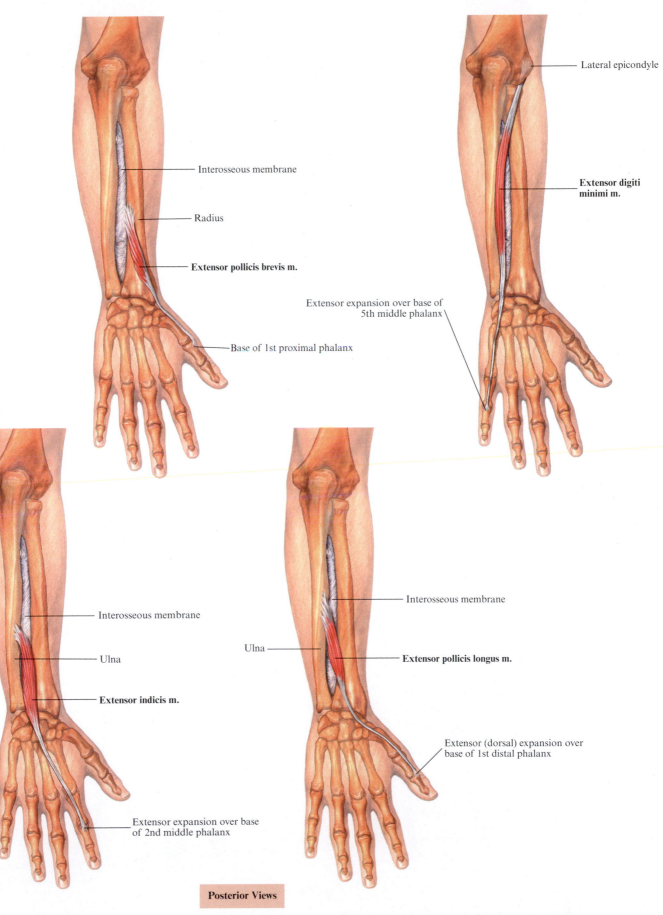

Interosseous membrane

Radius

Extensor pollicis brevis m.

Base of 1st proximal phalanx

Lateral epicondyle

Extensor digiti minimi m.

Extensor expansion over base of 5th middle phalanx

Interosseous membrane

Ulna

Extensor indicis m.

Extensor expansion over base of 2nd middle phalanx

Interosseous membrane

Ulna

Extensor pollicis longus m.

Extensor (dorsal) expansion over base of 1st distal phalanx

Posterior Views

TABLE 6.6   INTRINSIC HAND MUSCLES

Short Muscles of Hand

Muscle	Proximal Attachment	Distal Attachment	Innervation	Main Actions
Lumbricalis 1 & 2	Lateral two tendons of flex or digitorum profundus	Lateral sides of extensor expansions of digits 2 to 5	*Lumbricals 1 & 2,* median n. (C8 & **T1**)	Flex digits at metacarpophalangeal joints & extend interphalangeal joints
Lumbricalis 3 & 4	Medial three tendons of flex or digitorum profundus		*Lumbricals 3 & 4,* deep br. of ulnar n. (C8 & **T1**)	
Dorsal interossei 1–4	Adjacent sides of two metacarpal bones	Extensor expansion & bases of proximal phalanges of digits 2–4	Deep br. of ulnar n. (C8 & **T1**)	Abduct digits 2–4
Palmar interossei 1–3	Palmar surfaces of 1st, 2nd, 4th & 5th metacarpal bones	Extensor expansions of digits and bases of proximal phalanges of digits 1, 2, 4 & 5		Adduct digits 2–4
Abductor digiti minimi	Pisiform bone	Medial side of base of proximal phalanx of digit 5 (little finger)	Deep br. of ulnar n. (C8 & **T1**)	Abducts digit 5 (little finger)
Flexor digiti minimi brevis	Hook of hamate bone & flex or retinaculum			Flexes proximal phalanx of digit 5
Opponens digiti minimi		Medial border of 5th metacarpal bone		Draws 5th metacarpal bone anteriorly & rotates it, bringing digit 5 into opposition with thumb
Abductor pollicis brevis	Flexor retinaculum & tubercles of scaphoid & trapezium bones	Lateral side of base of proximal phalanx of thumb	Recurrent br. of median n. (**C8** & T1)	Abducts thumb & helps oppose it
Flexor pollicis brevis	Flexor retinaculum & tubercle of trapezium bone			Flexes thumb
Opponens pollicis		Lateral side of 1st metacarpal bone		Opposes thumb toward center of palm & rotates it medially
Adductor pollicis	*Oblique head:* Bases of 2nd & 3rd metacarpals, captate & adjacent carpal bones *Transverse head:* Ant. surface of body of 3rd metacarpal bone	Medial side of base of proximal phalanx of thumb	Deep br. of ulnar n. (C8 & **T1**)	Adducts thumb toward middle digit

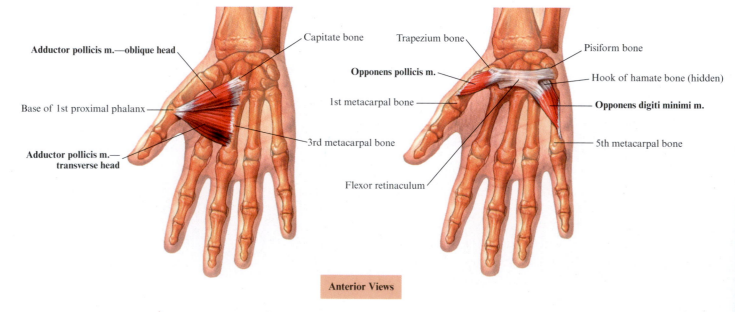

Anterior Views

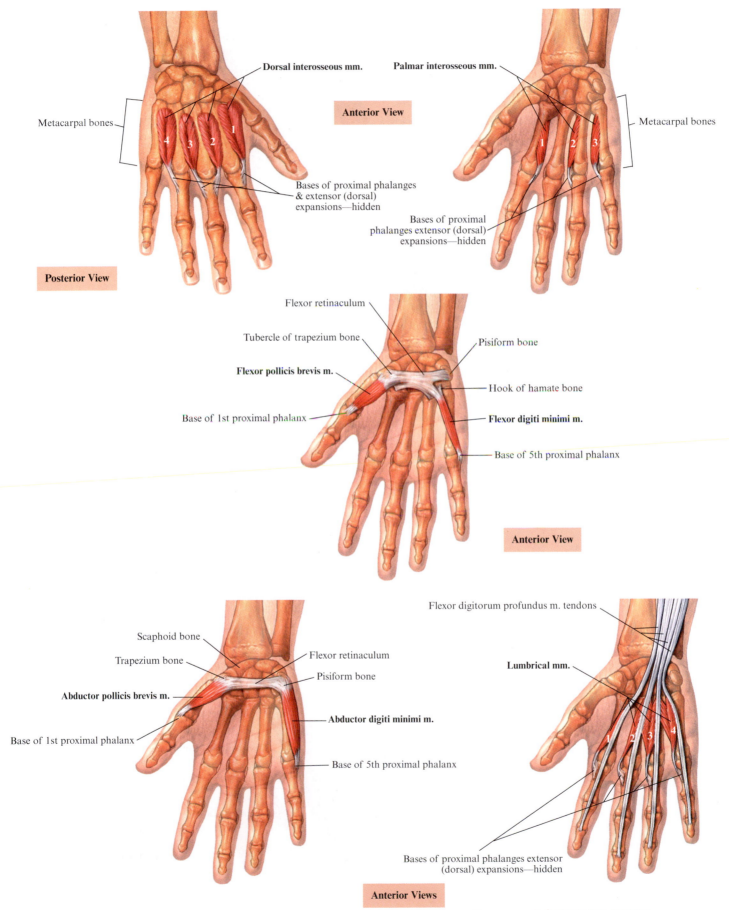

Dorsal interosseous mm.

Palmar interosseous mm.

Anterior View

Metacarpal bones

4 3 2 1

1 2 3

Metacarpal bones

Bases of proximal phalanges
& extensor (dorsal)
expansions—hidden

Bases of proximal
phalanges extensor (dorsal)
expansions—hidden

Posterior View

Flexor retinaculum

Tubercle of trapezium bone

Pisiform bone

Flexor pollicis brevis m.

Hook of hamate bone

Base of 1st proximal phalanx

Flexor digiti minimi m.

Base of 5th proximal phalanx

Anterior View

Scaphoid bone

Flexor digitorum profundus m. tendons

Trapezium bone

Flexor retinaculum

Lumbrical mm.

Pisiform bone

Abductor pollicis brevis m.

Abductor digiti minimi m.

Base of 1st proximal phalanx

1 2 3 4

Base of 5th proximal phalanx

Bases of proximal phalanges extensor
(dorsal) expansions—hidden

Anterior Views

CHAPTER 6 | **UPPER LIMB**   295

PLATE 6.15   VEINS OF UPPER LIMB

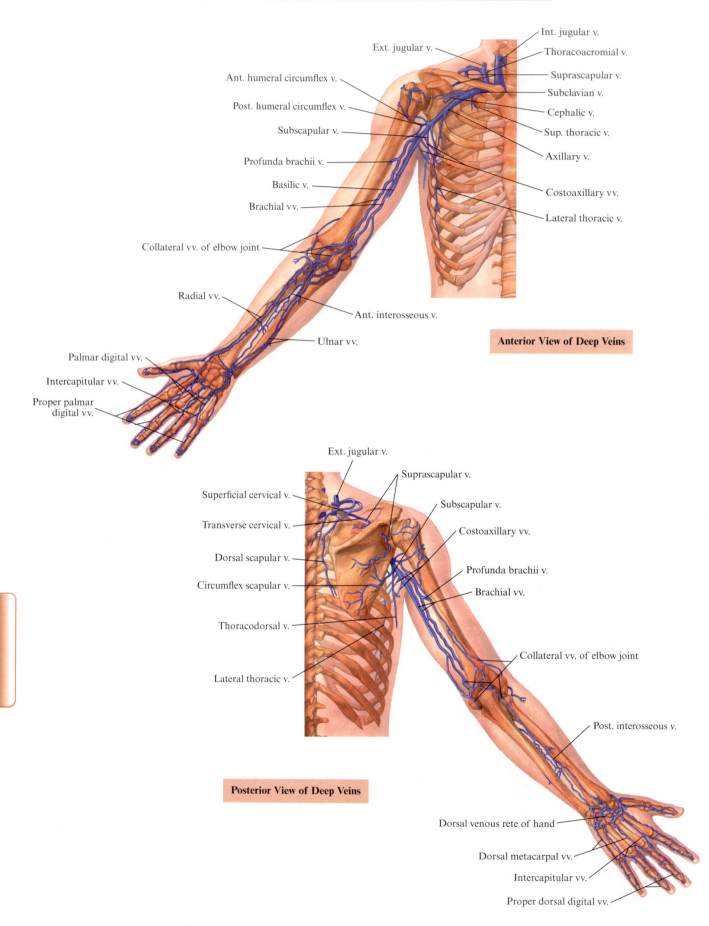

Int. jugular v.

Ext. jugular v.

Thoracoacromial v.

Ant. humeral circumflex v.

Suprascapular v.

Post. humeral circumflex v.

Subclavian v.

Subscapular v.

Cephalic v.

Profunda brachii v.

Sup. thoracic v.

Basilic v.

Axillary v.

Brachial vv.

Costoaxillary vv.

Collateral vv. of elbow joint

Lateral thoracic v.

Radial vv.

Ant. interosseous v.

Palmar digital vv.

Ulnar vv.

Intercapitular vv.

Proper palmar
digital vv.

Anterior View of Deep Veins

Ext. jugular v.

Suprascapular v.

Superficial cervical v.

Subscapular v.

Transverse cervical v.

Costoaxillary vv.

Dorsal scapular v.

Profunda brachii v.

Circumflex scapular v.

Brachial vv.

Thoracodorsal v.

Collateral vv. of elbow joint

Lateral thoracic v.

Post. interosseous v.

Posterior View of Deep Veins

Dorsal venous rete of hand

Dorsal metacarpal vv.

Intercapitular vv.

Proper dorsal digital vv.

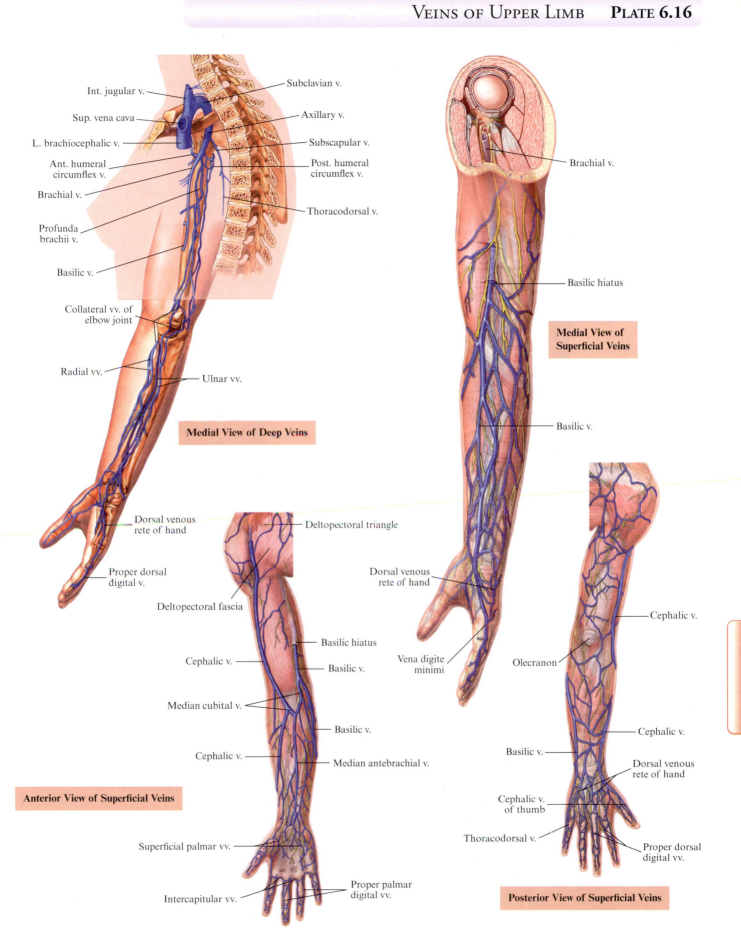

Int. jugular v.

Sup. vena cava

L. brachiocephalic v.

Ant. humeral circumflex v.

Brachial v.

Profunda brachii v.

Basilic v.

Collateral vv. of elbow joint

Radial vv.

Subclavian v.

Axillary v.

Subscapular v.

Post. humeral circumflex v.

Thoracodorsal v.

Ulnar vv.

Medial View of Deep Veins

Dorsal venous rete of hand

Proper dorsal digital v.

Brachial v.

Basilic hiatus

Medial View of Superficial Veins

Basilic v.

Deltopectoral triangle

Deltopectoral fascia

Cephalic v.

Median cubital v.

Cephalic v.

Basilic hiatus

Basilic v.

Basilic v.

Median antebrachial v.

Anterior View of Superficial Veins

Superficial palmar vv.

Intercapitular vv.

Proper palmar digital vv.

Dorsal venous rete of hand

Vena digite minimi

Cephalic v.

Olecranon

Basilic v.

Cephalic v. of thumb

Thoracodorsal v.

Cephalic v.

Cephalic v.

Dorsal venous rete of hand

Proper dorsal digital vv.

Posterior View of Superficial Veins

PLATE 6.19   DERMATOMES & CUTANEOUS NERVES

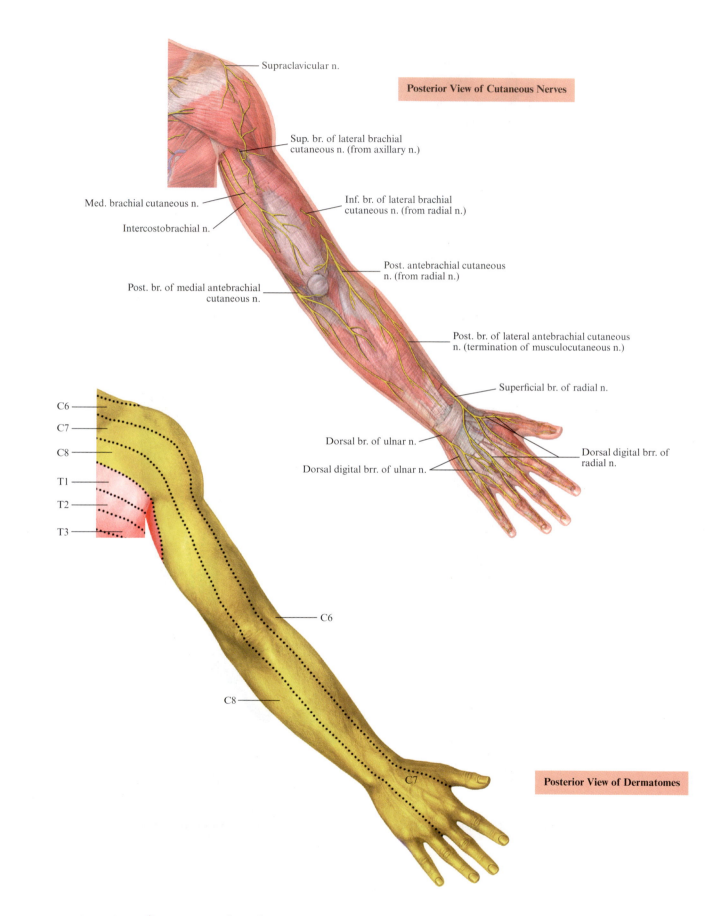

Supraclavicular n.

Posterior View of Cutaneous Nerves

Sup. br. of lateral brachial cutaneous n. (from axillary n.)

Med. brachial cutaneous n.

Intercostobrachial n.

Inf. br. of lateral brachial cutaneous n. (from radial n.)

Post. antebrachial cutaneous n. (from radial n.)

Post. br. of medial antebrachial cutaneous n.

Post. br. of lateral antebrachial cutaneous n. (termination of musculocutaneous n.)

Superficial br. of radial n.

Dorsal br. of ulnar n.

Dorsal digital brr. of ulnar n.

Dorsal digital brr. of radial n.

C6
C7
C8
T1
T2
T3

C6

C8

C7

Posterior View of Dermatomes

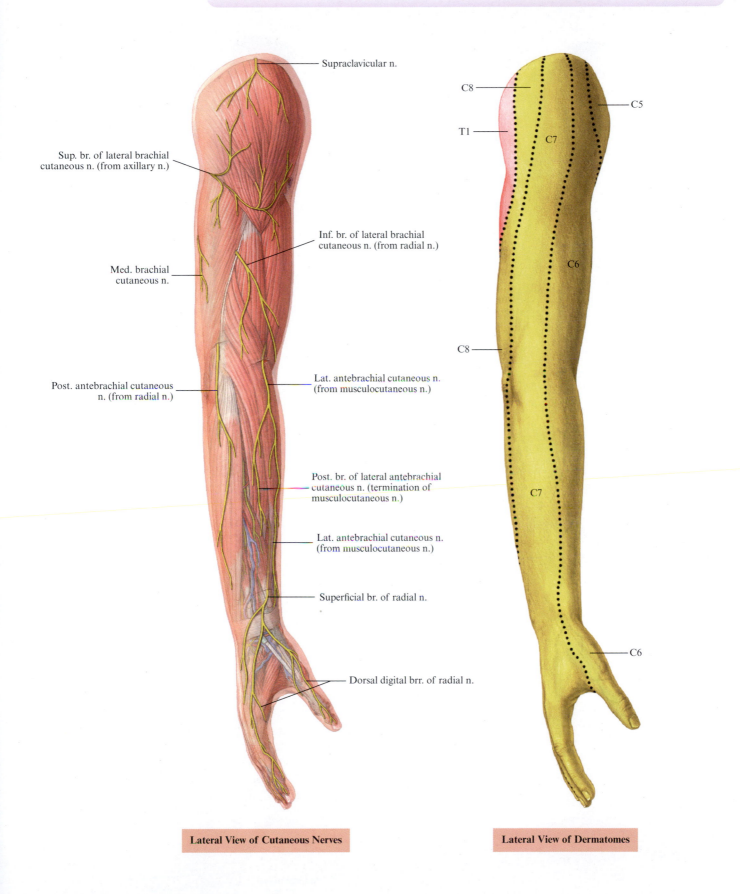

Supraclavicular n.

Sup. br. of lateral brachial
cutaneous n. (from axillary n.)

Inf. br. of lateral brachial
cutaneous n. (from radial n.)

Med. brachial
cutaneous n.

Lat. antebrachial cutaneous n.
(from musculocutaneous n.)

Post. antebrachial cutaneous
n. (from radial n.)

Post. br. of lateral antebrachial
cutaneous n. (termination of
musculocutaneous n.)

Lat. antebrachial cutaneous n.
(from musculocutaneous n.)

Superficial br. of radial n.

Dorsal digital brr. of radial n.

C8

T1

C5

C7

C6

C8

C7

C6

Lateral View of Cutaneous Nerves

Lateral View of Dermatomes

PLATE 6.21   SEGMENTAL INNERVATION OF JOINT ACTIONS

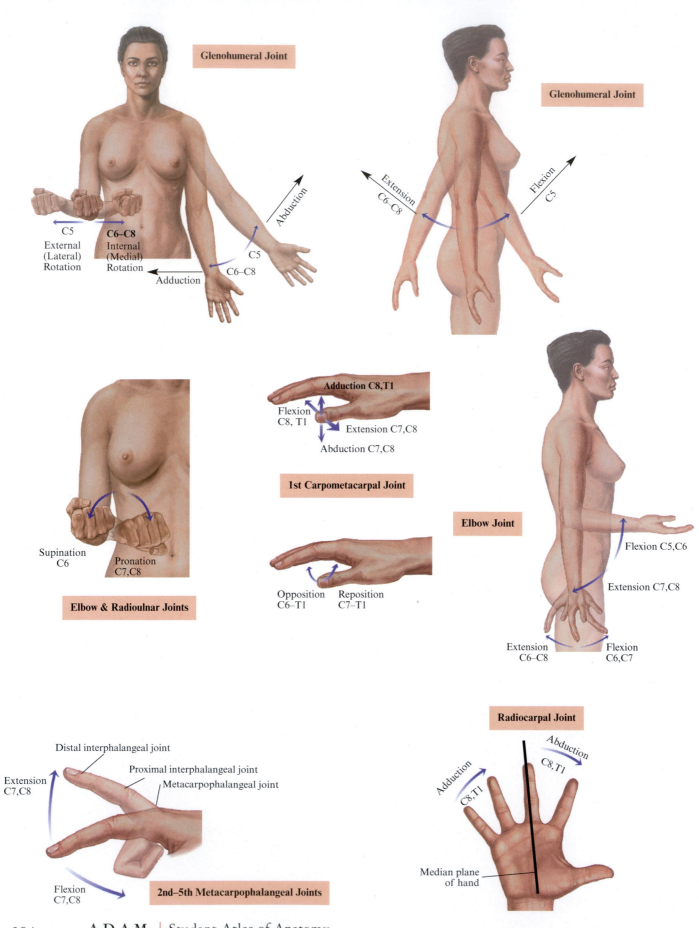

Glenohumeral Joint

Abduction

C5
External
(Lateral)
Rotation

C6–C8
Internal
(Medial)
Rotation

C5

C6–C8
Adduction

Glenohumeral Joint

Extension
C6–C8

Flexion
C5

Supination
C6

Pronation
C7,C8

Elbow & Radioulnar Joints

Adduction C8,T1

Flexion
C8, T1

Extension C7,C8

Abduction C7,C8

1st Carpometacarpal Joint

Opposition
C6–T1

Reposition
C7–T1

Elbow Joint

Flexion C5,C6

Extension C7,C8

Extension
C6–C8

Flexion
C6,C7

Distal interphalangeal joint

Proximal interphalangeal joint

Metacarpophalangeal joint

Extension
C7,C8

Flexion
C7,C8

2nd–5th Metacarpophalangeal Joints

Radiocarpal Joint

Abduction

C8,T1

Adduction

C8,T1

Median plane
of hand

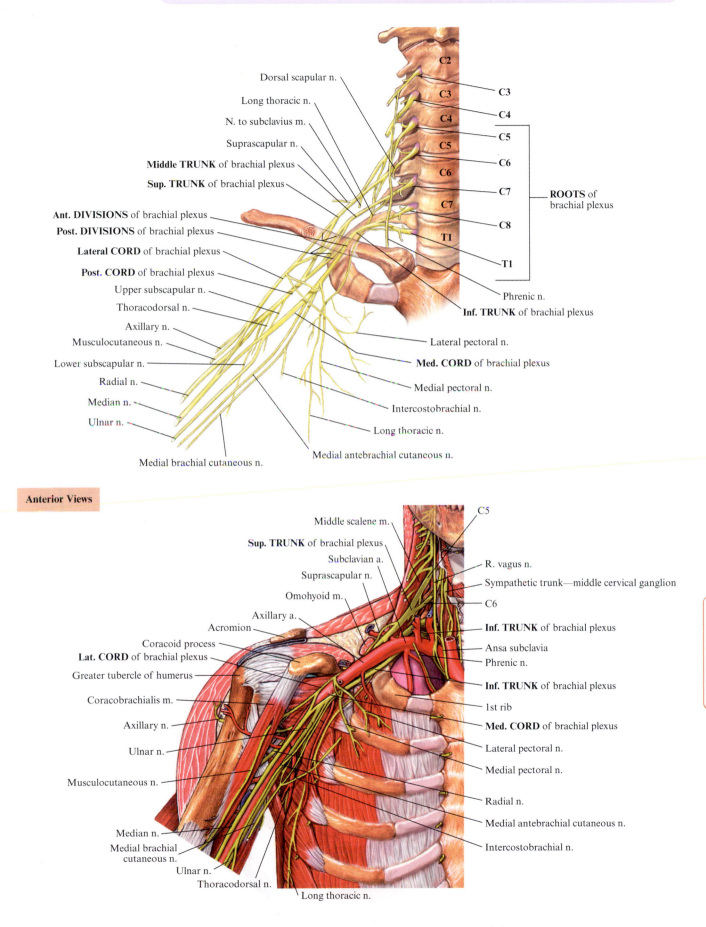

Dorsal scapular n.

Long thoracic n.

N. to subclavius m.

Suprascapular n.

Middle TRUNK of brachial plexus

Sup. TRUNK of brachial plexus

Ant. DIVISIONS of brachial plexus

Post. DIVISIONS of brachial plexus

Lateral CORD of brachial plexus

Post. CORD of brachial plexus

Upper subscapular n.

Thoracodorsal n.

Axillary n.

Musculocutaneous n.

Lower subscapular n.

Radial n.

Median n.

Ulnar n.

Medial brachial cutaneous n.

C2

C3

C4

C5

C6

C7

C8

T1

C3
C4
C5
C6
C7
C8
T1

ROOTS of
brachial plexus

Phrenic n.

Inf. TRUNK of brachial plexus

Lateral pectoral n.

Med. CORD of brachial plexus

Medial pectoral n.

Intercostobrachial n.

Long thoracic n.

Medial antebrachial cutaneous n.

Anterior Views

Middle scalene m.

Sup. TRUNK of brachial plexus

Subclavian a.

Suprascapular n.

Omohyoid m.

Axillary a.

Acromion

Coracoid process

Lat. CORD of brachial plexus

Greater tubercle of humerus

Coracobrachialis m.

Axillary n.

Ulnar n.

Musculocutaneous n.

Median n.

Medial brachial
cutaneous n.

Ulnar n.

Thoracodorsal n.

Long thoracic n.

C5

R. vagus n.

Sympathetic trunk—middle cervical ganglion

C6

Inf. TRUNK of brachial plexus

Ansa subclavia

Phrenic n.

Inf. TRUNK of brachial plexus

1st rib

Med. CORD of brachial plexus

Lateral pectoral n.

Medial pectoral n.

Radial n.

Medial antebrachial cutaneous n.

Intercostobrachial n.

PLATE 6.25 SUPERFICIAL & DEEP LYMPHATICS

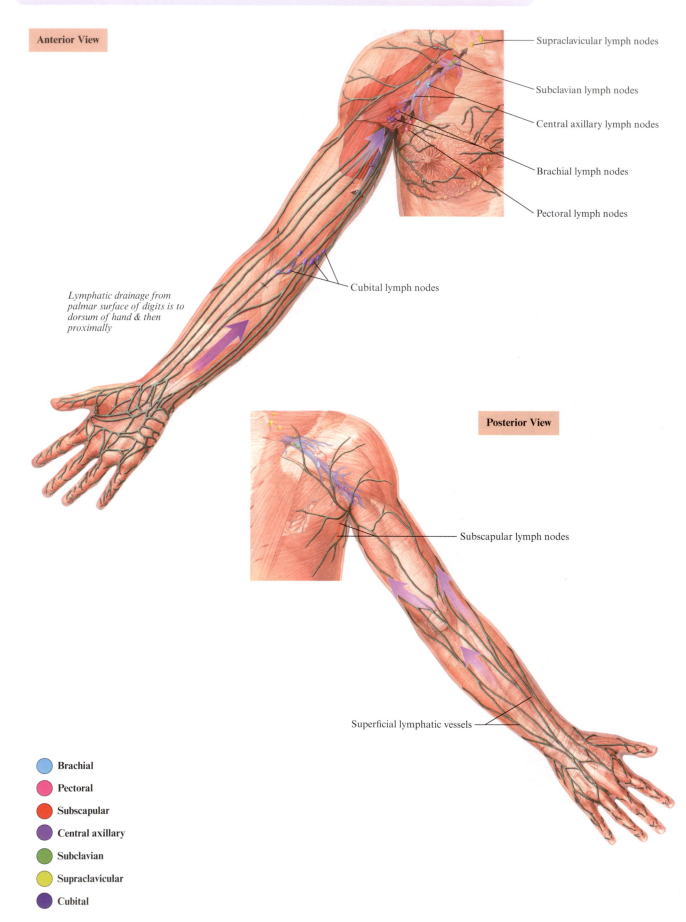

Anterior View

Supraclavicular lymph nodes

Subclavian lymph nodes

Central axillary lymph nodes

Brachial lymph nodes

Pectoral lymph nodes

Cubital lymph nodes

Lymphatic drainage from palmar surface of digits is to dorsum of hand & then proximally

Posterior View

Subscapular lymph nodes

Superficial lymphatic vessels

- ● Brachial
- ● Pectoral
- ● Subscapular
- ● Central axillary
- ● Subclavian
- ● Supraclavicular
- ● Cubital

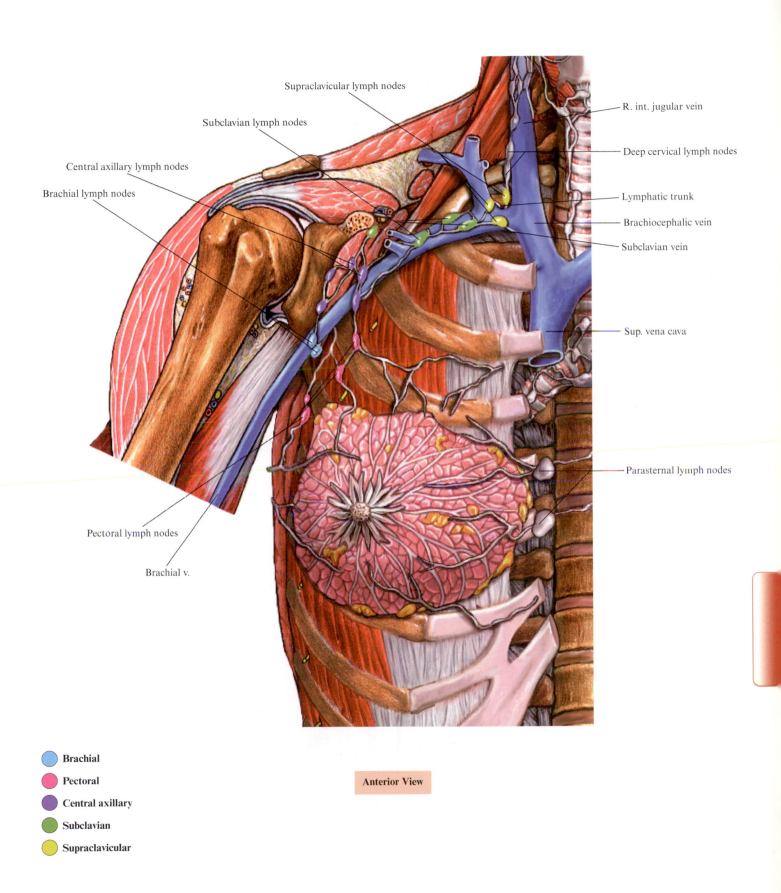

Supraclavicular lymph nodes

Subclavian lymph nodes

Central axillary lymph nodes

Brachial lymph nodes

R. int. jugular vein

Deep cervical lymph nodes

Lymphatic trunk

Brachiocephalic vein

Subclavian vein

Sup. vena cava

Parasternal lymph nodes

Pectoral lymph nodes

Brachial v.

Anterior View

● **Brachial**

● **Pectoral**

● **Central axillary**

● **Subclavian**

● **Supraclavicular**

PLATE 6.29 AXILLA—VASCULATURE

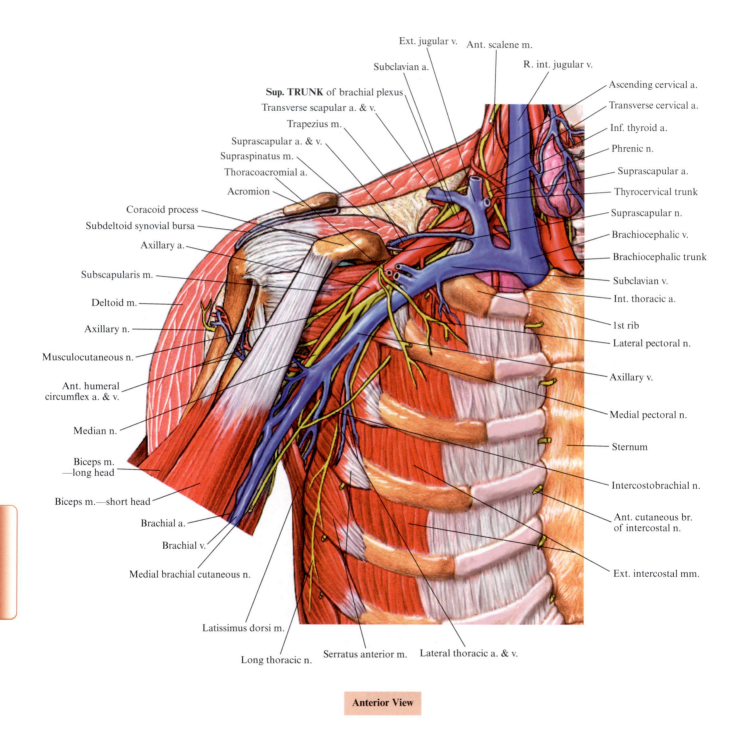

Ext. jugular v.   Ant. scalene m.

Subclavian a.

R. int. jugular v.

Sup. TRUNK of brachial plexus

Transverse scapular a. & v.

Trapezius m.

Suprascapular a. & v.

Supraspinatus m.

Thoracoacromial a.

Acromion

Coracoid process

Subdeltoid synovial bursa

Axillary a.

Subscapularis m.

Deltoid m.

Axillary n.

Musculocutaneous n.

Ant. humeral
circumflex a. & v.

Median n.

Biceps m.
—long head

Biceps m.—short head

Brachial a.

Brachial v.

Medial brachial cutaneous n.

Latissimus dorsi m.

Long thoracic n.   Serratus anterior m.   Lateral thoracic a. & v.

Ascending cervical a.

Transverse cervical a.

Inf. thyroid a.

Phrenic n.

Suprascapular a.

Thyrocervical trunk

Suprascapular n.

Brachiocephalic v.

Brachiocephalic trunk

Subclavian v.

Int. thoracic a.

1st rib

Lateral pectoral n.

Axillary v.

Medial pectoral n.

Sternum

Intercostobrachial n.

Ant. cutaneous br.
of intercostal n.

Ext. intercostal mm.

Anterior View

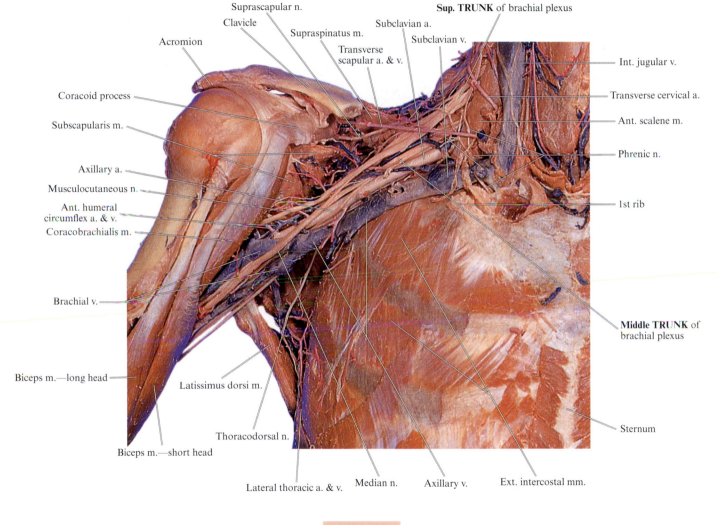

Suprascapular n.

Clavicle

Supraspinatus m.

Acromion

Transverse
scapular a. & v.

Sup. **TRUNK** of brachial plexus

Subclavian a.

Subclavian v.

Int. jugular v.

Coracoid process

Transverse cervical a.

Ant. scalene m.

Subscapularis m.

Phrenic n.

Axillary a.

Musculocutaneous n.

1st rib

Ant. humeral
circumflex a. & v.

Coracobrachialis m.

Brachial v.

Middle TRUNK of
brachial plexus

Biceps m.—long head

Latissimus dorsi m.

Sternum

Biceps m.—short head

Thoracodorsal n.

Lateral thoracic a. & v.   Median n.   Axillary v.   Ext. intercostal mm.

Anterior View

PLATE 6.33 ROTATOR CUFF MUSCLES

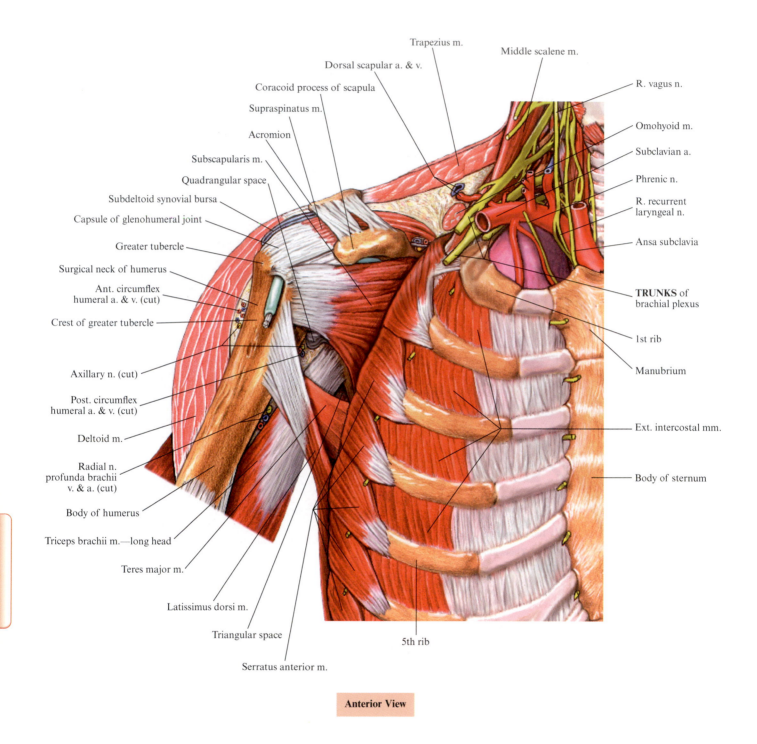

Trapezius m.

Middle scalene m.

Dorsal scapular a. & v.

R. vagus n.

Coracoid process of scapula

Omohyoid m.

Supraspinatus m.

Subclavian a.

Acromion

Phrenic n.

Subscapularis m.

R. recurrent laryngeal n.

Quadrangular space

Subdeltoid synovial bursa

Ansa subclavia

Capsule of glenohumeral joint

Greater tubercle

TRUNKS of brachial plexus

Surgical neck of humerus

1st rib

Ant. circumflex humeral a. & v. (cut)

Manubrium

Crest of greater tubercle

Axillary n. (cut)

Post. circumflex humeral a. & v. (cut)

Ext. intercostal mm.

Deltoid m.

Radial n. profunda brachii v. & a. (cut)

Body of sternum

Body of humerus

Triceps brachii m.—long head

Teres major m.

Latissimus dorsi m.

Triangular space

5th rib

Serratus anterior m.

Anterior View

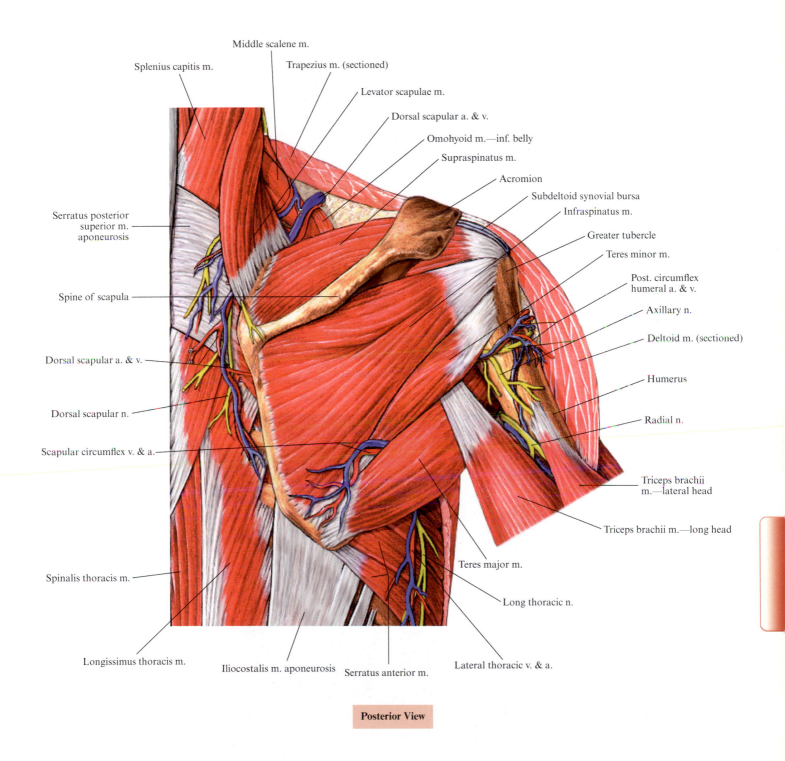

Middle scalene m.

Splenius capitis m.

Trapezius m. (sectioned)

Levator scapulae m.

Dorsal scapular a. & v.

Omohyoid m.—inf. belly

Supraspinatus m.

Acromion

Subdeltoid synovial bursa

Infraspinatus m.

Serratus posterior superior m. aponeurosis

Greater tubercle

Teres minor m.

Post. circumflex humeral a. & v.

Spine of scapula

Axillary n.

Deltoid m. (sectioned)

Dorsal scapular a. & v.

Humerus

Dorsal scapular n.

Radial n.

Scapular circumflex v. & a.

Triceps brachii m.—lateral head

Triceps brachii m.—long head

Teres major m.

Spinalis thoracis m.

Long thoracic n.

Longissimus thoracis m.

Iliocostalis m. aponeurosis   Serratus anterior m.

Lateral thoracic v. & a.

Posterior View

PLATE 6.37   ANTEROMEDIAL ARM

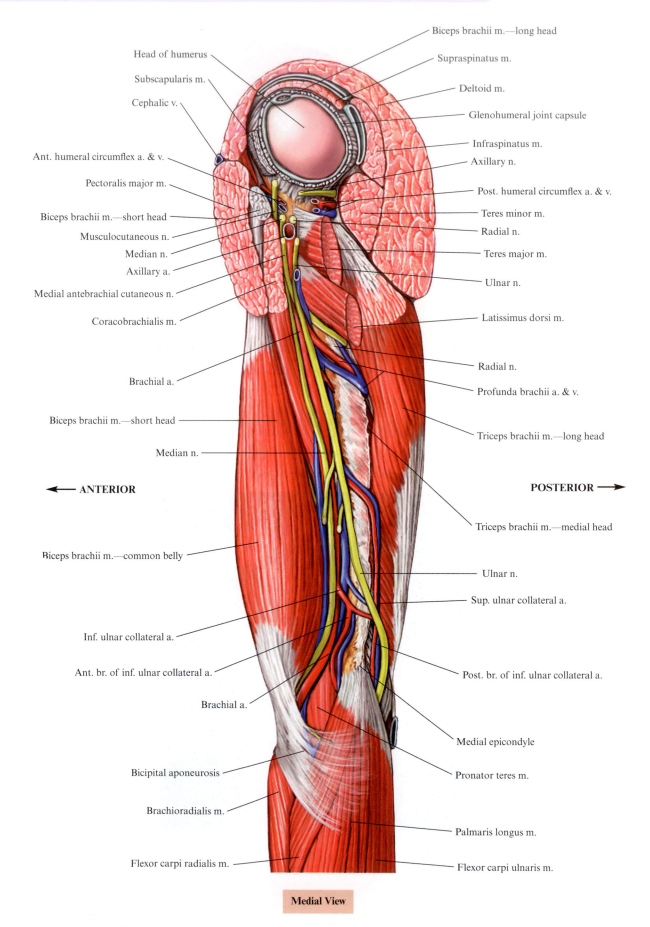

Head of humerus

Subscapularis m.

Cephalic v.

Ant. humeral circumflex a. & v.

Pectoralis major m.

Biceps brachii m.—short head

Musculocutaneous n.

Median n.

Axillary a.

Medial antebrachial cutaneous n.

Coracobrachialis m.

Brachial a.

Biceps brachii m.—short head

Median n.

◄— ANTERIOR

Biceps brachii m.—common belly

Inf. ulnar collateral a.

Ant. br. of inf. ulnar collateral a.

Brachial a.

Bicipital aponeurosis

Brachioradialis m.

Flexor carpi radialis m.

Biceps brachii m.—long head

Supraspinatus m.

Deltoid m.

Glenohumeral joint capsule

Infraspinatus m.

Axillary n.

Post. humeral circumflex a. & v.

Teres minor m.

Radial n.

Teres major m.

Ulnar n.

Latissimus dorsi m.

Radial n.

Profunda brachii a. & v.

Triceps brachii m.—long head

POSTERIOR —►

Triceps brachii m.—medial head

Ulnar n.

Sup. ulnar collateral a.

Post. br. of inf. ulnar collateral a.

Medial epicondyle

Pronator teres m.

Palmaris longus m.

Flexor carpi ulnaris m.

Medial View

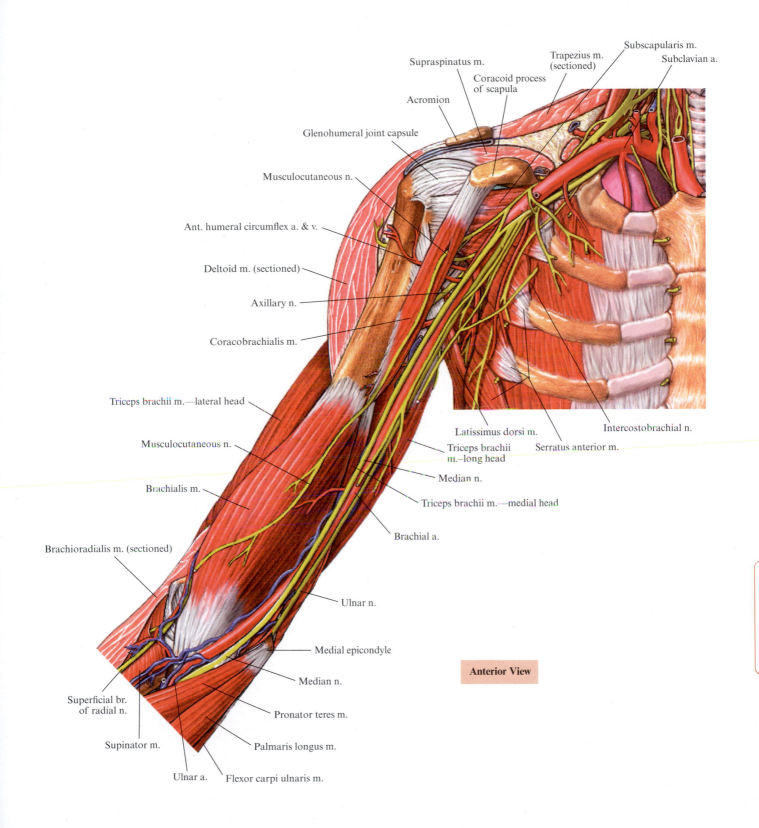

Supraspinatus m.

Coracoid process
of scapula

Acromion

Glenohumeral joint capsule

Musculocutaneous n.

Ant. humeral circumflex a. & v.

Deltoid m. (sectioned)

Axillary n.

Coracobrachialis m.

Triceps brachii m.—lateral head

Musculocutaneous n.

Brachialis m.

Brachioradialis m. (sectioned)

Ulnar n.

Medial epicondyle

Median n.

Superficial br.
of radial n.

Supinator m.

Pronator teres m.

Ulnar a.

Flexor carpi ulnaris m.

Palmaris longus m.

Trapezius m.
(sectioned)

Subscapularis m.

Subclavian a.

Latissimus dorsi m.

Triceps brachii
m.–long head

Median n.

Triceps brachii m.—medial head

Brachial a.

Intercostobrachial n.

Serratus anterior m.

Anterior View

PLATE **6.39**   ANTERIOR ARM

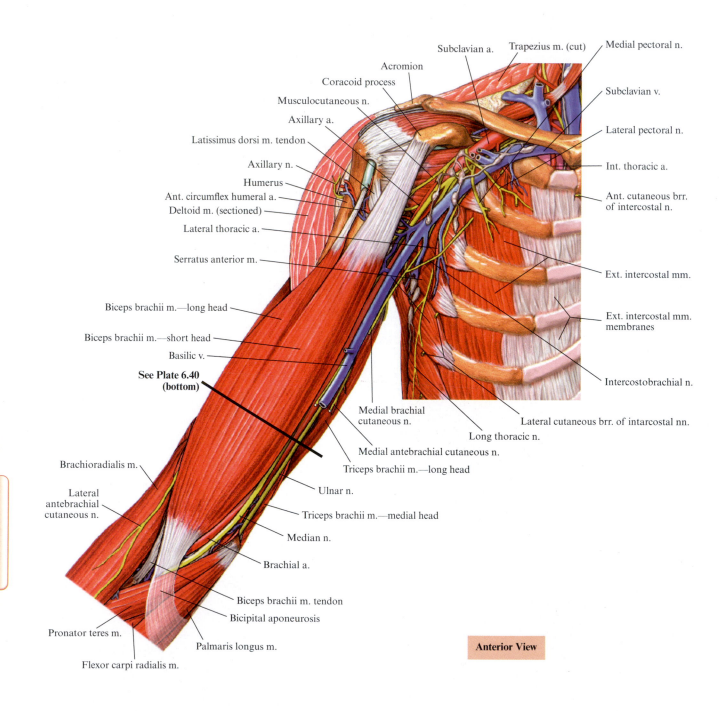

Subclavian a.

Trapezius m. (cut)

Medial pectoral n.

Acromion

Coracoid process

Musculocutaneous n.

Axillary a.

Latissimus dorsi m. tendon

Axillary n.

Humerus

Ant. circumflex humeral a.

Deltoid m. (sectioned)

Lateral thoracic a.

Serratus anterior m.

Biceps brachii m.—long head

Biceps brachii m.—short head

Basilic v.

See Plate 6.40 (bottom)

Brachioradialis m.

Lateral antebrachial cutaneous n.

Pronator teres m.

Flexor carpi radialis m.

Palmaris longus m.

Bicipital aponeurosis

Biceps brachii m. tendon

Brachial a.

Median n.

Triceps brachii m.—medial head

Ulnar n.

Triceps brachii m.—long head

Medial antebrachial cutaneous n.

Medial brachial cutaneous n.

Long thoracic n.

Lateral cutaneous brr. of intarcostal nn.

Intercostobrachial n.

Ext. intercostal mm. membranes

Ext. intercostal mm.

Ant. cutaneous brr. of intercostal n.

Int. thoracic a.

Lateral pectoral n.

Subclavian v.

Anterior View

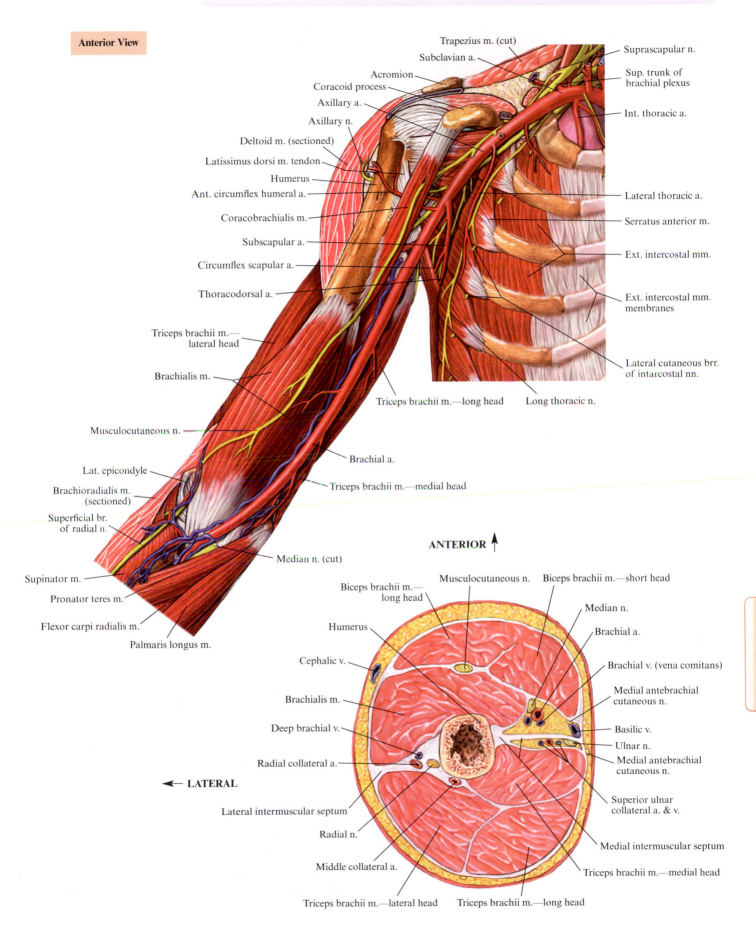

Anterior View

Trapezius m. (cut)
Subclavian a.
Acromion
Coracoid process
Axillary a.
Axillary n.
Deltoid m. (sectioned)
Latissimus dorsi m. tendon
Humerus
Ant. circumflex humeral a.
Coracobrachialis m.
Subscapular a.
Circumflex scapular a.
Thoracodorsal a.
Triceps brachii m.—lateral head
Brachialis m.
Musculocutaneous n.
Lat. epicondyle
Brachioradialis m. (sectioned)
Superficial br. of radial n.
Supinator m.
Pronator teres m.
Flexor carpi radialis m.
Palmaris longus m.

Suprascapular n.
Sup. trunk of brachial plexus
Int. thoracic a.
Lateral thoracic a.
Serratus anterior m.
Ext. intercostal mm.
Ext. intercostal mm. membranes
Lateral cutaneous brr. of intarcostal nn.

Triceps brachii m.—long head
Long thoracic n.
Brachial a.
Triceps brachii m.—medial head
Median n. (cut)

ANTERIOR ↑

Biceps brachii m.—long head
Musculocutaneous n.
Biceps brachii m.—short head
Median n.
Humerus
Brachial a.
Cephalic v.
Brachial v. (vena comitans)
Medial antebrachial cutaneous n.
Brachialis m.
Basilic v.
Deep brachial v.
Ulnar n.
Medial antebrachial cutaneous n.
Radial collateral a.
Superior ulnar collateral a. & v.
← **LATERAL**
Lateral intermuscular septum
Radial n.
Medial intermuscular septum
Middle collateral a.
Triceps brachii m.—medial head
Triceps brachii m.—lateral head
Triceps brachii m.—long head

PLATE 6.43   ANTERIOR FOREARM—DEEP

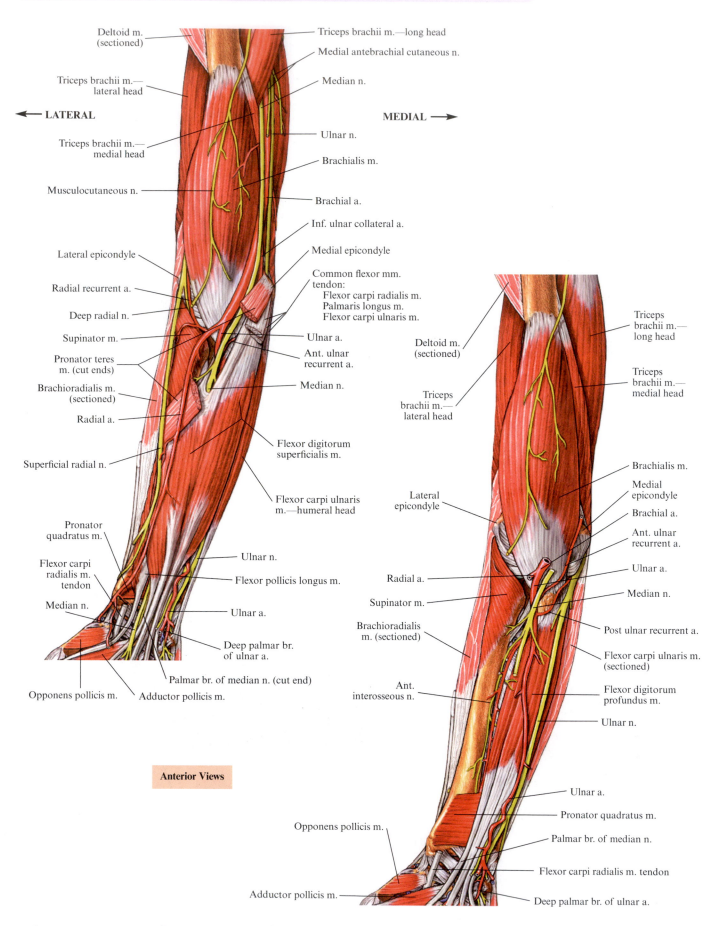

Deltoid m. (sectioned)

Triceps brachii m.—lateral head

Triceps brachii m.—medial head

Musculocutaneous n.

← LATERAL

Lateral epicondyle

Radial recurrent a.

Deep radial n.

Supinator m.

Pronator teres m. (cut ends)

Brachioradialis m. (sectioned)

Radial a.

Superficial radial n.

Pronator quadratus m.

Flexor carpi radialis m. tendon

Median n.

Opponens pollicis m.

Adductor pollicis m.

Triceps brachii m.—long head

Medial antebrachial cutaneous n.

Median n.

Ulnar n.

Brachialis m.

Brachial a.

Inf. ulnar collateral a.

MEDIAL →

Medial epicondyle

Common flexor mm. tendon:
    Flexor carpi radialis m.
    Palmaris longus m.
    Flexor carpi ulnaris m.

Ulnar a.

Ant. ulnar recurrent a.

Median n.

Flexor digitorum superficialis m.

Flexor carpi ulnaris m.—humeral head

Ulnar n.

Flexor pollicis longus m.

Ulnar a.

Deep palmar br. of ulnar a.

Palmar br. of median n. (cut end)

Anterior Views

Deltoid m. (sectioned)

Triceps brachii m.—lateral head

Lateral epicondyle

Radial a.

Supinator m.

Brachioradialis m. (sectioned)

Ant. interosseous n.

Opponens pollicis m.

Adductor pollicis m.

Triceps brachii m.—long head

Triceps brachii m.—medial head

Brachialis m.

Medial epicondyle

Brachial a.

Ant. ulnar recurrent a.

Ulnar a.

Median n.

Post ulnar recurrent a.

Flexor carpi ulnaris m. (sectioned)

Flexor digitorum profundus m.

Ulnar n.

Ulnar a.

Pronator quadratus m.

Palmar br. of median n.

Flexor carpi radialis m. tendon

Deep palmar br. of ulnar a.

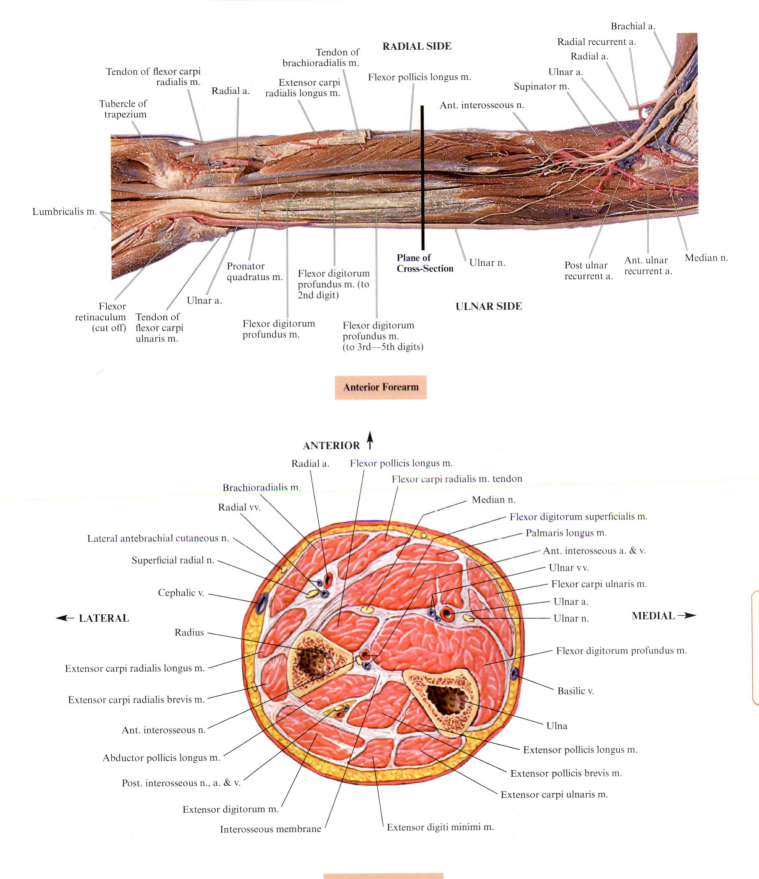

RADIAL SIDE

Tubercle of trapezium

Tendon of flexor carpi radialis m.

Radial a.

Tendon of brachioradialis m.

Extensor carpi radialis longus m.

Flexor pollicis longus m.

Ant. interosseous n.

Brachial a.

Radial recurrent a.

Radial a.

Ulnar a.

Supinator m.

Lumbricalis m.

Flexor retinaculum (cut off)

Tendon of flexor carpi ulnaris m.

Ulnar a.

Pronator quadratus m.

Flexor digitorum profundus m.

Flexor digitorum profundus m. (to 2nd digit)

Flexor digitorum profundus m. (to 3rd—5th digits)

Plane of Cross-Section

Ulnar n.

Post ulnar recurrent a.

Ant. ulnar recurrent a.

Median n.

ULNAR SIDE

Anterior Forearm

ANTERIOR ↑

Radial a.

Flexor pollicis longus m.

Brachioradialis m.

Flexor carpi radialis m. tendon

Radial vv.

Median n.

Lateral antebrachial cutaneous n.

Flexor digitorum superficialis m.

Superficial radial n.

Palmaris longus m.

Cephalic v.

Ant. interosseous a. & v.

Ulnar vv.

Flexor carpi ulnaris m.

Ulnar a.

← **LATERAL**

Ulnar n.

MEDIAL →

Radius

Flexor digitorum profundus m.

Extensor carpi radialis longus m.

Basilic v.

Extensor carpi radialis brevis m.

Ulna

Ant. interosseous n.

Abductor pollicis longus m.

Extensor pollicis longus m.

Post. interosseous n., a. & v.

Extensor pollicis brevis m.

Extensor carpi ulnaris m.

Extensor digitorum m.

Interosseous membrane

Extensor digiti minimi m.

Section at Mid-Forearm

PLATE 6.49 POSTERIOR ARM

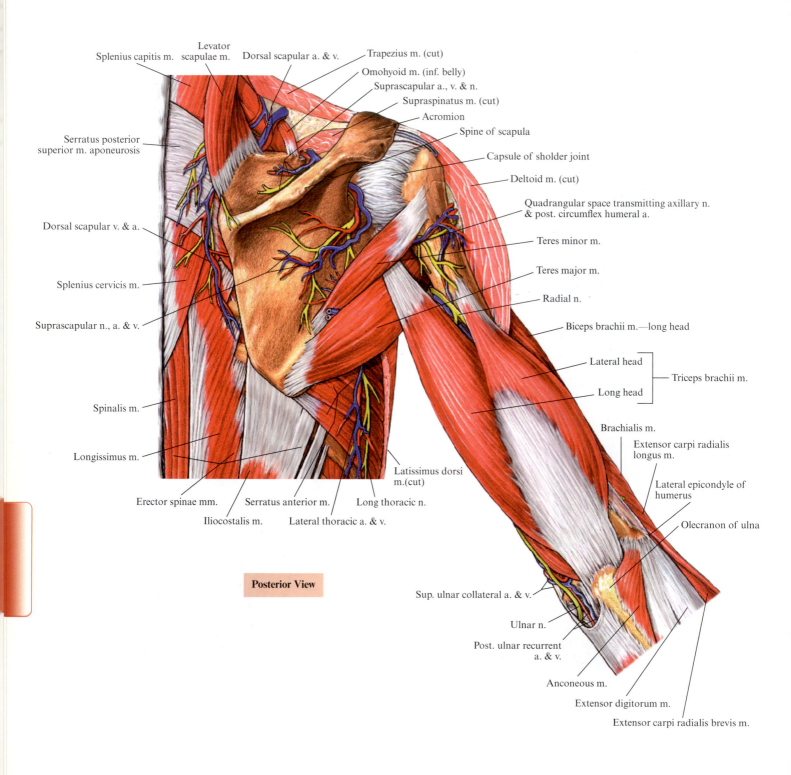

Levator
Splenius capitis m. scapulae m. Dorsal scapular a. & v. Trapezius m. (cut)

Omohyoid m. (inf. belly)

Suprascapular a., v. & n.

Supraspinatus m. (cut)

Acromion

Serratus posterior Spine of scapula
superior m. aponeurosis
Capsule of sholder joint

Deltoid m. (cut)

Quadrangular space transmitting axillary n.
& post. circumflex humeral a.

Dorsal scapular v. & a. Teres minor m.

Teres major m.

Splenius cervicis m. Radial n.

Suprascapular n., a. & v. Biceps brachii m.—long head

Lateral head
Triceps brachii m.
Long head

Brachialis m.

Spinalis m. Extensor carpi radialis
longus m.

Lateral epicondyle of
Longissimus m. humerus

Latissimus dorsi Olecranon of ulna
m.(cut)

Erector spinae mm. Serratus anterior m. Long thoracic n.

Iliocostalis m. Lateral thoracic a. & v.

Posterior View

Sup. ulnar collateral a. & v.

Ulnar n.

Post. ulnar recurrent
a. & v.

Anconeous m.

Extensor digitorum m.

Extensor carpi radialis brevis m.

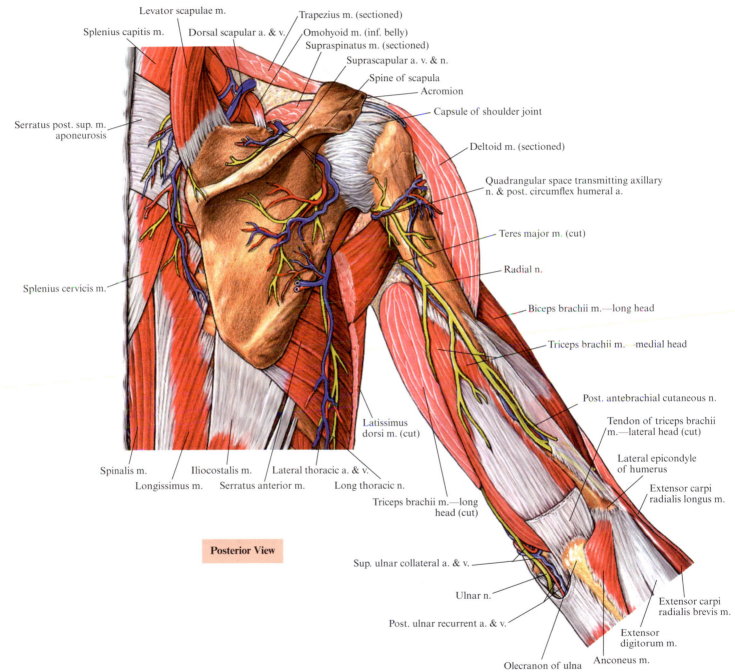

Levator scapulae m.

Splenius capitis m.

Dorsal scapular a. & v.

Trapezius m. (sectioned)

Omohyoid m. (inf. belly)

Supraspinatus m. (sectioned)

Suprascapular a. v. & n.

Spine of scapula

Acromion

Capsule of shoulder joint

Serratus post. sup. m. aponeurosis

Deltoid m. (sectioned)

Quadrangular space transmitting axillary n. & post. circumflex humeral a.

Teres major m. (cut)

Radial n.

Biceps brachii m.—long head

Splenius cervicis m.

Triceps brachii m.—medial head

Post. antebrachial cutaneous n.

Tendon of triceps brachii m.—lateral head (cut)

Latissimus dorsi m. (cut)

Lateral epicondyle of humerus

Extensor carpi radialis longus m.

Spinalis m.   Iliocostalis m.   Lateral thoracic a. & v.

Longissimus m.   Serratus anterior m.   Long thoracic n.

Triceps brachii m.—long head (cut)

Posterior View

Sup. ulnar collateral a. & v.

Ulnar n.

Extensor carpi radialis brevis m.

Post. ulnar recurrent a. & v.

Extensor digitorum m.

Olecranon of ulna   Anconeus m.

7 HEAD AND NECK

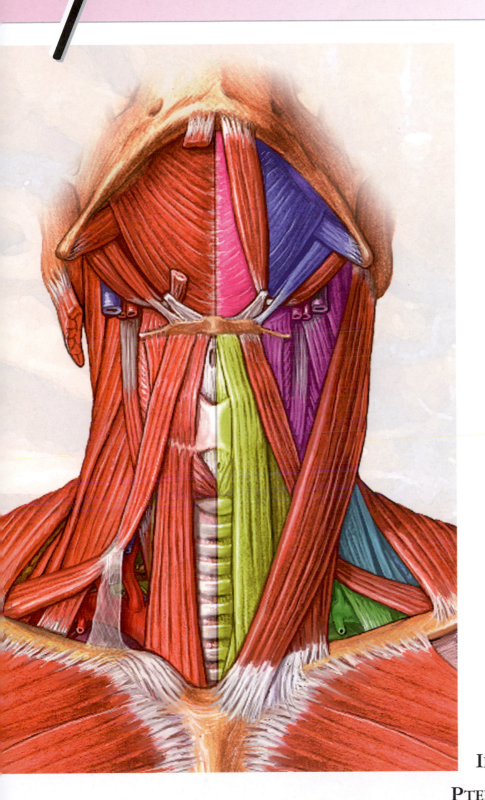

PLATE 7.1   TOPOGRAPHY

Anterior View

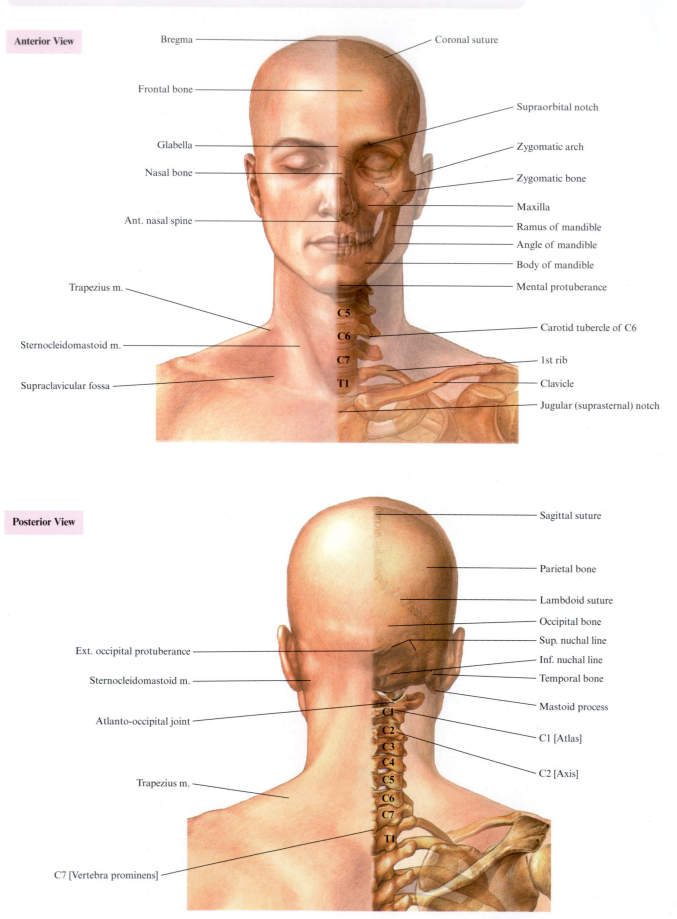

Bregma

Coronal suture

Frontal bone

Supraorbital notch

Glabella

Zygomatic arch

Nasal bone

Zygomatic bone

Maxilla

Ant. nasal spine

Ramus of mandible

Angle of mandible

Body of mandible

Trapezius m.

Mental protuberance

C5

C6

Carotid tubercle of C6

Sternocleidomastoid m.

C7

1st rib

T1

Supraclavicular fossa

Clavicle

Jugular (suprasternal) notch

Posterior View

Sagittal suture

Parietal bone

Lambdoid suture

Occipital bone

Sup. nuchal line

Ext. occipital protuberance

Inf. nuchal line

Sternocleidomastoid m.

Temporal bone

Mastoid process

C1

Atlanto-occipital joint

C2

C1 [Atlas]

C3

C4

C2 [Axis]

C5

Trapezius m.

C6

C7

T1

C7 [Vertebra prominens]

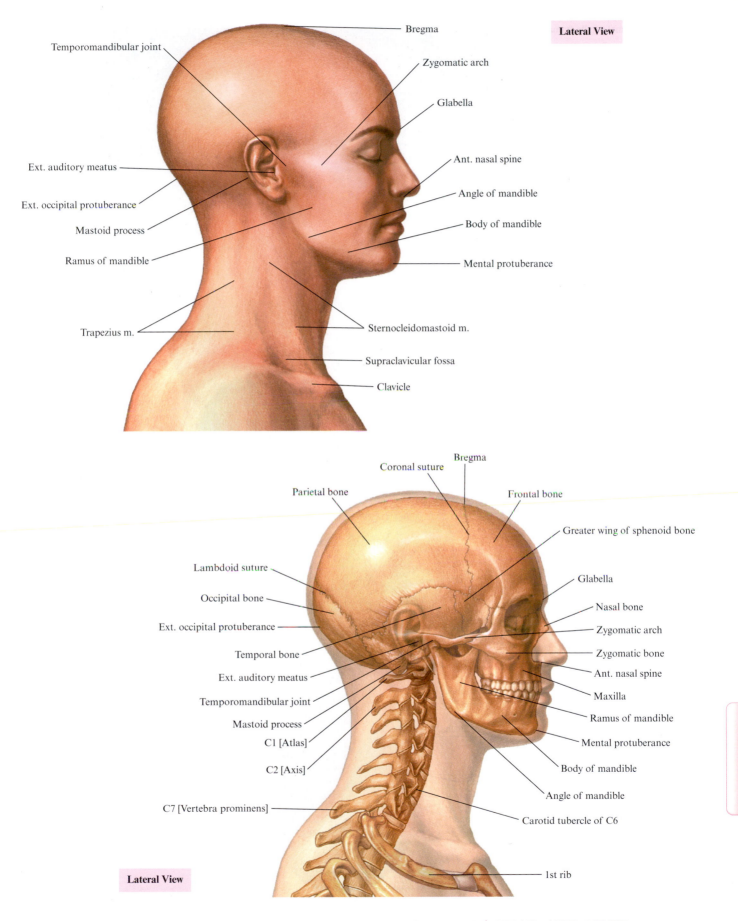

Lateral View

Bregma

Temporomandibular joint

Zygomatic arch

Glabella

Ant. nasal spine

Ext. auditory meatus

Angle of mandible

Ext. occipital protuberance

Body of mandible

Mastoid process

Mental protuberance

Ramus of mandible

Trapezius m.

Sternocleidomastoid m.

Supraclavicular fossa

Clavicle

Bregma

Coronal suture

Parietal bone

Frontal bone

Greater wing of sphenoid bone

Lambdoid suture

Glabella

Occipital bone

Nasal bone

Ext. occipital protuberance

Zygomatic arch

Temporal bone

Zygomatic bone

Ext. auditory meatus

Ant. nasal spine

Temporomandibular joint

Maxilla

Mastoid process

Ramus of mandible

C1 [Atlas]

Mental protuberance

C2 [Axis]

Body of mandible

C7 [Vertebra prominens]

Angle of mandible

Carotid tubercle of C6

1st rib

Lateral View

PLATE 7.5   CRANIUM—ANTERIOR

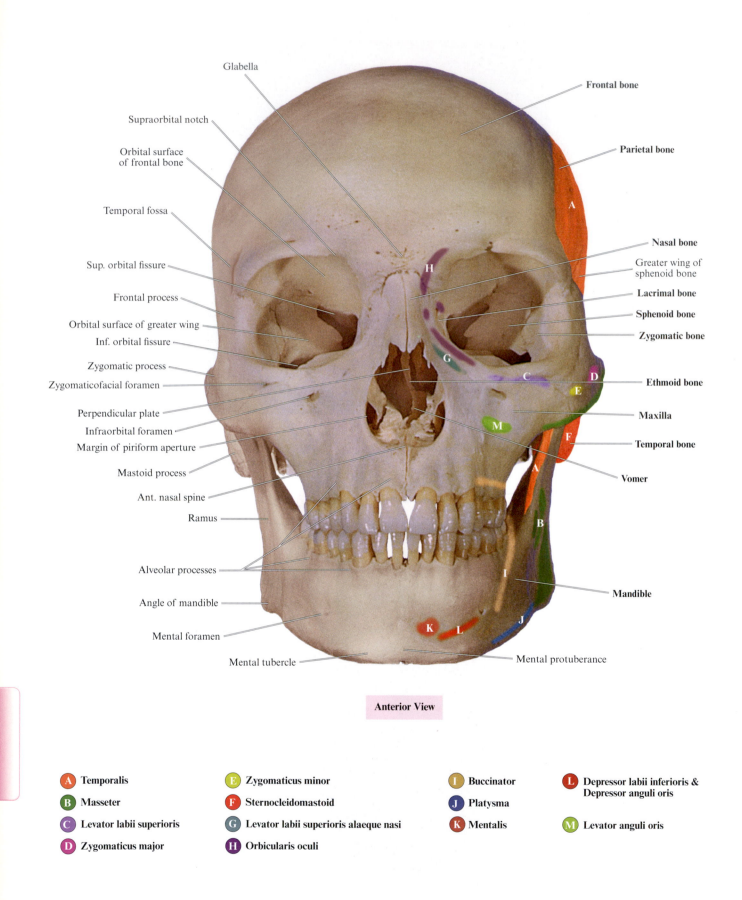

Glabella

Frontal bone

Supraorbital notch

Parietal bone

Orbital surface
of frontal bone

A

Temporal fossa

Nasal bone

Greater wing of
sphenoid bone

Sup. orbital fissure

H

Lacrimal bone

Frontal process

Sphenoid bone

Orbital surface of greater wing

G

Zygomatic bone

Inf. orbital fissure

Zygomatic process

C

D

Ethmoid bone

Zygomaticofacial foramen

E

Perpendicular plate

M

Maxilla

Infraorbital foramen

F

Temporal bone

Margin of piriform aperture

Mastoid process

A

Vomer

Ant. nasal spine

Ramus

B

Alveolar processes

I

Angle of mandible

Mandible

Mental foramen

J

K   L

Mental tubercle

Mental protuberance

Anterior View

A Temporalis	**E** Zygomaticus minor	**I** Buccinator	**L** Depressor labii inferioris & Depressor anguli oris
B Masseter	**F** Sternocleidomastoid	**J** Platysma	
C Levator labii superioris	**G** Levator labii superioris alaeque nasi	**K** Mentalis	**M** Levator anguli oris
D Zygomaticus major	**H** Orbicularis oculi		

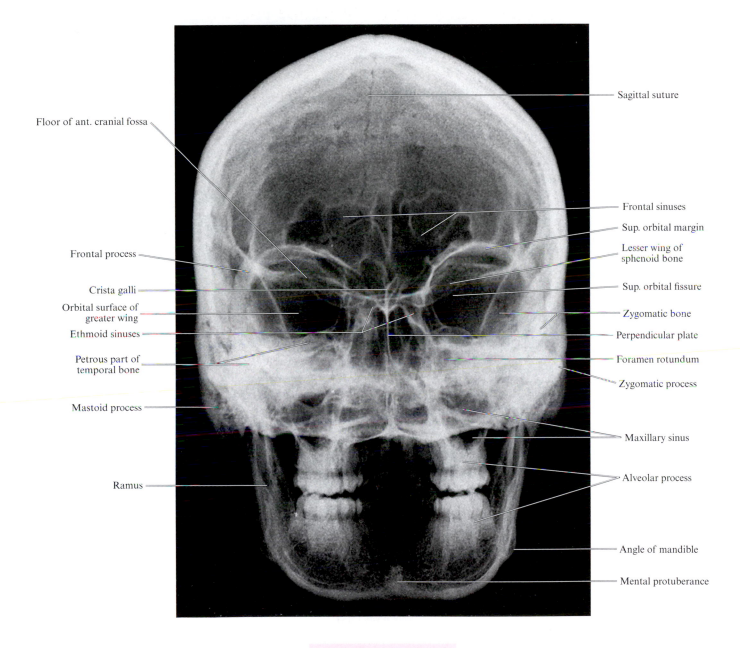

Floor of ant. cranial fossa

Sagittal suture

Frontal sinuses

Sup. orbital margin

Frontal process

Lesser wing of sphenoid bone

Crista galli

Sup. orbital fissure

Orbital surface of greater wing

Zygomatic bone

Ethmoid sinuses

Perpendicular plate

Petrous part of temporal bone

Foramen rotundum

Zygomatic process

Mastoid process

Maxillary sinus

Ramus

Alveolar process

Angle of mandible

Mental protuberance

Anteroposterior View of Skull

TABLE 7.2 INTERNAL NEUROCRANIAL FORAMINA, FISSURES & CANALS

Foramina/Openings	Contents
ANTERIOR CRANIAL FOSSA	
Foramen cecum	Inconsistent passage for nasal emissary vv. tributaries of superior sagittal sinus
Foramina in cribriform plates	CN I — Sensory axons from olfactory epithelium that collectively constitute the olfactory nn.
Anterior ethmoidal foramen	CN V^1 — anterior ethmoidal br. of nasociliary n. & vessels
Posterior ethmoidal foramen	CN V^1 — posterior ethmoidal br. of nasociliary n. & vessels
MIDDLE CRANIAL FOSSA	
Optic canal	CN II, & ophthalmic a.
Superior orbital fissure	Passage between middle cranial fossa & orbit for CN III, IV, VI, V1 — lacrimal n., V1 — frontal n., V^1 — nasociliary n., postganglionic sympathetic n. fibers, & ophthalmic v.
Foramen rotundum	CN V^2 — maxillary n.
Foramen ovale	CN V^3 — mandibular n., CN IX - lesser petrosal n. & accessory meningeal a.
Foramen spinosum	CN V^3 — meningeal br. & middle meningeal vessels
Foramen lacerum	Internal carotid a., sympathetic nn. & venous plexi from carotid canal, & CN VII — greater petrosal n. Closed inferoexternally by fibrocartilage
Hiatus for greater petrosal n. (Facial hiatus)	CN VII — greater petrosal n., & petrosal br. of middle meningeal a.
Hiatus for lesser petrosal n.	CN IX — lesser petrosal n.
POSTERIOR CRANIAL FOSSA	
Internal acoustic meatus	CN VII & VIII, labyrinthine a.
Jugular fossa & foramen	CN IX, X & XI, superior bulb of internal jugular v., inferior petrosal & sigmoid sinuses, & meningeal brr. of ascending pharyngeal & occipital aa.
Condylar fossa & canal	*Inconsistent* passage for condylar emissary v. between sigmoid sinus & vertebral venous plexi
Mastoid foramen	Mastoid br. of occipital a. & mastoid emissary v. to sigmoid sinus & diploic vv.
Hypoglossal canal	CN XII — hypoglossal n.
Foramen magnum	Medulla & meninges of spinal cord, CN XI, vertebral aa., ant. & post. spinal aa., & brr. of internal vertebral venous plexus

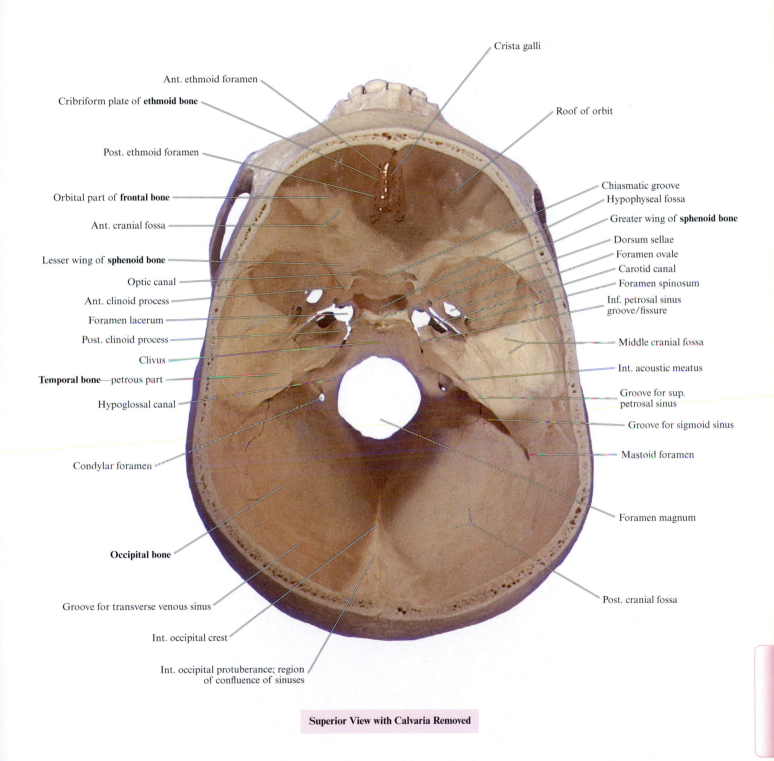

Crista galli

Ant. ethmoid foramen

Cribriform plate of **ethmoid bone**

Roof of orbit

Post. ethmoid foramen

Orbital part of **frontal bone**

Chiasmatic groove

Hypophyseal fossa

Ant. cranial fossa

Greater wing of **sphenoid bone**

Lesser wing of **sphenoid bone**

Dorsum sellae

Foramen ovale

Optic canal

Carotid canal

Ant. clinoid process

Foramen spinosum

Foramen lacerum

Inf. petrosal sinus groove/fissure

Post. clinoid process

Middle cranial fossa

Clivus

Int. acoustic meatus

Temporal bone—petrous part

Groove for sup. petrosal sinus

Hypoglossal canal

Groove for sigmoid sinus

Condylar foramen

Mastoid foramen

Occipital bone

Foramen magnum

Groove for transverse venous sinus

Post. cranial fossa

Int. occipital crest

Int. occipital protuberance; region of confluence of sinuses

Superior View with Calvaria Removed

PLATE 7.13   CRANIUM—SPHENOID BONE

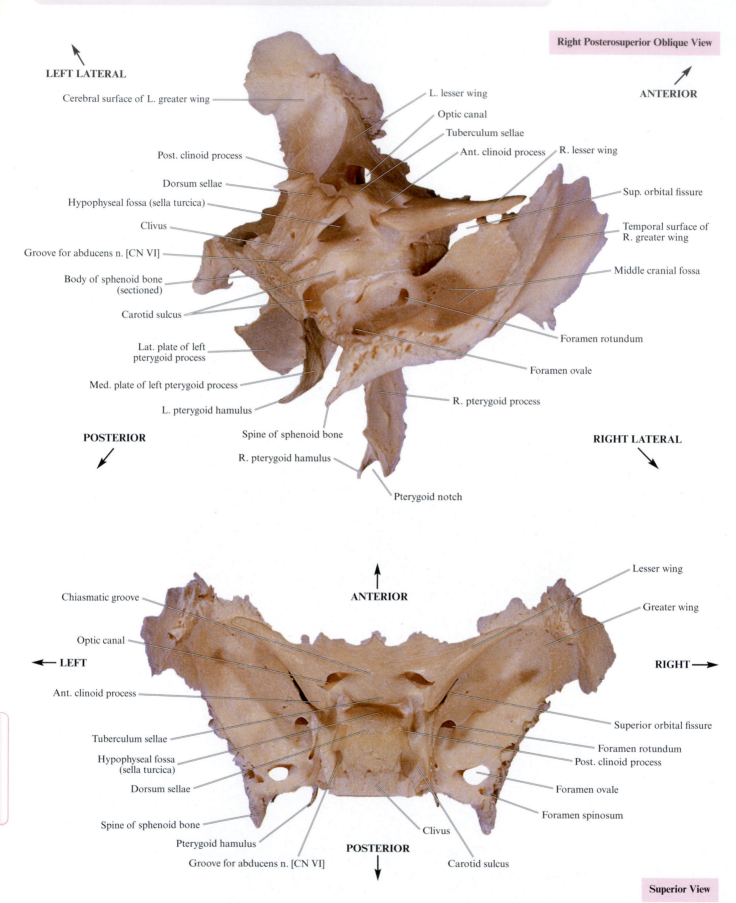

Right Posterosuperior Oblique View

LEFT LATERAL

Cerebral surface of L. greater wing

L. lesser wing

Optic canal

Tuberculum sellae

Ant. clinoid process

R. lesser wing

ANTERIOR

Post. clinoid process

Dorsum sellae

Sup. orbital fissure

Hypophyseal fossa (sella turcica)

Temporal surface of
R. greater wing

Clivus

Groove for abducens n. [CN VI]

Middle cranial fossa

Body of sphenoid bone
(sectioned)

Carotid sulcus

Foramen rotundum

Lat. plate of left
pterygoid process

Foramen ovale

Med. plate of left pterygoid process

L. pterygoid hamulus

R. pterygoid process

POSTERIOR

Spine of sphenoid bone

R. pterygoid hamulus

RIGHT LATERAL

Pterygoid notch

Chiasmatic groove

Lesser wing

ANTERIOR

Greater wing

Optic canal

LEFT

RIGHT

Ant. clinoid process

Superior orbital fissure

Tuberculum sellae

Foramen rotundum

Hypophyseal fossa
(sella turcica)

Post. clinoid process

Dorsum sellae

Foramen ovale

Spine of sphenoid bone

Foramen spinosum

Pterygoid hamulus

Clivus

Groove for abducens n. [CN VI]

POSTERIOR

Carotid sulcus

Superior View

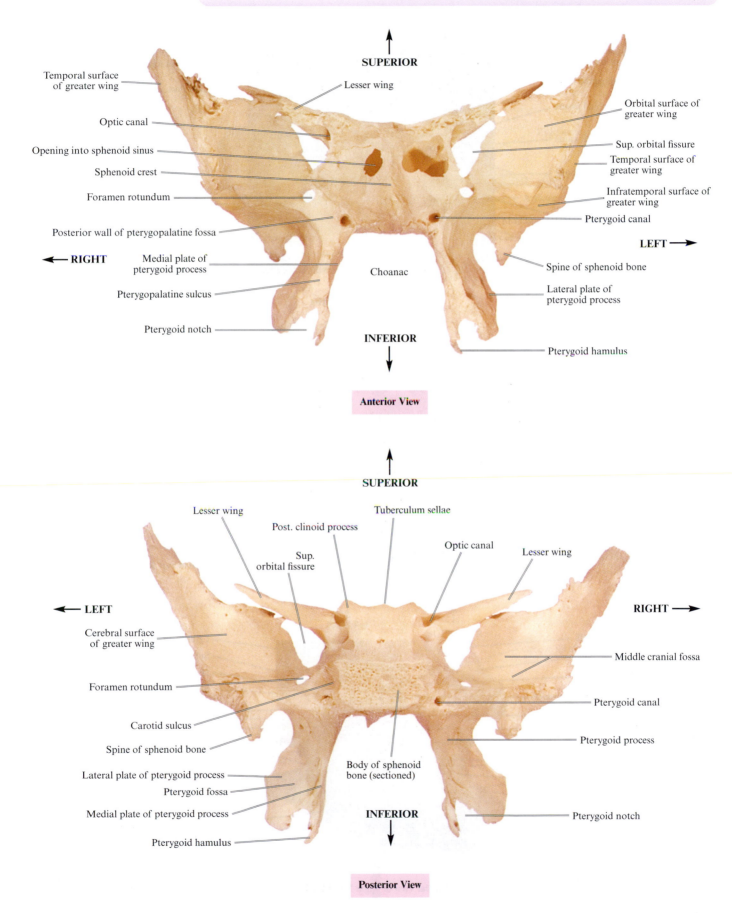

SUPERIOR

Temporal surface of greater wing

Lesser wing

Optic canal

Orbital surface of greater wing

Opening into sphenoid sinus

Sup. orbital fissure

Sphenoid crest

Temporal surface of greater wing

Foramen rotundum

Infratemporal surface of greater wing

Posterior wall of pterygopalatine fossa

Pterygoid canal

← RIGHT

LEFT →

Medial plate of pterygoid process

Spine of sphenoid bone

Choanac

Pterygopalatine sulcus

Lateral plate of pterygoid process

Pterygoid notch

INFERIOR

Pterygoid hamulus

Anterior View

SUPERIOR

Lesser wing

Tuberculum sellae

Post. clinoid process

Optic canal

Lesser wing

Sup. orbital fissure

← LEFT

RIGHT →

Cerebral surface of greater wing

Middle cranial fossa

Foramen rotundum

Pterygoid canal

Carotid sulcus

Pterygoid process

Spine of sphenoid bone

Lateral plate of pterygoid process

Body of sphenoid bone (sectioned)

Pterygoid fossa

Medial plate of pterygoid process

Pterygoid notch

Pterygoid hamulus

INFERIOR

Posterior View

PLATE 7.17 PALATE & PHARYNGEAL REGION

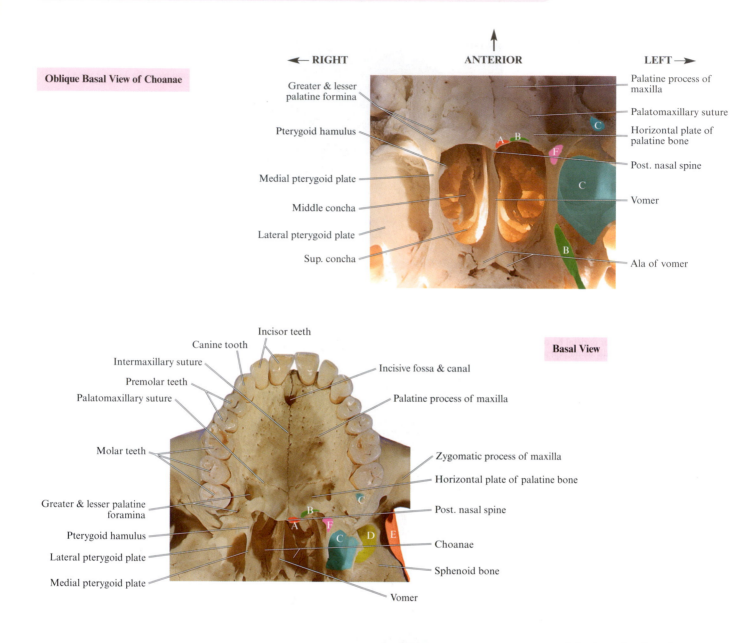

Oblique Basal View of Choanae

← RIGHT   ANTERIOR   LEFT →

Greater & lesser palatine formina
Pterygoid hamulus
Medial pterygoid plate
Middle concha
Lateral pterygoid plate
Sup. concha

Palatine process of maxilla
Palatomaxillary suture
Horizontal plate of palatine bone
Post. nasal spine
Vomer
Ala of vomer

Basal View

Incisor teeth
Canine tooth
Intermaxillary suture
Premolar teeth
Palatomaxillary suture
Molar teeth
Greater & lesser palatine foramina
Pterygoid hamulus
Lateral pterygoid plate
Medial pterygoid plate

Incisive fossa & canal
Palatine process of maxilla
Zygomatic process of maxilla
Horizontal plate of palatine bone
Post. nasal spine
Choanae
Sphenoid bone
Vomer

Basal View of Left Mandibular Fossa

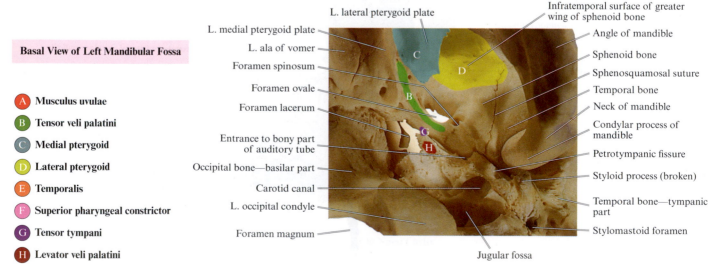

L. lateral pterygoid plate
L. medial pterygoid plate
L. ala of vomer
Foramen spinosum
Foramen ovale
Foramen lacerum
Entrance to bony part of auditory tube
Occipital bone—basilar part
Carotid canal
L. occipital condyle
Foramen magnum

Infratemporal surface of greater wing of sphenoid bone
Angle of mandible
Sphenoid bone
Sphenosquamosal suture
Temporal bone
Neck of mandible
Condylar process of mandible
Petrotympanic fissure
Styloid process (broken)
Temporal bone—tympanic part
Stylomastoid foramen
Jugular fossa

A **Musculus uvulae**
B **Tensor veli palatini**
C **Medial pterygoid**
D **Lateral pterygoid**
E **Temporalis**
F **Superior pharyngeal constrictor**
G **Tensor tympani**
H **Levator veli palatini**

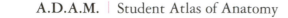

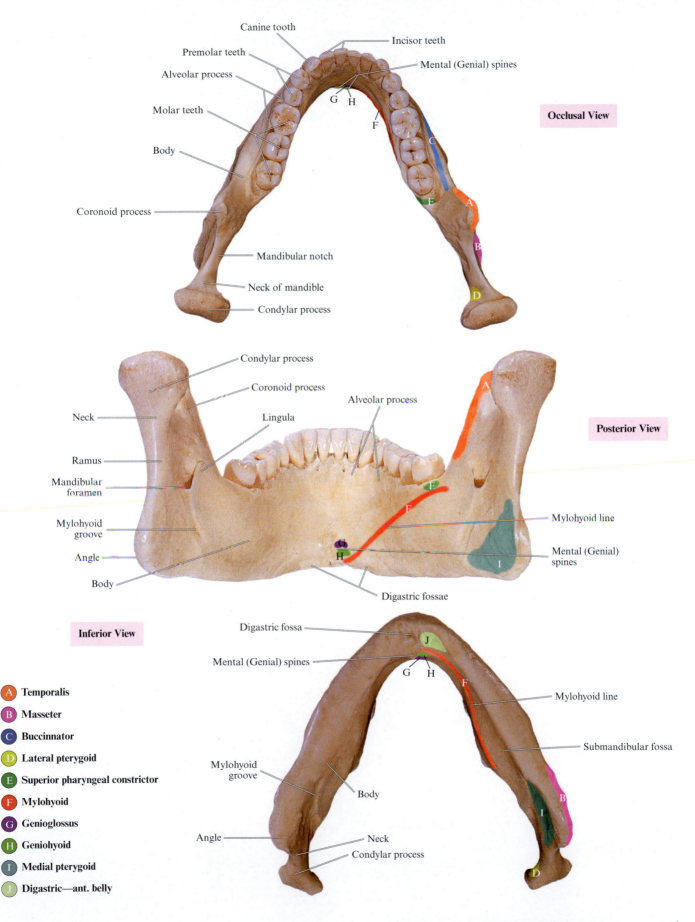

Canine tooth

Incisor teeth

Premolar teeth

Mental (Genial) spines

Alveolar process

Molar teeth

G H

Occlusal View

F

Body

C

E

A

Coronoid process

B

Mandibular notch

D

Neck of mandible

Condylar process

Condylar process

Coronoid process

Alveolar process

A

Neck

Lingula

Posterior View

Ramus

Mandibular
foramen

E

E

Mylohyoid line

Mylohyoid
groove

Mental (Genial)
spines

Angle

G

I

Body

H

Digastric fossae

Inferior View

Digastric fossa

J

Mental (Genial) spines

G   H

F

Mylohyoid line

A **Temporalis**

Mylohyoid
groove

Submandibular fossa

B **Masseter**

Body

C **Buccinnator**

D **Lateral pterygoid**

E **Superior pharyngeal constrictor**

Angle

B

Neck

F **Mylohyoid**

I

Condylar process

G **Genioglossus**

H **Geniohyoid**

D

I **Medial pterygoid**

J **Digastric—ant. belly**

PLATE 7.19   SKELETON—LARYNGEAL

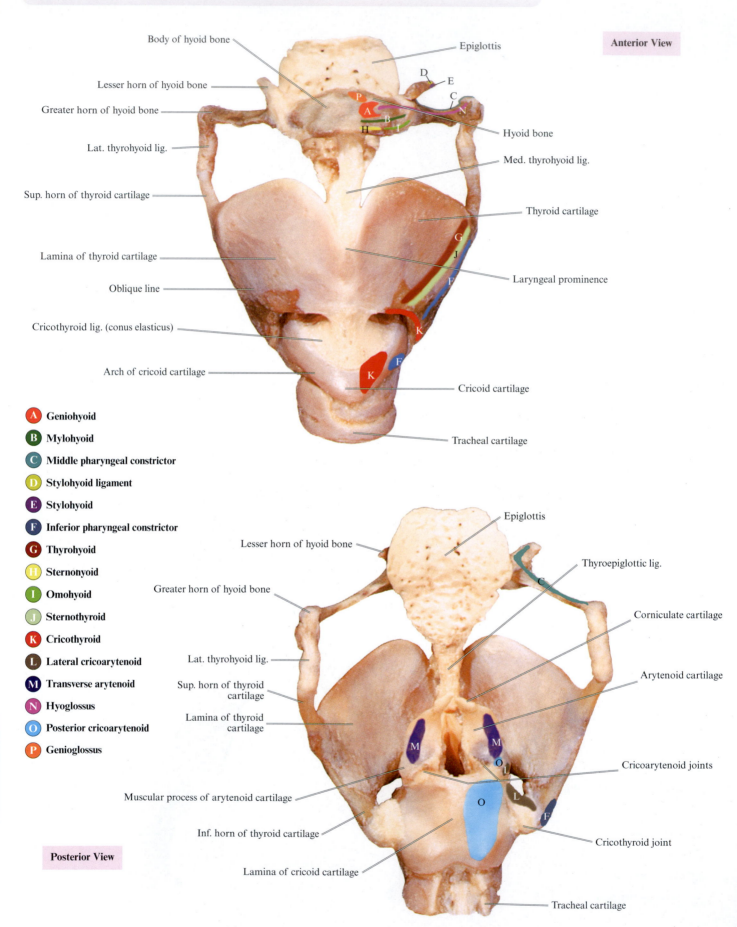

Anterior View

Body of hyoid bone

Epiglottis

Lesser horn of hyoid bone

D

E

C

N

Lat. thyrohyoid lig.

Greater horn of hyoid bone

Hyoid bone

P

A

B

H

I

Med. thyrohyoid lig.

Sup. horn of thyroid cartilage

Thyroid cartilage

G

Lamina of thyroid cartilage

J

F

Oblique line

Laryngeal prominence

Cricothyroid lig. (conus elasticus)

K

Arch of cricoid cartilage

F

K

Cricoid cartilage

Tracheal cartilage

A Geniohyoid

B Mylohyoid

C Middle pharyngeal constrictor

D Stylohyoid ligament

E Stylohyoid

F Inferior pharyngeal constrictor

G Thyrohyoid

H Sternonyoid

I Omohyoid

J Sternothyroid

K Cricothyroid

L Lateral cricoarytenoid

M Transverse arytenoid

N Hyoglossus

O Posterior cricoarytenoid

P Genioglossus

Epiglottis

Lesser horn of hyoid bone

Thyroepiglottic lig.

C

Greater horn of hyoid bone

Corniculate cartilage

Lat. thyrohyoid lig.

Arytenoid cartilage

Sup. horn of thyroid cartilage

Lamina of thyroid cartilage

M

M

O

L

Cricoarytenoid joints

Muscular process of arytenoid cartilage

O

L

Inf. horn of thyroid cartilage

F

Cricothyroid joint

Lamina of cricoid cartilage

Tracheal cartilage

Posterior View

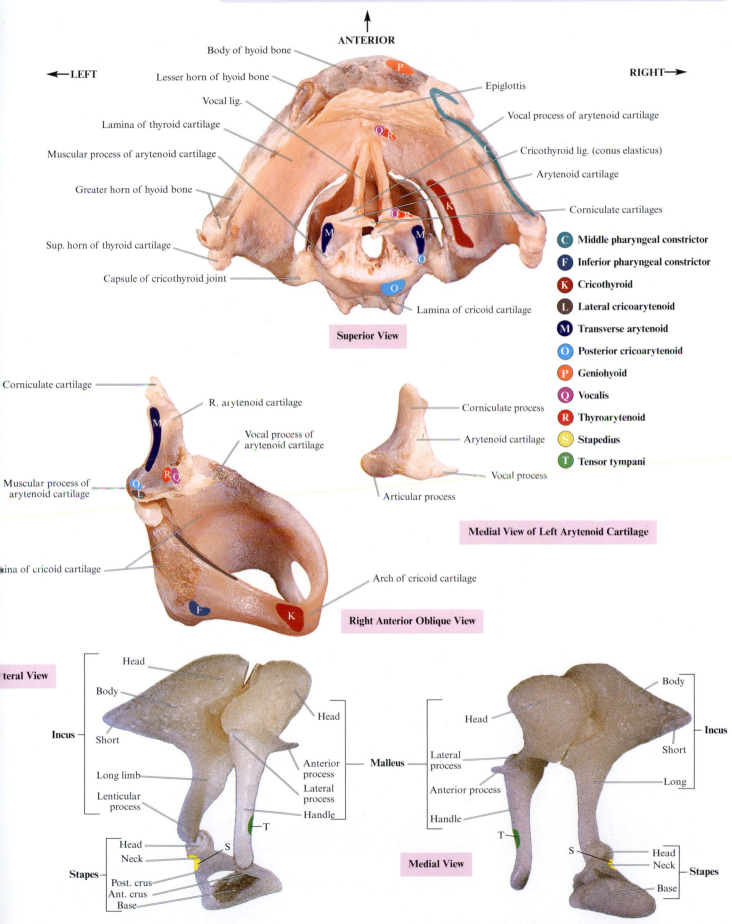

ANTERIOR

←**LEFT**

RIGHT→

Body of hyoid bone

Lesser horn of hyoid bone

Vocal lig.

Epiglottis

Lamina of thyroid cartilage

Vocal process of arytenoid cartilage

Muscular process of arytenoid cartilage

Cricothyroid lig. (conus elasticus)

Greater horn of hyoid bone

Arytenoid cartilage

Corniculate cartilages

Sup. horn of thyroid cartilage

Capsule of cricothyroid joint

Lamina of cricoid cartilage

Superior View

C **Middle pharyngeal constrictor**

F **Inferior pharyngeal constrictor**

K **Cricothyroid**

L **Lateral cricoarytenoid**

M **Transverse arytenoid**

O **Posterior cricoarytenoid**

P **Geniohyoid**

Q **Vocalis**

R **Thyroarytenoid**

S **Stapedius**

T **Tensor tympani**

Corniculate cartilage

R. arytenoid cartilage

Vocal process of arytenoid cartilage

Corniculate process

Arytenoid cartilage

Muscular process of arytenoid cartilage

Vocal process

Articular process

Medial View of Left Arytenoid Cartilage

...ina of cricoid cartilage

Arch of cricoid cartilage

Right Anterior Oblique View

...teral View

Head

Body

Head

Incus

Short

Anterior process

Malleus

Long limb

Lateral process

Lenticular process

Handle

Head

Neck

S

Stapes

Post. crus

Ant. crus

Base

T

Body

Head

Incus

Lateral process

Short

Anterior process

Long

Handle

Head

T

S

Neck

Stapes

Base

Medial View

PLATE 7.21   MUSCLES—SUPERFICIAL

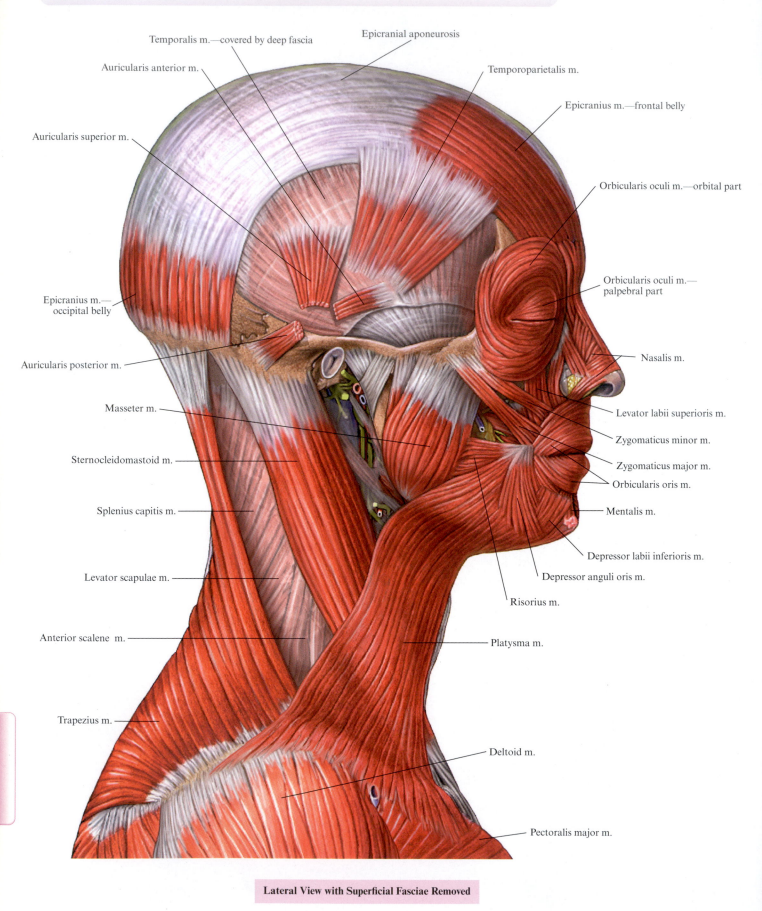

Temporalis m.—covered by deep fascia

Epicranial aponeurosis

Auricularis anterior m.

Temporoparietalis m.

Epicranius m.—frontal belly

Auricularis superior m.

Orbicularis oculi m.—orbital part

Epicranius m.—
occipital belly

Orbicularis oculi m.—
palpebral part

Auricularis posterior m.

Nasalis m.

Masseter m.

Levator labii superioris m.

Sternocleidomastoid m.

Zygomaticus minor m.

Zygomaticus major m.

Orbicularis oris m.

Splenius capitis m.

Mentalis m.

Depressor labii inferioris m.

Levator scapulae m.

Depressor anguli oris m.

Risorius m.

Anterior scalene m.

Platysma m.

Trapezius m.

Deltoid m.

Pectoralis major m.

Lateral View with Superficial Fasciae Removed

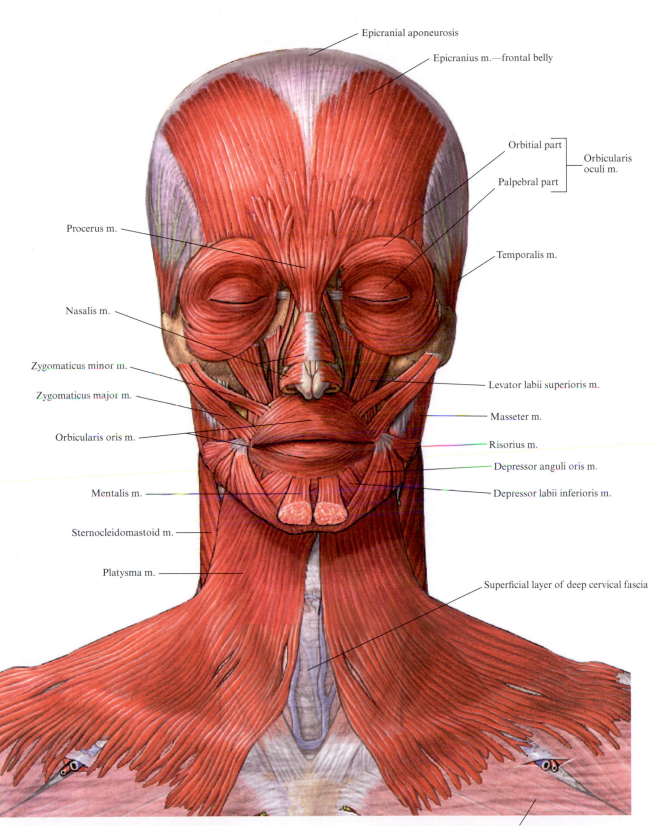

Epicranial aponeurosis

Epicranius m.—frontal belly

Orbitial part

Orbicularis
oculi m.

Palpebral part

Procerus m.

Temporalis m.

Nasalis m.

Zygomaticus minor m.

Levator labii superioris m.

Zygomaticus major m.

Masseter m.

Orbicularis oris m.

Risorius m.

Depressor anguli oris m.

Mentalis m.

Depressor labii inferioris m.

Sternocleidomastoid m.

Platysma m.

Superficial layer of deep cervical fascia

Deep layer of superficial fascia

Anterior View

TABLE 7.3   MUSCLES—MASTICATORY

Muscles Acting on the Temporomandibular Joint

Muscle	Stable Attachment	Mobile Attachment	Innervation	Main Actions
Temporalis	Floor of temporal fossa & deep surface of temporal fascia	Tip & medial surface of coronoid process & ant. border of ramus of mandible	Deep temporal br. of mandibular n. (CN V³)	Elevates mandible, closing jaws; its posterior fibers retrude mandible after protrusion
Masseter	Inf. border & medial surface of zygomatic arch	Lateral surface of ramus of mandible & its coronoid process	Mandibular n. (CN V³) via masseteric nerve that enters its deep surface	Elevates & protrudes mandible, thus closing jaws
Lateral pterygoid	*Superior head:* Infratemporal surface & infratemporal crest of greater wing of sphenoid bone *Inferior head:* Lateral surface of lateral pterygoid plate	Articular disc & capsule of temporomandibular joint Neck of mandible	Mandibular n. (CN V³) via lateral petrygoid n. from ant. trunk, which enters it unilaterally deep surface	*Acting bilaterally,* they protrude mandible & depress chin *Acting unilaterally* & alternately, they produce side-to-side movements of mandible
Medial pterygoid	*Deep head:* Medial surface of lateral pterygoid plate & pyramidal process of palatine bone *Superficial head:* Tuberosity of maxilla	Medial surface of ramus of mandible, inf. to mandibular foramen	Mandibular n. (CN V³) via medial pterygoid n.	Helps to elevate mandible, closing jaws *Acting bilaterally,* they help to protrude mandible *Acting unilaterally,* it protrudes side of jaw *Acting alternately,* they produce a grinding motion

Sup. temporal line
Temporalis m.
Fibrous capsule of temporomandibular joint
Temporomandibular lig.

Fibrous capsule of temporomandibular joint
Zygomatic arch
Temporomandibular lig.
Masseter m.—deep part
Masseter m.— superficial part
Angle of mandible

Articular disc of temporomandibular joint
Lateral pterygoid m.
Sup. head
Inf. head
Condyle of mandible

Lateral pterygoid plate
Medial pterygoid m.

Actions and Nerve Supply of the Ocular Muscles

Muscle	Abbreviations	Action(s) on the Eyeball	Nerve Supply
Medial rectus[a]	MR	Adducts	CN III
Lateral rectus[a]	LR	Abducts	CN VI[b]
Superior rectus	SR	Elevates, adducts & rotate medially	CN III
Inferior rectus	IR	Depresses, adducts & rotates laterally	CN III
Superior oblique[c]	SO	Abducts, depresses & rotates eye medially (intorsion), depresses adducted eye	CN IV[b]
Inferior oblique[c]	IO	Abducts, elevates & rotates eye laterally (extorsion), elevates adducted eye	CN III

[a]The medial and lateral rectus muscles move the eyeball in one axis only, whereas each of the other four muscles moves it in all three axes.
[b]CN IV and VI each supply one muscle, whereas CN III supplies the other four muscles.
[c]The superior and inferior oblique muscles are used with the medial rectus muscle in adducting both eyes medially for near vision. This movement, accompanied by pupillary construction, is known as accommodation.

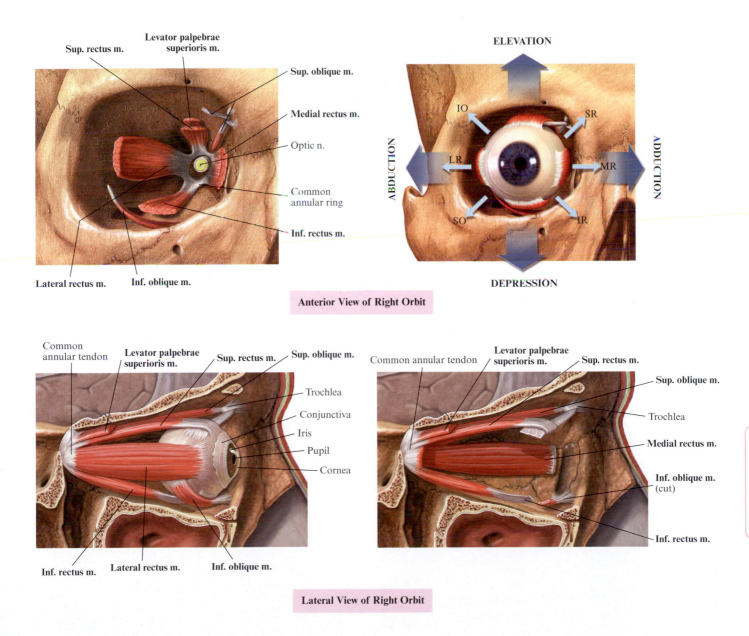

Anterior View of Right Orbit

Lateral View of Right Orbit

TABLE 7.5   MUSCLES—SOFT PALATE & TONGUE

Muscles of the Soft Palate

Muscle	Superior Attachment	Inferior Attachment	Innervation	Main Actions
Levator veli palatini	Cartilage of auditory tube & petrous part of temporal bone	Palatine aponeurosis	Pharyngeal br. of vagus n. via pharyngeal plexus (CN X)	Elevates soft palate during swallowing & yawning
Tensor veli palatini	Scaphoid fossa of medial pterygoid plate, spine of sphenoid bone & cartilage of auditory tube		Medial pterygoid n. (a br. of the mandibular n.) via otic ganglion (CN V^3)	Tenses soft palate & opens cartilagenous part of auditory tube during swallowing & yawning
Palatoglossus	Palatine aponeurosis	Side of tongue	Pharyngeal br. of vagus n. (CN X) via pharyngeal plexus	Elevates posterior part of tongue & draws soft palate onto tongue
Palatopharyngeus	Hard palate & palatine aponeurosis	Lateral wall of pharynx		Tenses soft palate & pulls walls of pharynx superiorly, anteriorly, and medially during swallowing
Musculus uvulae	Posterior nasal spine & palatine aponeurosis	Mucosa of uvula		Shortens uvula & pulls it superiorly

Extrinsic Muscles of the Tongue

Muscle	Stable Attachment	Mobile Attachment	Innervation	Actions
Genioglossus	Sup. part of mental spine of mandible	Dorsum of tongue & body of hyoid bone	Hypoglossal n. CN XII	Protrudes, retracts & depresses tongue; its post, part protrudes tongue
Hyoglossus	Body & greater horn of hyoid bone	Side of tongue		Depresses & retracts tongue
Styloglossus	Styloid process & stylohyoid lig.	Side & inf. aspect of tongue		Retracts tongue & draws it up to create a trough for swallowing
Palatoglossus	Palatine aponeurosis of soft palate	Side of tongue	Pharyngeal br. CN X & pharyngeal plexus	Elevates post. part of tongue

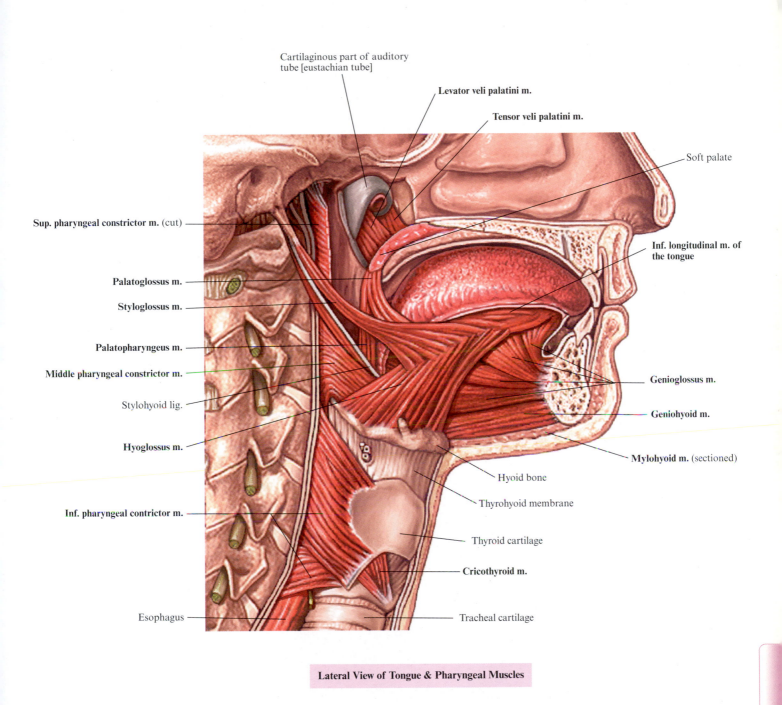

Cartilaginous part of auditory tube [eustachian tube]

Levator veli palatini m.

Tensor veli palatini m.

Soft palate

Sup. pharyngeal constrictor m. (cut)

Inf. longitudinal m. of the tongue

Palatoglossus m.

Styloglossus m.

Palatopharyngeus m.

Middle pharyngeal constrictor m.

Stylohyoid lig.

Genioglossus m.

Geniohyoid m.

Hyoglossus m.

Mylohyoid m. (sectioned)

Hyoid bone

Thyrohyoid membrane

Inf. pharyngeal contrictor m.

Thyroid cartilage

Cricothyroid m.

Esophagus

Tracheal cartilage

Lateral View of Tongue & Pharyngeal Muscles

TABLE 7.6   MUSCLES—HYOID

Suprahyoid Muscles[a]

Muscle	Superior Attachment	Inferior Attachment	Innervation	Main Actions
Mylohyoid	Mylohyoid line of mandible	Oral raphe & body of hyoid bone	Mylohyoid n., a br. of inf. alveolar n. (CN V³)	Elevates hyoid bone, floor of mouth & tongue during swallowing & speaking
Geniohyoid	Inf. mental spine of mandible	Body of hyoid bone	C1 via the hypoglossal n. (CN XII)	Pulls hyoid bone anterosuperiorly, shortens floor of mouth & widens pharynx
Stylohyoid	Styloid process of temporal bone		Facial n. (CN VII)	Elevates & retracts hyoid bone, thereby elongating floor of mouth
Digastric	*Anterior belly:* Digastric fossa of mandible *Posterior belly:* Mastoid notch of temporal bone	Intermediate tendon to body & greater horn of hyoid bone	*Anterior belly:* Mylohyoid n., a br. of inf. alveolar n. (CN V³) *Posterior belly:* Facial n. (CN VII)	Depresses mandible, raises hyoid bone & steadies it during swallowing & speaking

[a]These muscles connect the hyoid bone to the skull.

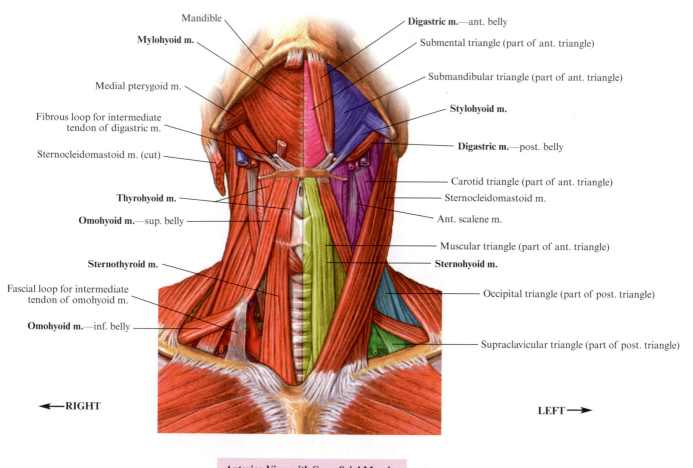

Anterior View with Superficial Muscles on Left & Deeper Muscles on Right

Infrahyoid Muscles[a]

Muscle	Origin	Insertion	Innervation	Actions
Sternohyoid	Manubrium of sternum & medial end of clavicle	Body of hyoid bone	C1, C2 & C3 from ansa cervicalis	Depresses hyoid bone after it has been elevated during swallowing
Sternothyroid	Post. surface of manubrium of sternum	Oblique line of thyroid cartilage	C2 & C3 by a br. of ansa cervicalis	Depresses hyoid bone & larynx
Thyrohyoid	Oblique line of thyroid cartilage	Inf. border of body & greater horn of hyoid bone	C1 via hypoglossal n. (CN XII)	Depresses hyoid bone & elevates larynx
Omohyoid	Sup. border of scapula near suprascapular notch	Inf. border of hyoid bone	C1, C2 & C3 by a br. of ansa cervicalis	Depresses, retracts & steadies hyoid bone

[a]These four step-like muscles anchor the hyoid bone (*ie.,* they fix and steady it). They are concerned with the suprahyoid muscles in movements of the tongue, hyoid bone, and larynx in both swallowing and speaking.

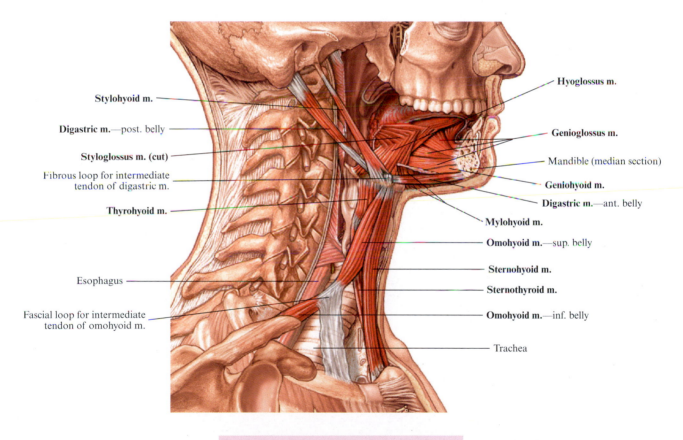

Lateral View with Right Half of Mandible Removed

TABLE 7.8   MUSCLES—PHARYNGEAL

Muscle	Lateral Attachments	Medial Attachments	Innervation	Main Actions
CIRCULAR PHARYNGEAL MUSCLES				
Superior constrictor	Pterygoid hamulus, ptergomandibular raphe, post. end of mylohyoid line of mandible & side of tongue	Median raphe of pharynx & pharyngeal tubercle	Pharyngeal & sup. laryngeal brr. of vagus n. [CN X] through pharyngeal plexus	Constrict wall of pharynx during swallowing
Middle constrictor	Stylohyoid lig. and greater & lesser horns of hyoid bone	Median raphe of pharynx		
Inferior constrictor	Oblique line of thyroid cartilage & side of cricoid cartilage			
LONGITUDINAL PHARYNGEAL MUSCLES				
Palatopharyngeus	Hard palate & palatine aponeurosis	Post. border of lamina of thyroid cartilage & side of pharynx & esophagus		Elevate pharynx & larynx during swallowing speaking[a]
Salpingopharynegeus	Cartilaginous part of auditory tube	Blends with palatopharynegeus		
Stylopharyngeus	Styloid process of temporal bone	Post. & sup. borders of thyroid cartilage with palatopharynegus m.	Glossopharyngeal n. [CN IX]	

[a]The salpingopharyngeus muscle also opens the auditory tube.

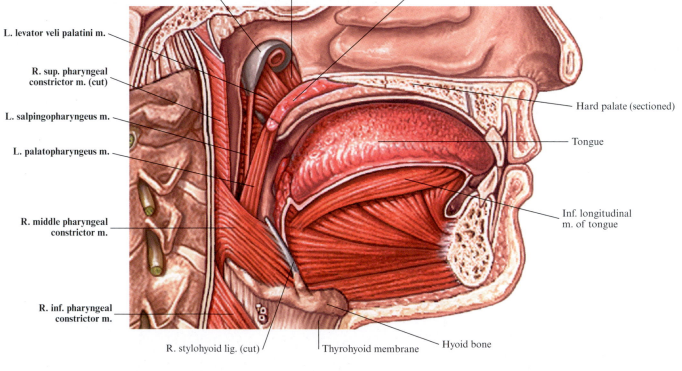

L. cartilaginous part of auditory tube [eustachian tube]

L. tensor veli palatini m.

Muscles of soft palate (sectioned)

L. levator veli palatini m.

R. sup. pharyngeal constrictor m. (cut)

L. salpingopharyngeus m.

L. palatopharyngeus m.

R. middle pharyngeal constrictor m.

R. inf. pharyngeal constrictor m.

Hard palate (sectioned)

Tongue

Inf. longitudinal m. of tongue

R. stylohyoid lig. (cut)

Thyrohyoid membrane

Hyoid bone

Lateral View of Neck & Median Sectioned Skull

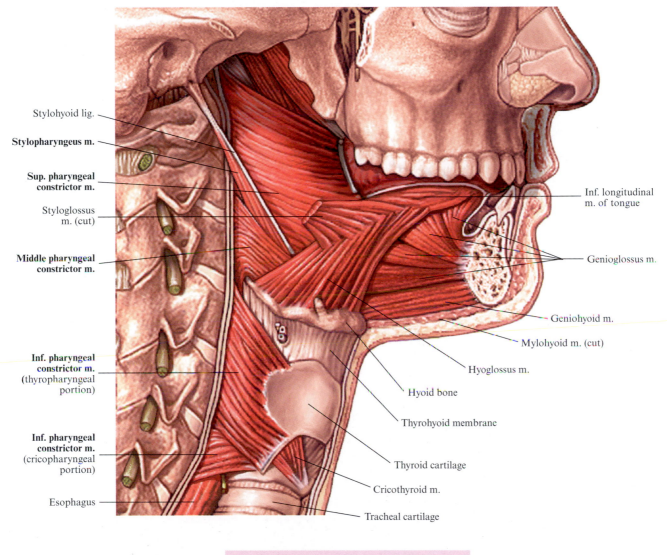

Stylohyoid lig.

Stylopharyngeus m.

Sup. pharyngeal constrictor m.

Styloglossus m. (cut)

Middle pharyngeal constrictor m.

Inf. pharyngeal constrictor m. (thyropharyngeal portion)

Inf. pharyngeal constrictor m. (cricopharyngeal portion)

Esophagus

Inf. longitudinal m. of tongue

Genioglossus m.

Geniohyoid m.

Mylohyoid m. (cut)

Hyoglossus m.

Hyoid bone

Thyrohyoid membrane

Thyroid cartilage

Cricothyroid m.

Tracheal cartilage

Lateral View with Right Half of Mandible Removed

TABLE 7.9   MUSCLES—LARYNGEAL

Muscles of the Larynx

Muscle	Origin	Insertion	Innervation	Main Actions
Cricothyroid	Anterolateral part of cricoid cartilage	Inf. margin & inf. horn of thyroid cartilage	Sup. larnyngeal n. [CN X]	Stretches & tenses the vocal fold
Posterior cricoarytenoid	Post. surface of laminae of cricoid cartilage	Muscular process of arytenoid cartilage		Abducts vocal fold
Lateral cricoarytenoid	Arch of cricoid cartilage			Adducts vocal fold
Thyroarytenoid[a]	Post. surface of thyroid cartilage	Muscular process of arytenoid process	Recurrent laryngeal n. [CN X]	Relaxes vocal fold
Transverse & oblique arytenoids	One arytenoid cartilage	Opposition arytenoid cartilage		Close laryngeal aditus by approximating arytenoid cartilages
Vocalis[b]	Angle between laminae of thyroid cartilage	Vocal process of arytenoid cartilage		Alters vocal fold during phonation

[a]The superior fibers of the thyroarytenoid muscle pass into the aryepiglottic fold, and some of them reach the epiglottic cartilage. These fibers constitute the *thyroepiglottic muscle*, which widens the inlet of the larynx.
[b]These short fine muscular slips are derived from the most medial fibers of the thyroarytenoid muscle.

Body of hyoid bone — **ANTERIOR** — Epiglottis

Lesser horn of hyoid bone — Vocal ligg.

Thyroepiglottic lig. — Vocalis m.

Thyroarytenoid m.

Greater horn of hyoid bone — Cricothyroid m.

Lateral cricoarytenoid m. — Transverse arytenoid m.

Cricothyroid joint (fibrous capsule) — Oblique arytenoid m.

Post. cricoarytenoid m.

Superior View

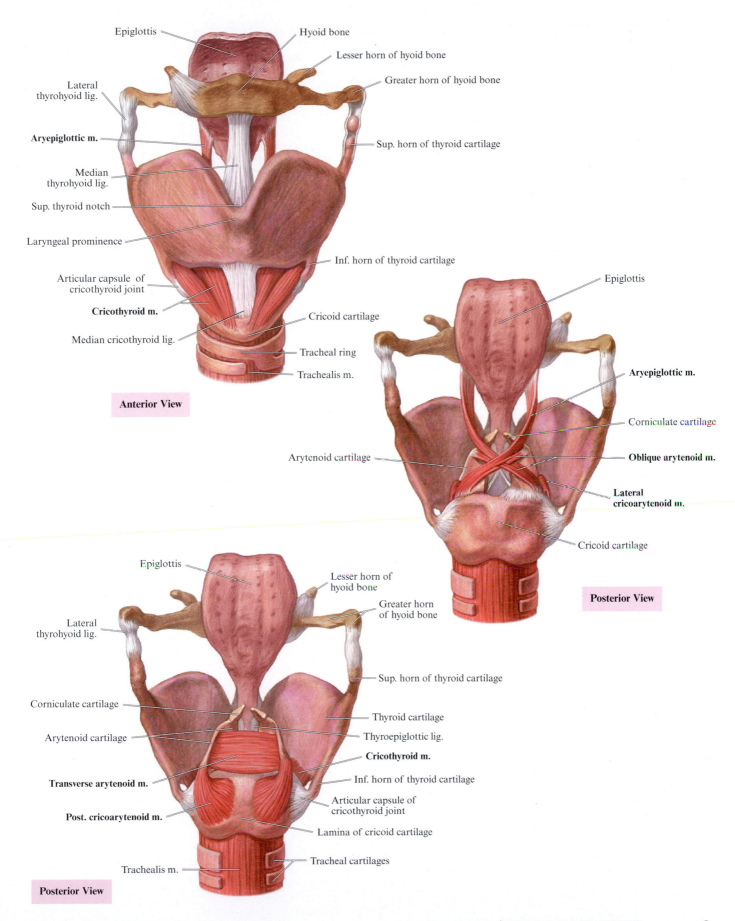

Epiglottis

Hyoid bone

Lesser horn of hyoid bone

Greater horn of hyoid bone

Lateral
thyrohyoid lig.

Aryepiglottic m.

Sup. horn of thyroid cartilage

Median
thyrohyoid lig.

Sup. thyroid notch

Laryngeal prominence

Inf. horn of thyroid cartilage

Articular capsule of
cricothyroid joint

Cricothyroid m.

Cricoid cartilage

Median cricothyroid lig.

Tracheal ring

Trachealis m.

Anterior View

Epiglottis

Aryepiglottic m.

Corniculate cartilage

Arytenoid cartilage

Oblique arytenoid m.

**Lateral
cricoarytenoid m.**

Cricoid cartilage

Posterior View

Epiglottis

Lesser horn of
hyoid bone

Greater horn
of hyoid bone

Lateral
thyrohyoid lig.

Sup. horn of thyroid cartilage

Corniculate cartilage

Thyroid cartilage

Arytenoid cartilage

Thyroepiglottic lig.

Cricothyroid m.

Transverse arytenoid m.

Inf. horn of thyroid cartilage

Articular capsule of
cricothyroid joint

Post. cricoarytenoid m.

Lamina of cricoid cartilage

Trachealis m.

Tracheal cartilages

Posterior View

TABLE 7.10   MUSCLES—LATERAL & PREVERTEBRAL

Muscle	Inferior Attachment	Superior Attachment	Innervation	Main Actions
Sternocleidomastoid				
Sternal head	Ventral surface of the manubrium sterni	Lateral surface of mastoid process; sup. nuchal line of occipital bone	Accessory n. [CN XI] (motor); sensory fibers of C2 cervical spinal n.	Various: both sides together support head, move chin upward, and pull back of head down. One side alone turns chin upward and to opposite side.
Clavicular head	Cranial surface of medial third of clavicle			
Splenius capitis	Inf. half of ligamentum nuchae & spinous process of sup. six thoracic vertebrae	Lateral aspect of mastoid process & lateral third of sup. nuchal line	Dorsal rami of middle cervical spinal nn.	Laterally flexes & rotates head & neck to same side; acting bilaterally, they extend head & neck
Splenius cervicis	Spines of 3rd (or 4th) to 6th thoracic vertebrae	Posterior tubercles of the transverse process of the upper three cervical vertebrae	Dorsal rami of nn. (C2-C5) lateral brr. (same as splenius capitis m.)	
Posterior scalene	Post. tubercles of transverse processes of C4-C6	Ext. border of second rib	Ventral rami of cervical spinal nn. (C7 & C8)	Flexes neck laterally; elevates second rib during forced inspiration
Middle scalene	Posterior tubercles of transverse processes of C2-C7	Sup. surface of first rib, posterior to groove for subclavian a.	Ventral rami of cervical spinal nn. (C3-C8)	Flexes neck laterally; elevates first rib during forced inspiration
Anterior scalene	Ant. tubercles of transverse processes of C3-C6	Scalene tubercle of 1st rib	Long thoracic n. (C5-C7)	
Longus colli				
Vertical portion	Body of first three thoracic & last three cervical vertebrae	Bodies of C2-C4	Ventral rami of cervical spinal nn. (C2-C6)	Bilaterally acting to flex neck and head anteriorly, unilaterally to flex head and neck laterally and to rotate the head toward the same side
Superior oblique	Ant. tubercles of transverse process of C3-C5	Tubercle on ant. arch of the atlas & body axis		
Inferior oblique	Ant. surface of bodies of first two or three thoracic vertebrae	Ant. tubercles of the transverse processes of C5 & C6	Ventral rami of cervical spinal nn. (C1-C4)	
Longus capitis	Ant. tubercle of transverse processes of C3-C6	Inf. border of basilar part of occipital		

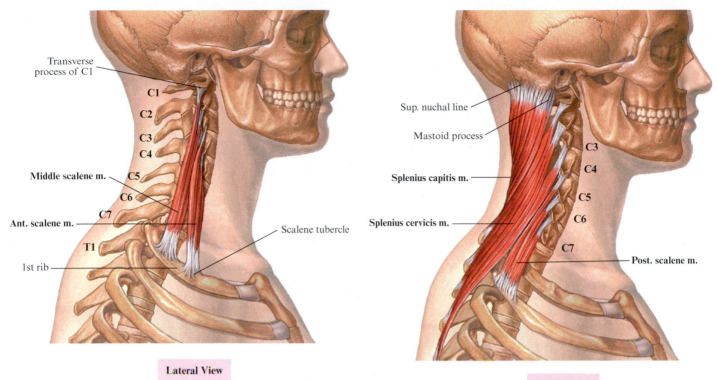

Lateral View

Lateral View

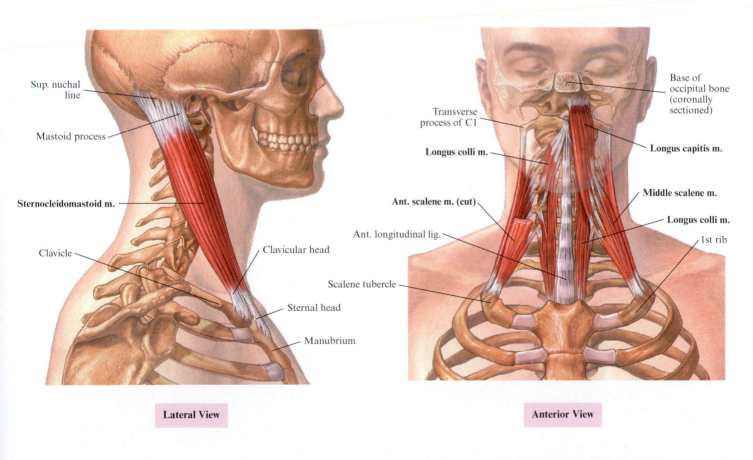

Lateral View

Anterior View

PLATE 7.27   CERVICAL FASCIAL PLANES

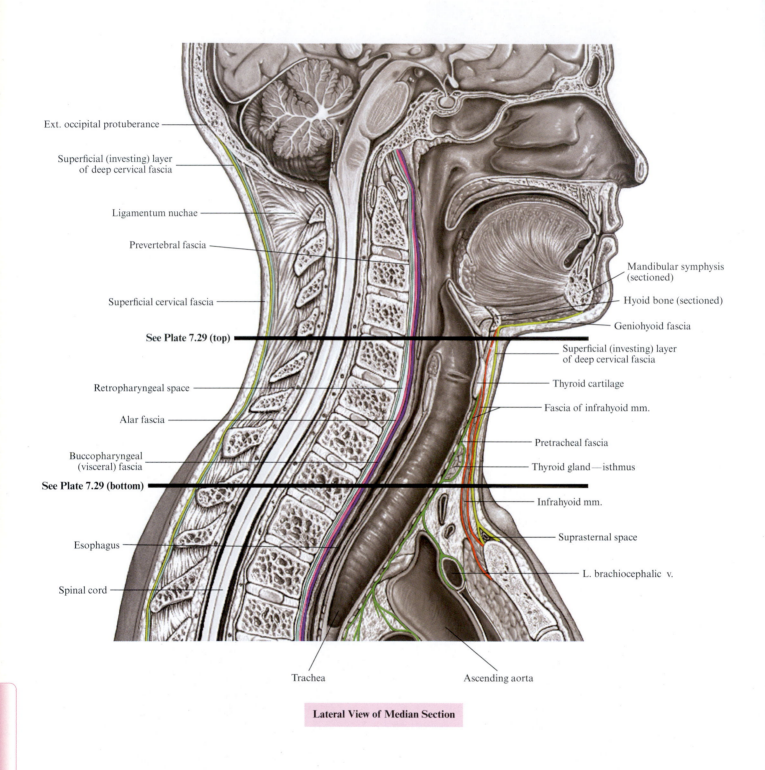

Ext. occipital protuberance

Superficial (investing) layer of deep cervical fascia

Ligamentum nuchae

Prevertebral fascia

Superficial cervical fascia

See Plate 7.29 (top)

Retropharyngeal space

Alar fascia

Buccopharyngeal (visceral) fascia

See Plate 7.29 (bottom)

Esophagus

Spinal cord

Mandibular symphysis (sectioned)

Hyoid bone (sectioned)

Geniohyoid fascia

Superficial (investing) layer of deep cervical fascia

Thyroid cartilage

Fascia of infrahyoid mm.

Pretracheal fascia

Thyroid gland—isthmus

Infrahyoid mm.

Suprasternal space

L. brachiocephalic v.

Trachea

Ascending aorta

Lateral View of Median Section

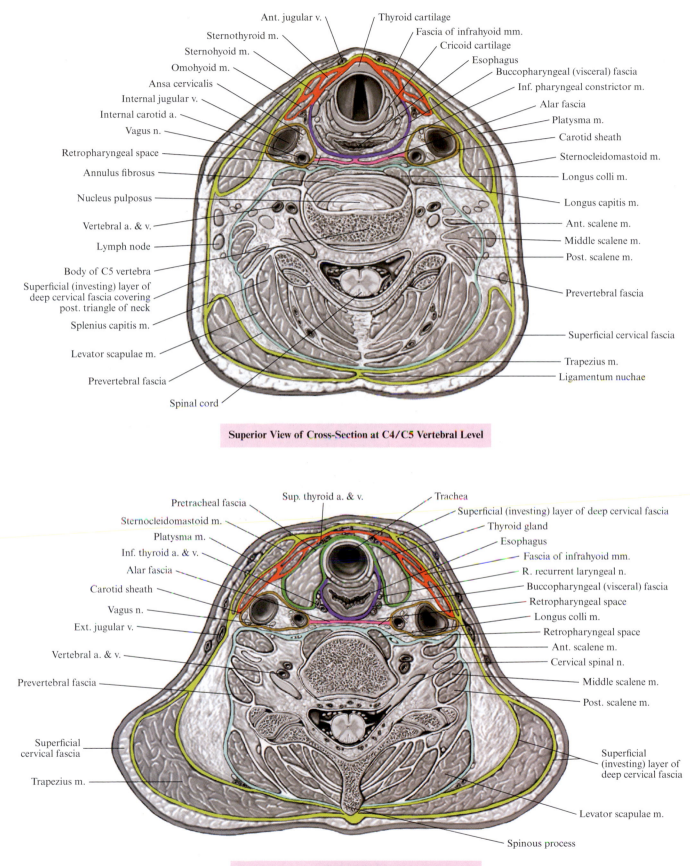

Ant. jugular v.
Sternothyroid m.
Sternohyoid m.
Omohyoid m.
Ansa cervicalis
Internal jugular v.
Internal carotid a.
Vagus n.
Retropharyngeal space
Annulus fibrosus
Nucleus pulposus
Vertebral a. & v.
Lymph node
Body of C5 vertebra
Superficial (investing) layer of deep cervical fascia covering post. triangle of neck
Splenius capitis m.
Levator scapulae m.
Prevertebral fascia
Spinal cord

Thyroid cartilage
Fascia of infrahyoid mm.
Cricoid cartilage
Esophagus
Buccopharyngeal (visceral) fascia
Inf. pharyngeal constrictor m.
Alar fascia
Platysma m.
Carotid sheath
Sternocleidomastoid m.
Longus colli m.
Longus capitis m.
Ant. scalene m.
Middle scalene m.
Post. scalene m.
Prevertebral fascia
Superficial cervical fascia
Trapezius m.
Ligamentum nuchae

Superior View of Cross-Section at C4/C5 Vertebral Level

Pretracheal fascia
Sternocleidomastoid m.
Platysma m.
Inf. thyroid a. & v.
Alar fascia
Carotid sheath
Vagus n.
Ext. jugular v.
Vertebral a. & v.
Prevertebral fascia
Superficial cervical fascia
Trapezius m.

Sup. thyroid a. & v.
Trachea

Trachea
Superficial (investing) layer of deep cervical fascia
Thyroid gland
Esophagus
Fascia of infrahyoid mm.
R. recurrent laryngeal n.
Buccopharyngeal (visceral) fascia
Retropharyngeal space
Longus colli m.
Retropharyngeal space
Ant. scalene m.
Cervical spinal n.
Middle scalene m.
Post. scalene m.
Superficial (investing) layer of deep cervical fascia
Levator scapulae m.
Spinous process

Superior View of Cross-Section at T1 Vertebral Level

PLATE 7.31   ARTERIES—BRAIN & BRAINSTEM

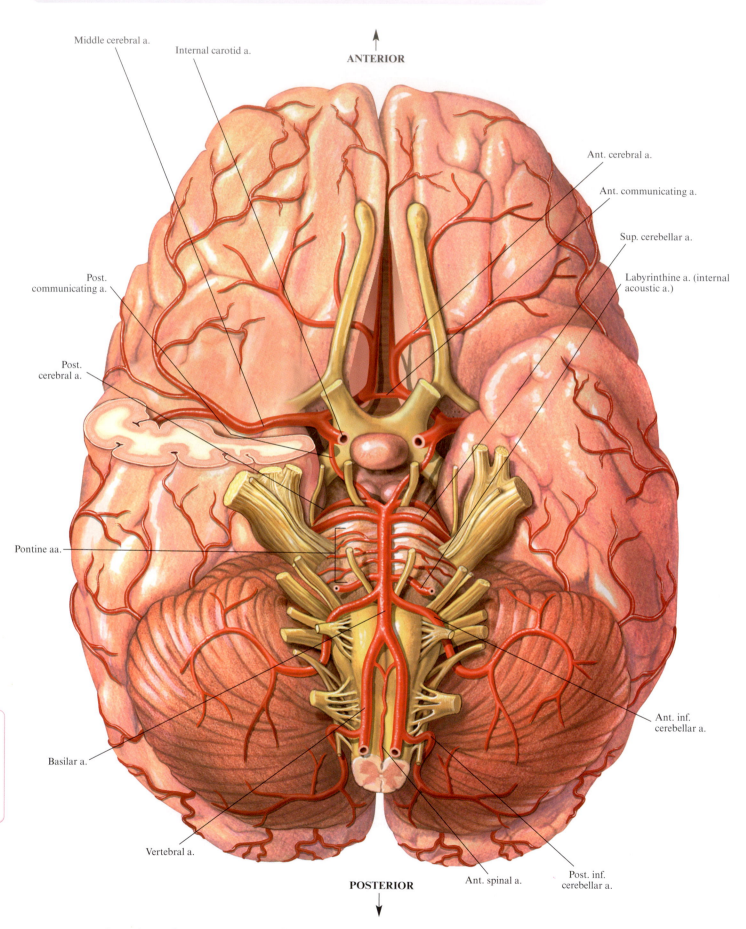

Middle cerebral a.

Internal carotid a.

ANTERIOR

Ant. cerebral a.

Ant. communicating a.

Sup. cerebellar a.

Labyrinthine a. (internal acoustic a.)

Post. communicating a.

Post. cerebral a.

Pontine aa.

Ant. inf. cerebellar a.

Basilar a.

Vertebral a.

Ant. spinal a.

Post. inf. cerebellar a.

POSTERIOR

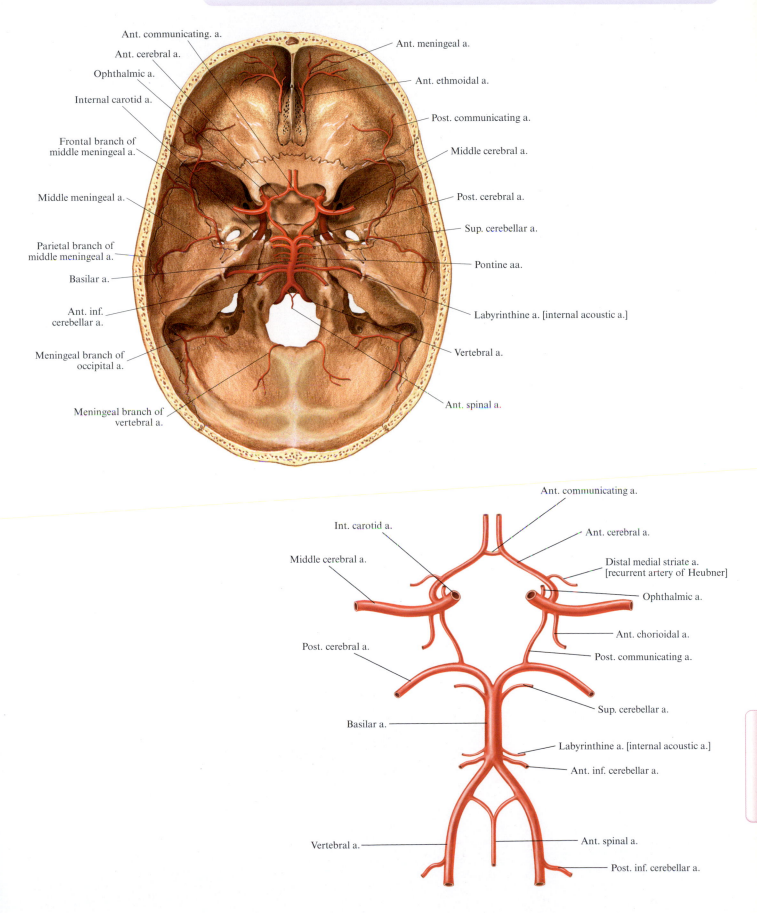

Ant. communicating. a.

Ant. cerebral a.

Ophthalmic a.

Internal carotid a.

Frontal branch of
middle meningeal a.

Middle meningeal a.

Parietal branch of
middle meningeal a.

Basilar a.

Ant. inf.
cerebellar a.

Meningeal branch of
occipital a.

Meningeal branch of
vertebral a.

Ant. meningeal a.

Ant. ethmoidal a.

Post. communicating a.

Middle cerebral a.

Post. cerebral a.

Sup. cerebellar a.

Pontine aa.

Labyrinthine a. [internal acoustic a.]

Vertebral a.

Ant. spinal a.

Ant. communicating a.

Int. carotid a.

Middle cerebral a.

Post. cerebral a.

Basilar a.

Vertebral a.

Ant. cerebral a.

Distal medial striate a.
[recurrent artery of Heubner]

Ophthalmic a.

Ant. chorioidal a.

Post. communicating a.

Sup. cerebellar a.

Labyrinthine a. [internal acoustic a.]

Ant. inf. cerebellar a.

Ant. spinal a.

Post. inf. cerebellar a.

PLATE 7.33   VEINS—SUPERFICIAL

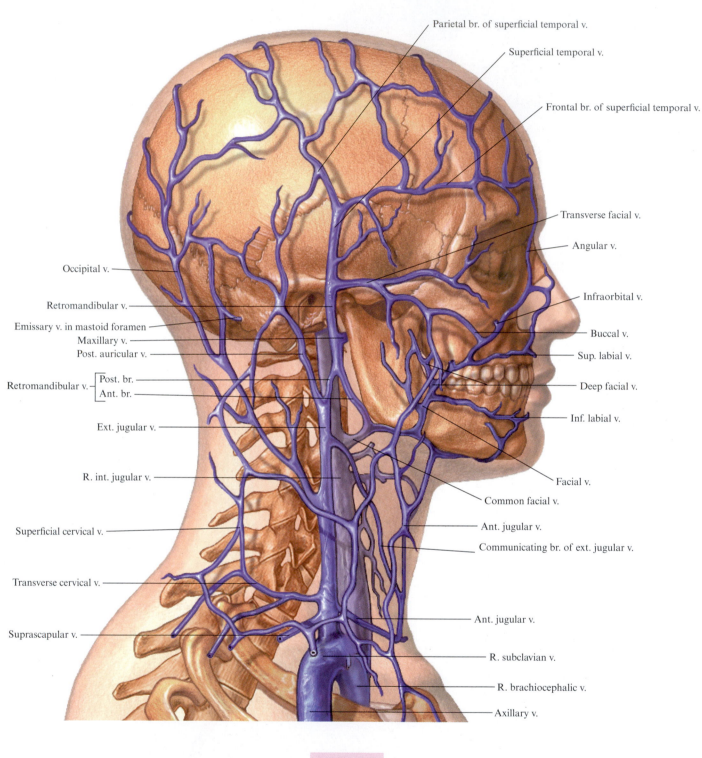

Parietal br. of superficial temporal v.

Superficial temporal v.

Frontal br. of superficial temporal v.

Transverse facial v.

Angular v.

Occipital v.

Infraorbital v.

Retromandibular v.

Emissary v. in mastoid foramen

Buccal v.

Maxillary v.

Post. auricular v.

Sup. labial v.

Retromandibular v. — Post. br.

Ant. br.

Deep facial v.

Inf. labial v.

Ext. jugular v.

R. int. jugular v.

Facial v.

Common facial v.

Superficial cervical v.

Ant. jugular v.

Communicating br. of ext. jugular v.

Transverse cervical v.

Ant. jugular v.

Suprascapular v.

R. subclavian v.

R. brachiocephalic v.

Axillary v.

Lateral View

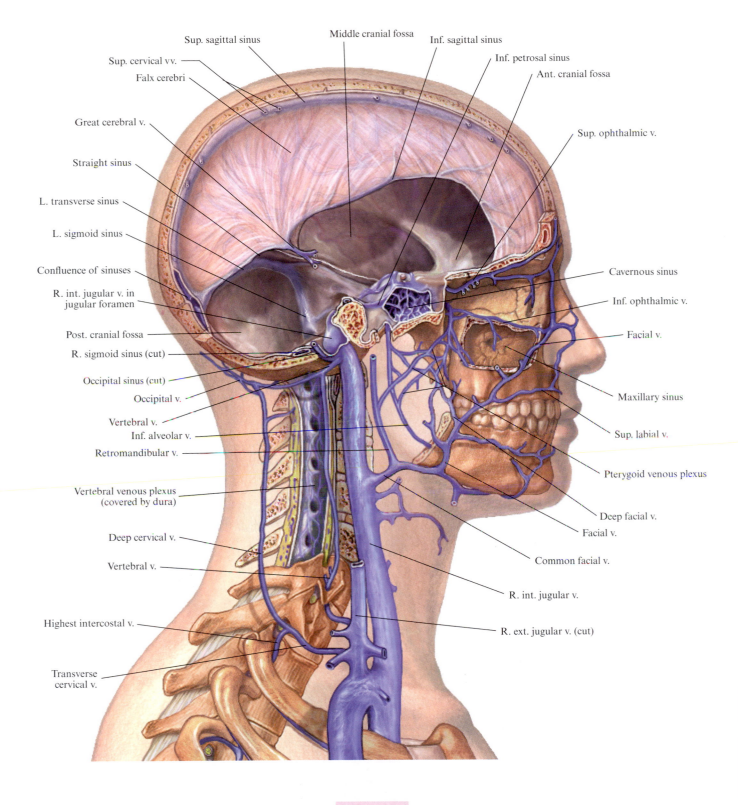

Sup. cervical vv.

Falx cerebri

Great cerebral v.

Straight sinus

L. transverse sinus

L. sigmoid sinus

Confluence of sinuses

R. int. jugular v. in
jugular foramen

Post. cranial fossa

R. sigmoid sinus (cut)

Occipital sinus (cut)

Occipital v.

Vertebral v.

Inf. alveolar v.

Retromandibular v.

Vertebral venous plexus
(covered by dura)

Deep cervical v.

Vertebral v.

Highest intercostal v.

Transverse
cervical v.

Sup. sagittal sinus

Middle cranial fossa

Inf. sagittal sinus

Inf. petrosal sinus

Ant. cranial fossa

Sup. ophthalmic v.

Cavernous sinus

Inf. ophthalmic v.

Facial v.

Maxillary sinus

Sup. labial v.

Pterygoid venous plexus

Deep facial v.

Facial v.

Common facial v.

R. int. jugular v.

R. ext. jugular v. (cut)

Lateral View

PLATE 7.37   DERMATOMES & CUTANEOUS INNERVATION

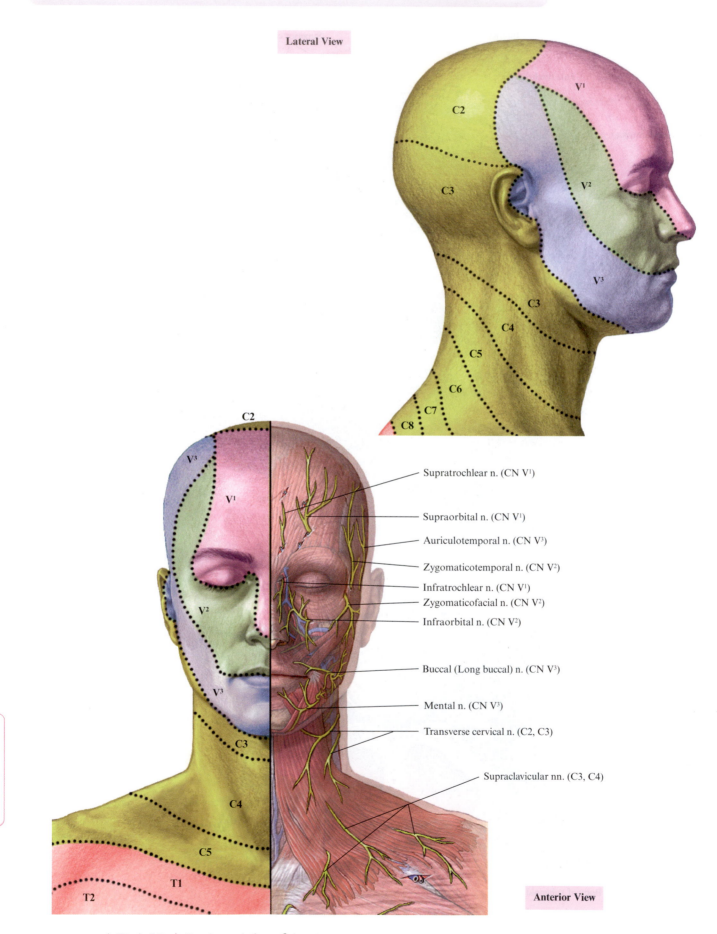

Lateral View

V¹
C2
V²
C3
V³
C3
C4
C5
C6
C7
C8

C2
V³
V¹
V²
V³
C3
C4
C5
T1
T2

Supratrochlear n. (CN V¹)

Supraorbital n. (CN V¹)

Auriculotemporal n. (CN V³)

Zygomaticotemporal n. (CN V²)

Infratrochlear n. (CN V¹)

Zygomaticofacial n. (CN V²)

Infraorbital n. (CN V²)

Buccal (Long buccal) n. (CN V³)

Mental n. (CN V³)

Transverse cervical n. (C2, C3)

Supraclavicular nn. (C3, C4)

Anterior View

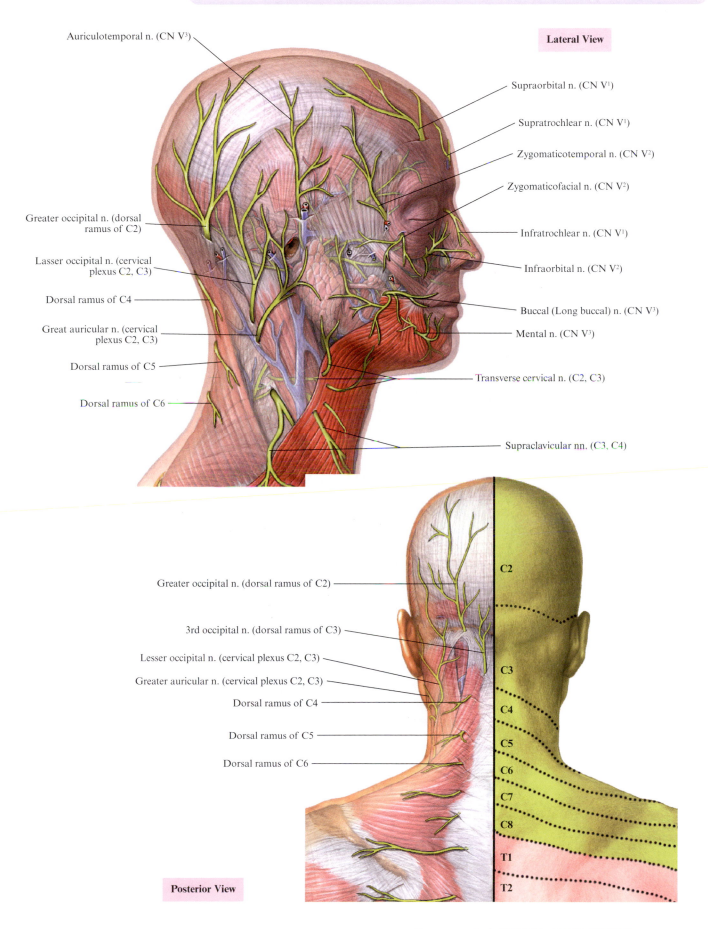

Lateral View

Auriculotemporal n. (CN V³)

Supraorbital n. (CN V¹)

Supratrochlear n. (CN V¹)

Zygomaticotemporal n. (CN V²)

Zygomaticofacial n. (CN V²)

Greater occipital n. (dorsal ramus of C2)

Infratrochlear n. (CN V¹)

Lasser occipital n. (cervical plexus C2, C3)

Infraorbital n. (CN V²)

Dorsal ramus of C4

Buccal (Long buccal) n. (CN V³)

Great auricular n. (cervical plexus C2, C3)

Mental n. (CN V³)

Dorsal ramus of C5

Dorsal ramus of C6

Transverse cervical n. (C2, C3)

Supraclavicular nn. (C3, C4)

Greater occipital n. (dorsal ramus of C2)

C2

3rd occipital n. (dorsal ramus of C3)

Lesser occipital n. (cervical plexus C2, C3)

C3

Greater auricular n. (cervical plexus C2, C3)

Dorsal ramus of C4

C4

Dorsal ramus of C5

C5

Dorsal ramus of C6

C6

C7

C8

T1

Posterior View

T2

PLATE 7.43   LYMPHATICS

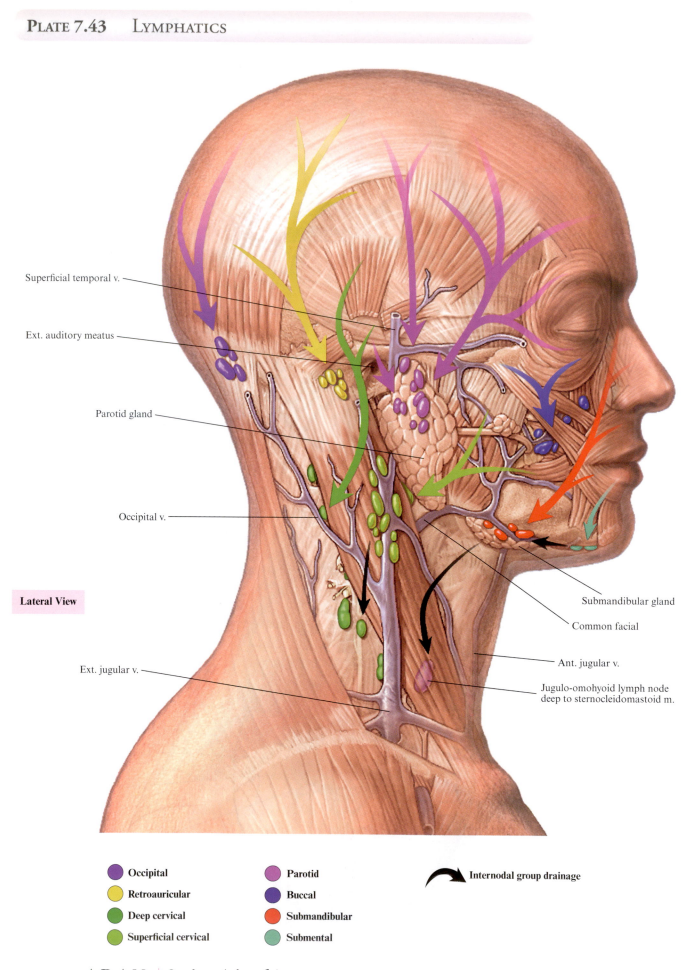

Superficial temporal v.

Ext. auditory meatus

Parotid gland

Occipital v.

Lateral View

Ext. jugular v.

Submandibular gland

Common facial

Ant. jugular v.

Jugulo-omohyoid lymph node
deep to sternocleidomastoid m.

● Occipital   ● Parotid   ➤ Internodal group drainage

● Retroauricular   ● Buccal

● Deep cervical   ● Submandibular

● Superficial cervical   ● Submental

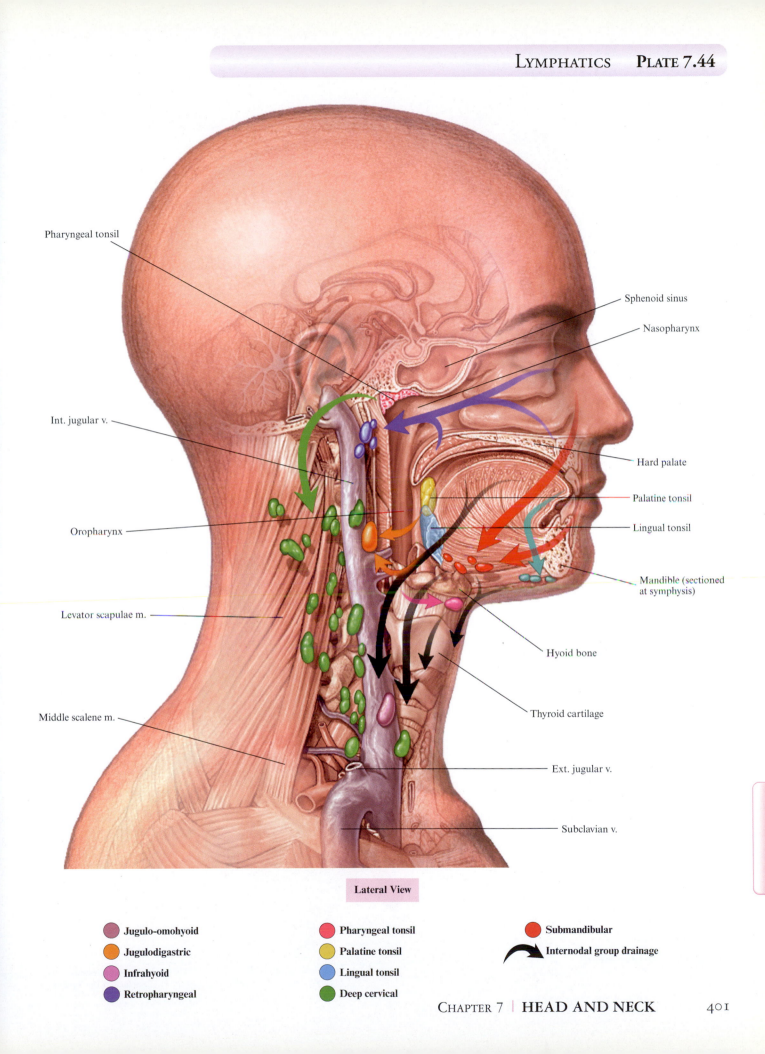

Pharyngeal tonsil

Sphenoid sinus

Nasopharynx

Int. jugular v.

Hard palate

Palatine tonsil

Oropharynx

Lingual tonsil

Mandible (sectioned at symphysis)

Levator scapulae m.

Hyoid bone

Thyroid cartilage

Middle scalene m.

Ext. jugular v.

Subclavian v.

Lateral View

● **Jugulo-omohyoid**   ● **Pharyngeal tonsil**   ● **Submandibular**

● **Jugulodigastric**   ● **Palatine tonsil**   ⮎ **Internodal group drainage**

● **Infrahyoid**   ● **Lingual tonsil**

● **Retropharyngeal**   ● **Deep cervical**

CHAPTER 7 ∣ **HEAD AND NECK**   401

PLATE 7.45 LYMPHATICS

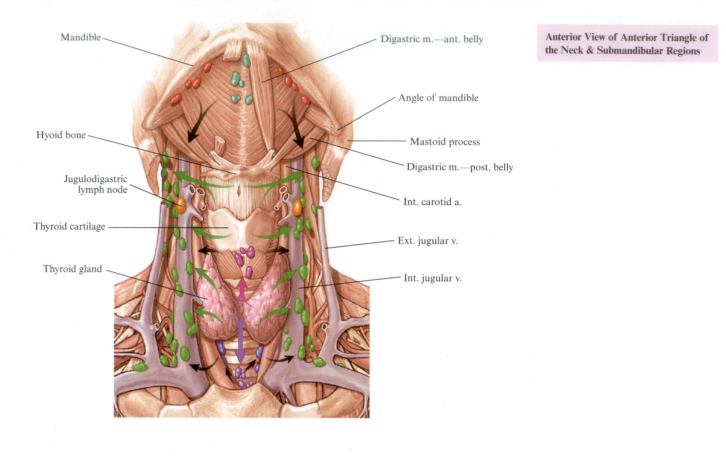

Mandible

Digastric m.—ant. belly

Anterior View of Anterior Triangle of the Neck & Submandibular Regions

Angle of mandible

Hyoid bone

Mastoid process

Digastric m.—post. belly

Jugulodigastric lymph node

Int. carotid a.

Thyroid cartilage

Ext. jugular v.

Thyroid gland

Int. jugular v.

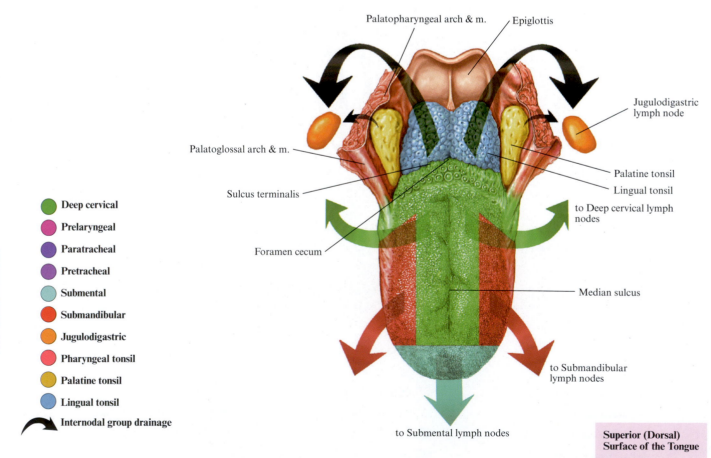

Palatopharyngeal arch & m.

Epiglottis

Jugulodigastric lymph node

Palatoglossal arch & m.

Palatine tonsil

Lingual tonsil

Sulcus terminalis

to Deep cervical lymph nodes

Foramen cecum

Median sulcus

to Submandibular lymph nodes

to Submental lymph nodes

Superior (Dorsal) Surface of the Tongue

- 🟢 **Deep cervical**
- 🟣 **Prelaryngeal**
- 🟣 **Paratracheal**
- 🟣 **Pretracheal**
- 🔵 **Submental**
- 🔴 **Submandibular**
- 🟠 **Jugulodigastric**
- 🔴 **Pharyngeal tonsil**
- 🟡 **Palatine tonsil**
- 🔵 **Lingual tonsil**
- ⬛ **Internodal group drainage**

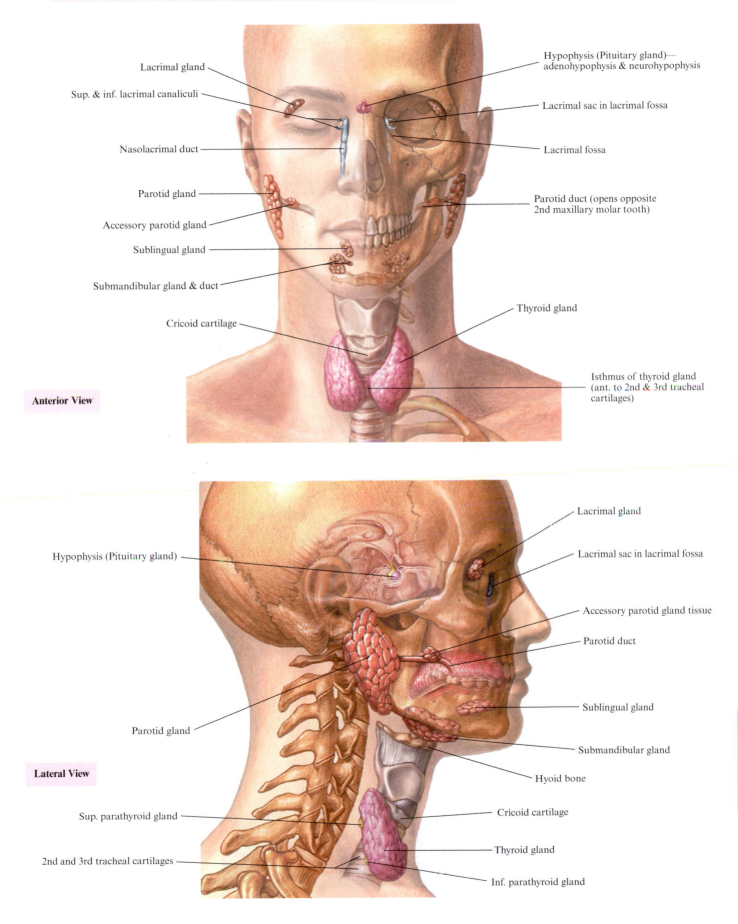

Lacrimal gland

Sup. & inf. lacrimal canaliculi

Nasolacrimal duct

Parotid gland

Accessory parotid gland

Sublingual gland

Submandibular gland & duct

Cricoid cartilage

Hypophysis (Pituitary gland)—
adenohypophysis & neurohypophysis

Lacrimal sac in lacrimal fossa

Lacrimal fossa

Parotid duct (opens opposite
2nd maxillary molar tooth)

Thyroid gland

Isthmus of thyroid gland
(ant. to 2nd & 3rd tracheal
cartilages)

Anterior View

Hypophysis (Pituitary gland)

Parotid gland

Sup. parathyroid gland

2nd and 3rd tracheal cartilages

Lacrimal gland

Lacrimal sac in lacrimal fossa

Accessory parotid gland tissue

Parotid duct

Sublingual gland

Submandibular gland

Hyoid bone

Cricoid cartilage

Thyroid gland

Inf. parathyroid gland

Lateral View

PLATE 7.53   NECK—DEEP ANTERIOR

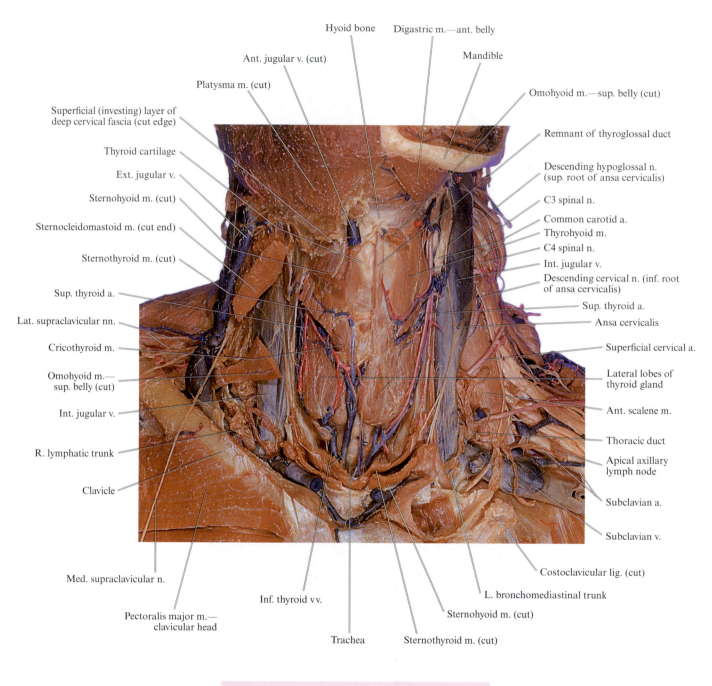

Hyoid bone

Digastric m.—ant. belly

Ant. jugular v. (cut)

Mandible

Platysma m. (cut)

Omohyoid m.—sup. belly (cut)

Superficial (investing) layer of
deep cervical fascia (cut edge)

Remnant of thyroglossal duct

Thyroid cartilage

Descending hypoglossal n.
(sup. root of ansa cervicalis)

Ext. jugular v.

C3 spinal n.

Sternohyoid m. (cut)

Common carotid a.

Sternocleidomastoid m. (cut end)

Thyrohyoid m.

C4 spinal n.

Sternothyroid m. (cut)

Int. jugular v.

Descending cervical n. (inf. root
of ansa cervicalis)

Sup. thyroid a.

Sup. thyroid a.

Lat. supraclavicular nn.

Ansa cervicalis

Cricothyroid m.

Superficial cervical a.

Omohyoid m.—
sup. belly (cut)

Lateral lobes of
thyroid gland

Int. jugular v.

Ant. scalene m.

R. lymphatic trunk

Thoracic duct

Apical axillary
lymph node

Clavicle

Subclavian a.

Subclavian v.

Med. supraclavicular n.

Costoclavicular lig. (cut)

L. bronchomediastinal trunk

Pectoralis major m.—
clavicular head

Sternohyoid m. (cut)

Inf. thyroid vv.

Sternothyroid m. (cut)

Trachea

Anterior View of Neck with Deep Structures on Right Side

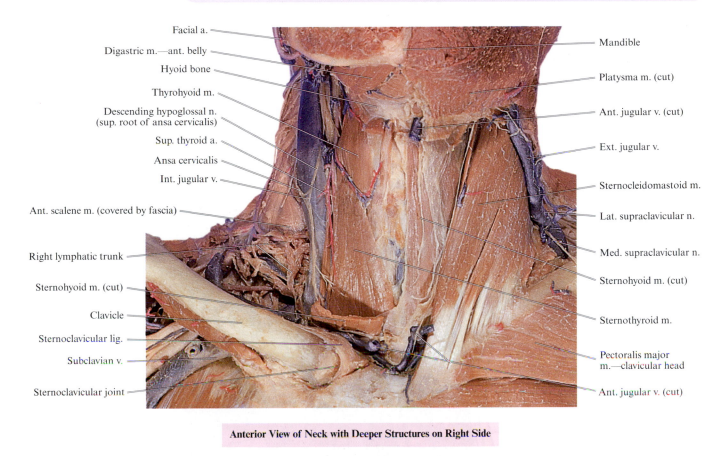

Facial a.

Digastric m.—ant. belly

Hyoid bone

Thyrohyoid m.

Descending hypoglossal n.
(sup. root of ansa cervicalis)

Sup. thyroid a.

Ansa cervicalis

Int. jugular v.

Ant. scalene m. (covered by fascia)

Right lymphatic trunk

Sternohyoid m. (cut)

Clavicle

Sternoclavicular lig.

Subclavian v.

Sternoclavicular joint

Mandible

Platysma m. (cut)

Ant. jugular v. (cut)

Ext. jugular v.

Sternocleidomastoid m.

Lat. supraclavicular n.

Med. supraclavicular n.

Sternohyoid m. (cut)

Sternothyroid m.

Pectoralis major
m.—clavicular head

Ant. jugular v. (cut)

Anterior View of Neck with Deeper Structures on Right Side

Mandible

Int. carotid a.

Int. jugular v.

Thyrohyoid m.

Descending hypoglossal n.
(sup. root of ansa cervicalis)

Sup. thyroid a.

Phrenic n.

Ansa cervicalis

Int. jugular v.

Ant. scalene m.

Superficial cervical a.

Descending cervical n.
(inf. root of ansa cervicalis)

Lateral lobes of thyroid
gland

Right lymphatic trunk

Sternohyoid m. (cut)

Subclavian v.

Clavicle

Depressor anguli oris m.

Mylohyoid m.

Hyoid bone

Omohyoid m.—sup.
belly (cut)

Sternohyoid m.

Sternocleidomastoid m.

Sternohyoid m.

Clavicle

Isthmus of thyroid gland

Sternothyroid m. (cut)

Pectoralis major m.—
clavicular head

Ant. jugular v.

Anterolateral View of Right Side of Neck

PLATE 7.57   LARYNX—SUPERFICIAL ANTERIOR

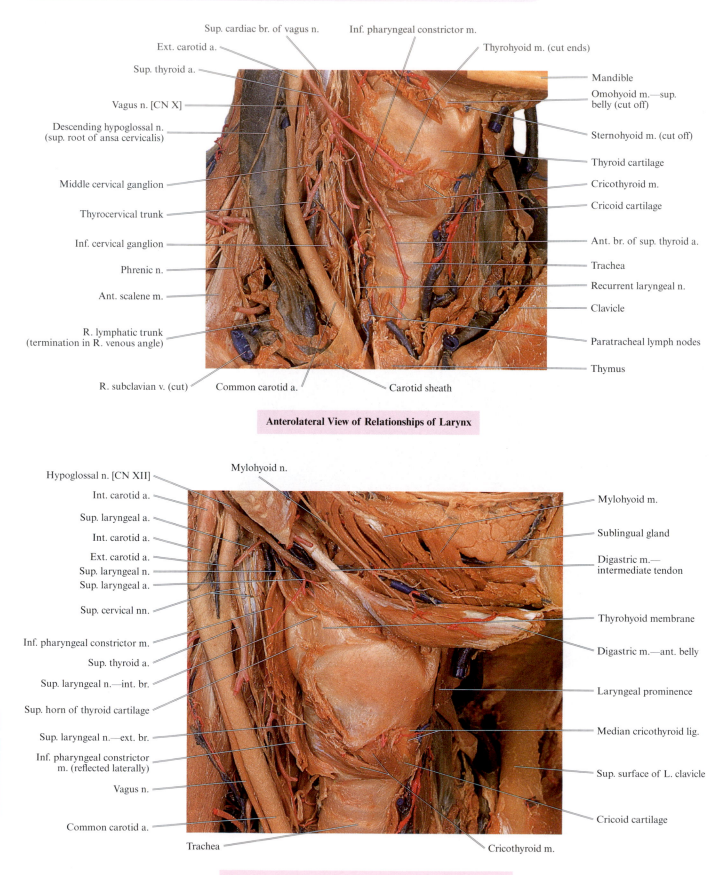

Sup. cardiac br. of vagus n.

Inf. pharyngeal constrictor m.

Ext. carotid a.

Thyrohyoid m. (cut ends)

Sup. thyroid a.

Mandible

Omohyoid m.—sup. belly (cut off)

Vagus n. [CN X]

Descending hypoglossal n. (sup. root of ansa cervicalis)

Sternohyoid m. (cut off)

Thyroid cartilage

Middle cervical ganglion

Cricothyroid m.

Thyrocervical trunk

Cricoid cartilage

Inf. cervical ganglion

Ant. br. of sup. thyroid a.

Phrenic n.

Trachea

Ant. scalene m.

Recurrent laryngeal n.

Clavicle

R. lymphatic trunk (termination in R. venous angle)

Paratracheal lymph nodes

Thymus

R. subclavian v. (cut)   Common carotid a.   Carotid sheath

Anterolateral View of Relationships of Larynx

Mylohyoid n.

Hypoglossal n. [CN XII]

Int. carotid a.

Mylohyoid m.

Sup. laryngeal a.

Sublingual gland

Int. carotid a.

Ext. carotid a.

Digastric m.— intermediate tendon

Sup. laryngeal n.

Sup. laryngeal a.

Sup. cervical nn.

Inf. pharyngeal constrictor m.

Thyrohyoid membrane

Sup. thyroid a.

Digastric m.—ant. belly

Sup. laryngeal n.—int. br.

Laryngeal prominence

Sup. horn of thyroid cartilage

Sup. laryngeal n.—ext. br.

Median cricothyroid lig.

Inf. pharyngeal constrictor m. (reflected laterally)

Sup. surface of L. clavicle

Vagus n.

Common carotid a.

Cricoid cartilage

Trachea   Cricothyroid m.

Anterolateral View of Larynx with Body of Mandible Removed

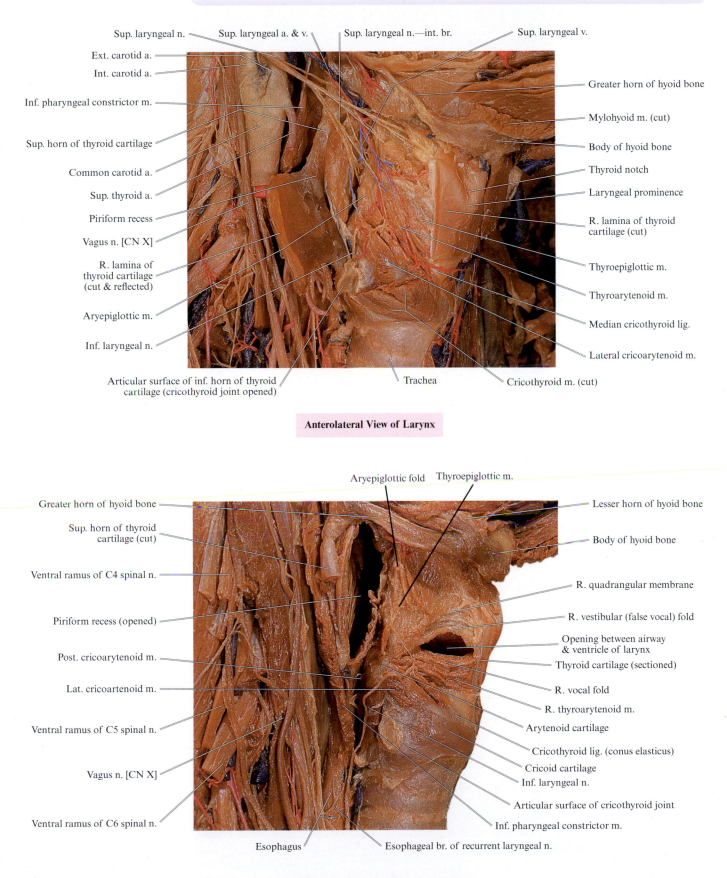

Sup. laryngeal n.   Sup. laryngeal a. & v.   Sup. laryngeal n.—int. br.   Sup. laryngeal v.

Ext. carotid a.

Int. carotid a.

Inf. pharyngeal constrictor m.

Sup. horn of thyroid cartilage

Common carotid a.

Sup. thyroid a.

Piriform recess

Vagus n. [CN X]

R. lamina of
thyroid cartilage
(cut & reflected)

Aryepiglottic m.

Inf. laryngeal n.

Articular surface of inf. horn of thyroid
cartilage (cricothyroid joint opened)

Greater horn of hyoid bone

Mylohyoid m. (cut)

Body of hyoid bone

Thyroid notch

Laryngeal prominence

R. lamina of thyroid
cartilage (cut)

Thyroepiglottic m.

Thyroarytenoid m.

Median cricothyroid lig.

Lateral cricoarytenoid m.

Trachea

Cricothyroid m. (cut)

Anterolateral View of Larynx

Aryepiglottic fold   Thyroepiglottic m.

Greater horn of hyoid bone

Sup. horn of thyroid
cartilage (cut)

Ventral ramus of C4 spinal n.

Piriform recess (opened)

Post. cricoarytenoid m.

Lat. cricoartenoid m.

Ventral ramus of C5 spinal n.

Vagus n. [CN X]

Ventral ramus of C6 spinal n.

Esophagus

Lesser horn of hyoid bone

Body of hyoid bone

R. quadrangular membrane

R. vestibular (false vocal) fold

Opening between airway
& ventricle of larynx

Thyroid cartilage (sectioned)

R. vocal fold

R. thyroarytenoid m.

Arytenoid cartilage

Cricothyroid lig. (conus elasticus)

Cricoid cartilage

Inf. laryngeal n.

Articular surface of cricothyroid joint

Inf. pharyngeal constrictor m.

Esophageal br. of recurrent laryngeal n.

Lateral View of Larynx & R. Vocal Folds

PLATE 7.59   LARYNX—POSTERIOR & SUPERIOR

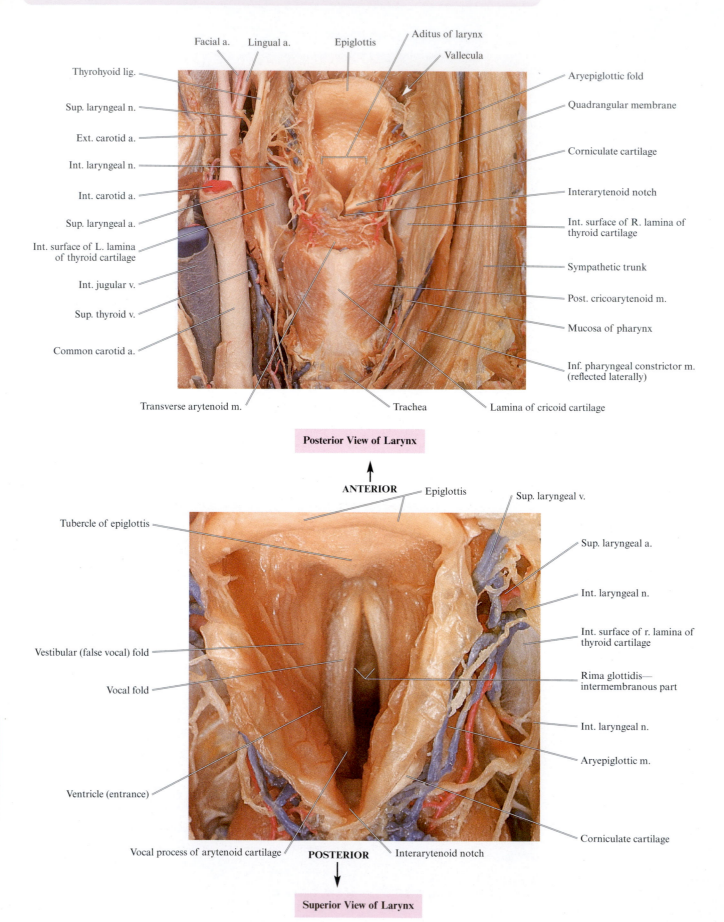

Facial a.   Lingual a.   Epiglottis   Aditus of larynx
Vallecula

Thyrohyoid lig.   Aryepiglottic fold

Sup. laryngeal n.   Quadrangular membrane

Ext. carotid a.   Corniculate cartilage

Int. laryngeal n.   Interarytenoid notch

Int. carotid a.   Int. surface of R. lamina of thyroid cartilage

Sup. laryngeal a.   Sympathetic trunk

Int. surface of L. lamina of thyroid cartilage   Post. cricoarytenoid m.

Int. jugular v.   Mucosa of pharynx

Sup. thyroid v.   Inf. pharyngeal constrictor m. (reflected laterally)

Common carotid a.

Transverse arytenoid m.   Trachea   Lamina of cricoid cartilage

Posterior View of Larynx

ANTERIOR   Epiglottis   Sup. laryngeal v.

Tubercle of epiglottis   Sup. laryngeal a.

Int. laryngeal n.

Int. surface of r. lamina of thyroid cartilage

Vestibular (false vocal) fold   Rima glottidis—intermembranous part

Vocal fold   Int. laryngeal n.

Aryepiglottic m.

Ventricle (entrance)

Corniculate cartilage

Vocal process of arytenoid cartilage   **POSTERIOR**   Interarytenoid notch

Superior View of Larynx

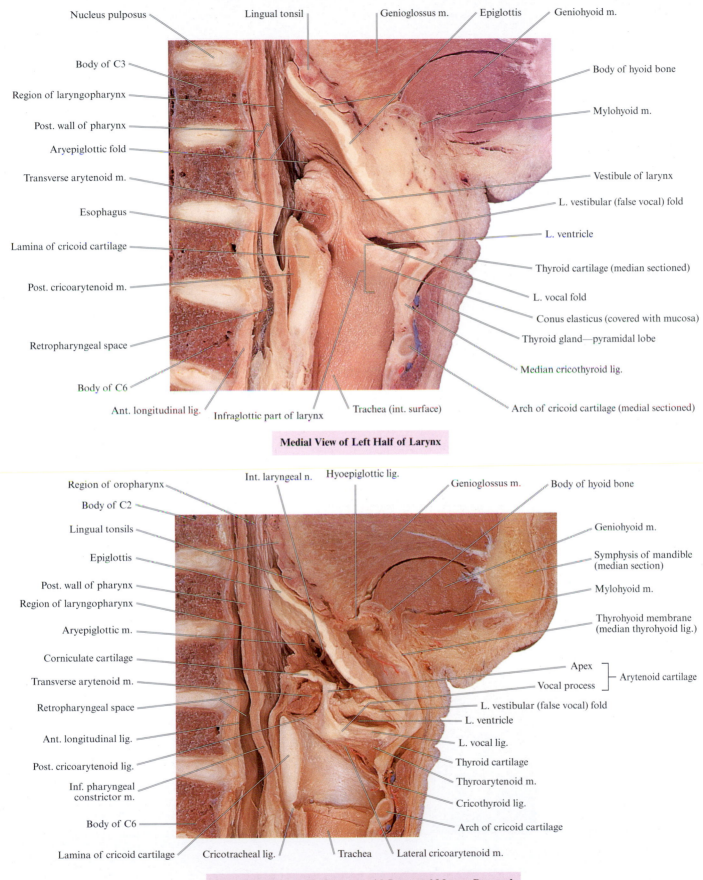

Nucleus pulposus

Lingual tonsil

Genioglossus m.

Epiglottis

Geniohyoid m.

Body of C3

Region of laryngopharynx

Post. wall of pharynx

Aryepiglottic fold

Transverse arytenoid m.

Esophagus

Lamina of cricoid cartilage

Post. cricoarytenoid m.

Retropharyngeal space

Body of C6

Ant. longitudinal lig.

Infraglottic part of larynx

Trachea (int. surface)

Body of hyoid bone

Mylohyoid m.

Vestibule of larynx

L. vestibular (false vocal) fold

L. ventricle

Thyroid cartilage (median sectioned)

L. vocal fold

Conus elasticus (covered with mucosa)

Thyroid gland—pyramidal lobe

Median cricothyroid lig.

Arch of cricoid cartilage (medial sectioned)

Medial View of Left Half of Larynx

Region of oropharynx

Int. laryngeal n.

Hyoepiglottic lig.

Genioglossus m.

Body of hyoid bone

Body of C2

Lingual tonsils

Epiglottis

Post. wall of pharynx

Region of laryngopharynx

Aryepiglottic m.

Corniculate cartilage

Transverse arytenoid m.

Retropharyngeal space

Ant. longitudinal lig.

Post. cricoarytenoid lig.

Inf. pharyngeal constrictor m.

Body of C6

Lamina of cricoid cartilage

Cricotracheal lig.

Trachea

Lateral cricoarytenoid m.

Geniohyoid m.

Symphysis of mandible (median section)

Mylohyoid m.

Thyrohyoid membrane (median thyrohyoid lig.)

Apex

Vocal process

Arytenoid cartilage

L. vestibular (false vocal) fold

L. ventricle

L. vocal lig.

Thyroid cartilage

Thyroarytenoid m.

Cricothyroid lig.

Arch of cricoid cartilage

Medial View of Left Half Larynx with Laryngeal Mucosa Removed

PLATE 7.61   POSTERIOR PHARYNX

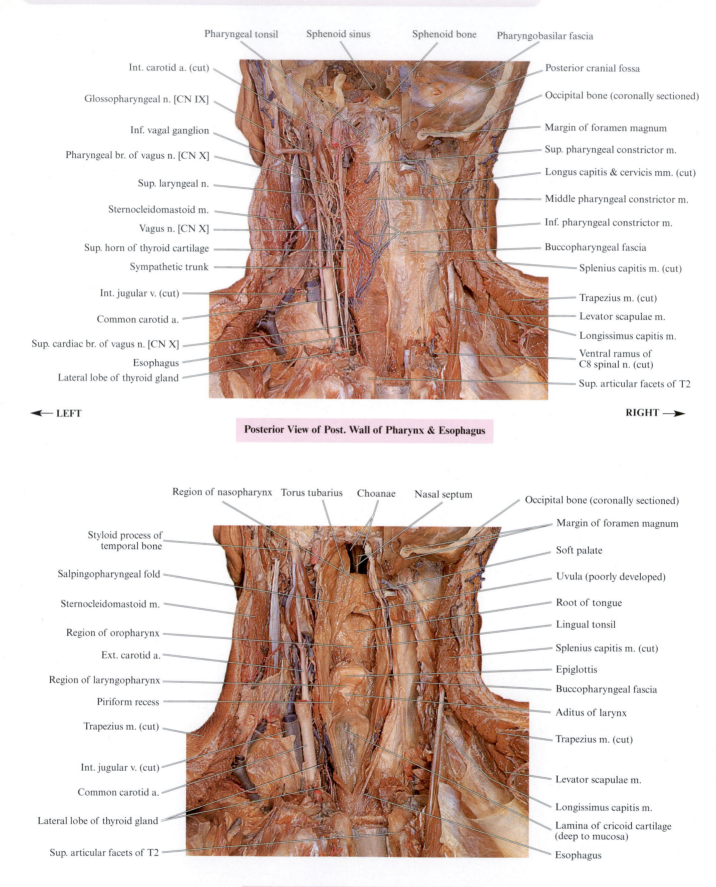

Pharyngeal tonsil   Sphenoid sinus   Sphenoid bone   Pharyngobasilar fascia

Int. carotid a. (cut)

Glossopharyngeal n. [CN IX]

Inf. vagal ganglion

Pharyngeal br. of vagus n. [CN X]

Sup. laryngeal n.

Sternocleidomastoid m.

Vagus n. [CN X]

Sup. horn of thyroid cartilage

Sympathetic trunk

Int. jugular v. (cut)

Common carotid a.

Sup. cardiac br. of vagus n. [CN X]

Esophagus

Lateral lobe of thyroid gland

Posterior cranial fossa

Occipital bone (coronally sectioned)

Margin of foramen magnum

Sup. pharyngeal constrictor m.

Longus capitis & cervicis mm. (cut)

Middle pharyngeal constrictor m.

Inf. pharyngeal constrictor m.

Buccopharyngeal fascia

Splenius capitis m. (cut)

Trapezius m. (cut)

Levator scapulae m.

Longissimus capitis m.

Ventral ramus of
C8 spinal n. (cut)

Sup. articular facets of T2

← LEFT   RIGHT →

Posterior View of Post. Wall of Pharynx & Esophagus

Region of nasopharynx   Torus tubarius   Choanae   Nasal septum

Styloid process of
temporal bone

Salpingopharyngeal fold

Sternocleidomastoid m.

Region of oropharynx

Ext. carotid a.

Region of laryngopharynx

Piriform recess

Trapezius m. (cut)

Int. jugular v. (cut)

Common carotid a.

Lateral lobe of thyroid gland

Sup. articular facets of T2

Occipital bone (coronally sectioned)

Margin of foramen magnum

Soft palate

Uvula (poorly developed)

Root of tongue

Lingual tonsil

Splenius capitis m. (cut)

Epiglottis

Buccopharyngeal fascia

Aditus of larynx

Trapezius m. (cut)

Levator scapulae m.

Longissimus capitis m.

Lamina of cricoid cartilage
(deep to mucosa)

Esophagus

Ant. Wall of Pharynx & Posterior View of Larynx

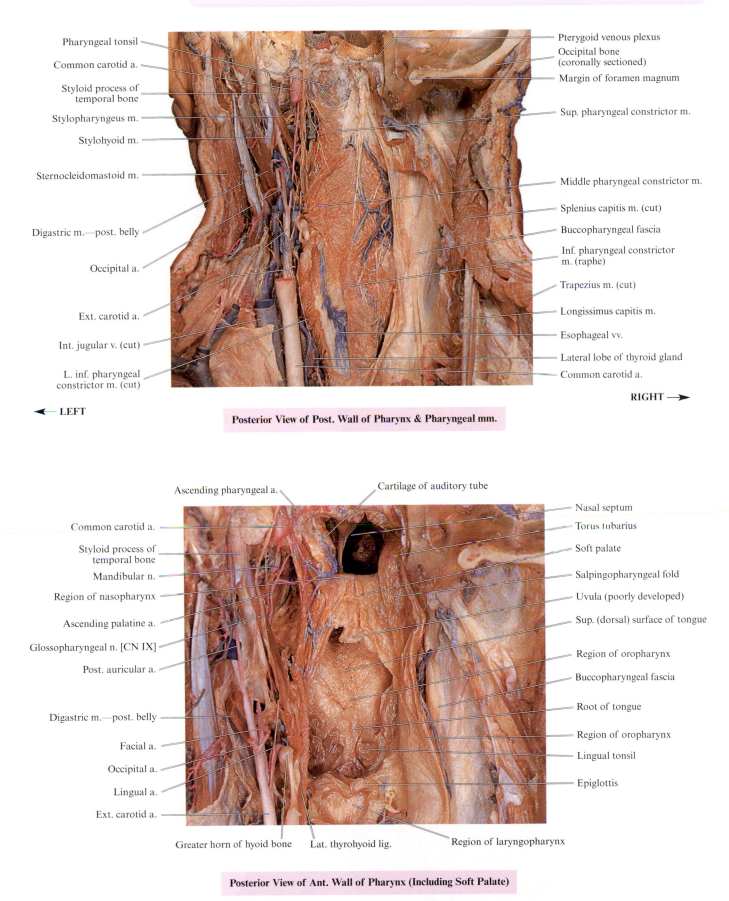

Pharyngeal tonsil

Common carotid a.

Styloid process of
temporal bone

Stylopharyngeus m.

Stylohyoid m.

Sternocleidomastoid m.

Digastric m.—post. belly

Occipital a.

Ext. carotid a.

Int. jugular v. (cut)

L. inf. pharyngeal
constrictor m. (cut)

Pterygoid venous plexus

Occipital bone
(coronally sectioned)

Margin of foramen magnum

Sup. pharyngeal constrictor m.

Middle pharyngeal constrictor m.

Splenius capitis m. (cut)

Buccopharyngeal fascia

Inf. pharyngeal constrictor
m. (raphe)

Trapezius m. (cut)

Longissimus capitis m.

Esophageal vv.

Lateral lobe of thyroid gland

Common carotid a.

◄— LEFT

RIGHT —►

Posterior View of Post. Wall of Pharynx & Pharyngeal mm.

Ascending pharyngeal a.

Common carotid a.

Styloid process of
temporal bone

Mandibular n.

Region of nasopharynx

Ascending palatine a.

Glossopharyngeal n. [CN IX]

Post. auricular a.

Digastric m.—post. belly

Facial a.

Occipital a.

Lingual a.

Ext. carotid a.

Cartilage of auditory tube

Nasal septum

Torus tubarius

Soft palate

Salpingopharyngeal fold

Uvula (poorly developed)

Sup. (dorsal) surface of tongue

Region of oropharynx

Buccopharyngeal fascia

Root of tongue

Region of oropharynx

Lingual tonsil

Epiglottis

Greater horn of hyoid bone   Lat. thyrohyoid lig.   Region of laryngopharynx

Posterior View of Ant. Wall of Pharynx (Including Soft Palate)

PLATE 7.67   ORAL CAVITY

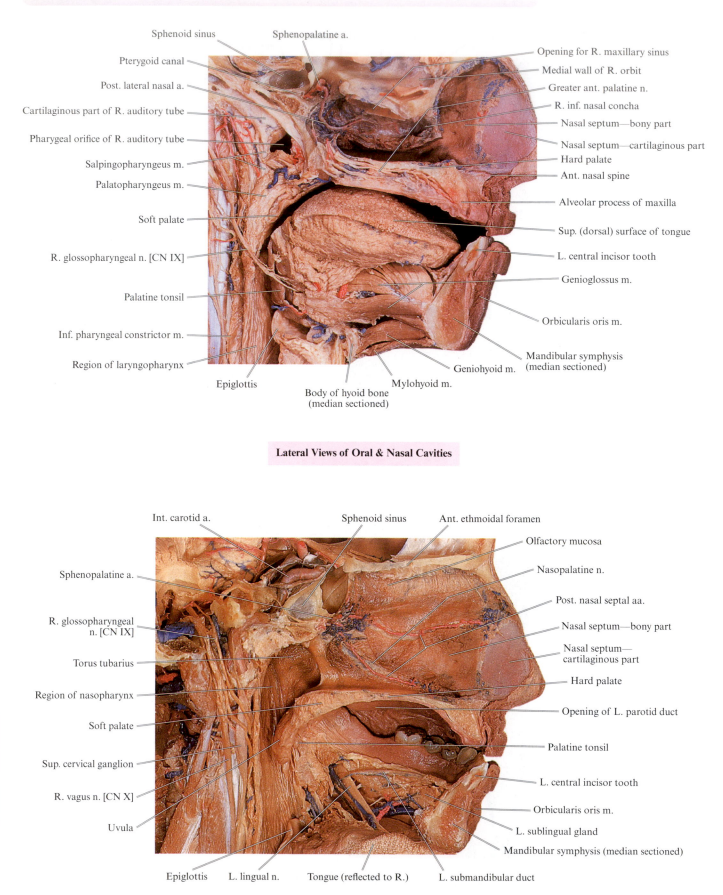

Sphenoid sinus

Sphenopalatine a.

Pterygoid canal

Post. lateral nasal a.

Cartilaginous part of R. auditory tube

Pharygeal orifice of R. auditory tube

Salpingopharyngeus m.

Palatopharyngeus m.

Soft palate

R. glossopharyngeal n. [CN IX]

Palatine tonsil

Inf. pharyngeal constrictor m.

Region of laryngopharynx

Epiglottis

Body of hyoid bone (median sectioned)

Opening for R. maxillary sinus

Medial wall of R. orbit

Greater ant. palatine n.

R. inf. nasal concha

Nasal septum—bony part

Nasal septum—cartilaginous part

Hard palate

Ant. nasal spine

Alveolar process of maxilla

Sup. (dorsal) surface of tongue

L. central incisor tooth

Genioglossus m.

Orbicularis oris m.

Mandibular symphysis (median sectioned)

Geniohyoid m.

Mylohyoid m.

Lateral Views of Oral & Nasal Cavities

Int. carotid a.

Sphenoid sinus

Ant. ethmoidal foramen

Sphenopalatine a.

R. glossopharyngeal n. [CN IX]

Torus tubarius

Region of nasopharynx

Soft palate

Sup. cervical ganglion

R. vagus n. [CN X]

Uvula

Epiglottis

L. lingual n.

Tongue (reflected to R.)

L. submandibular duct

Olfactory mucosa

Nasopalatine n.

Post. nasal septal aa.

Nasal septum—bony part

Nasal septum—cartilaginous part

Hard palate

Opening of L. parotid duct

Palatine tonsil

L. central incisor tooth

Orbicularis oris m.

L. sublingual gland

Mandibular symphysis (median sectioned)

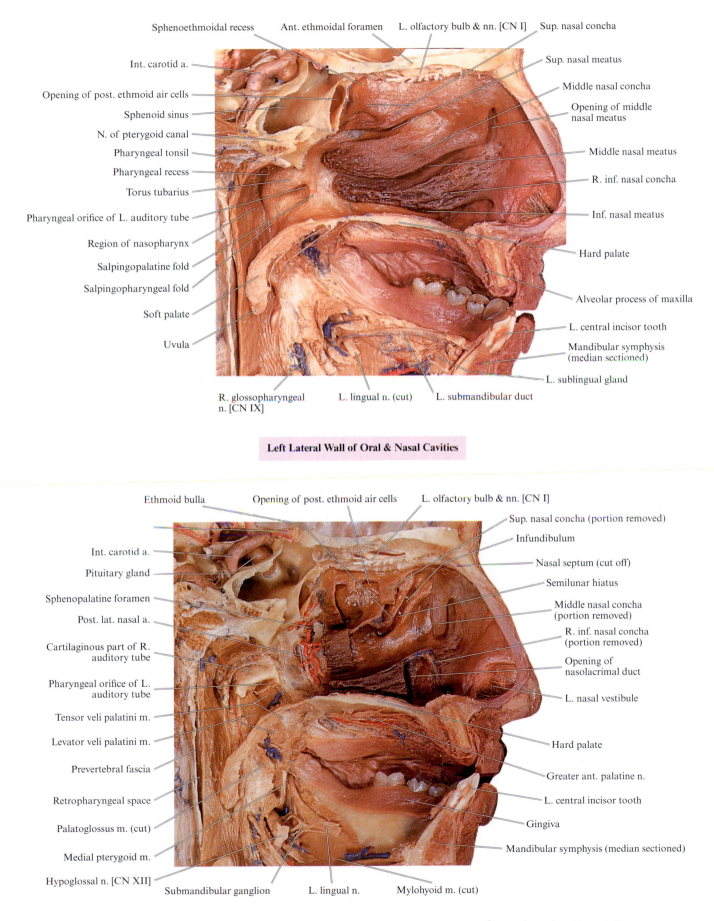

Sphenoethmoidal recess
Ant. ethmoidal foramen
L. olfactory bulb & nn. [CN I]
Sup. nasal concha

Int. carotid a.
Opening of post. ethmoid air cells
Sphenoid sinus
N. of pterygoid canal
Pharyngeal tonsil
Pharyngeal recess
Torus tubarius
Pharyngeal orifice of L. auditory tube
Region of nasopharynx
Salpingopalatine fold
Salpingopharyngeal fold
Soft palate
Uvula

Sup. nasal meatus
Middle nasal concha
Opening of middle nasal meatus
Middle nasal meatus
R. inf. nasal concha
Inf. nasal meatus
Hard palate
Alveolar process of maxilla
L. central incisor tooth
Mandibular symphysis (median sectioned)
L. sublingual gland

R. glossopharyngeal n. [CN IX]
L. lingual n. (cut)
L. submandibular duct

Left Lateral Wall of Oral & Nasal Cavities

Ethmoid bulla
Opening of post. ethmoid air cells
L. olfactory bulb & nn. [CN I]

Int. carotid a.
Pituitary gland
Sphenopalatine foramen
Post. lat. nasal a.
Cartilaginous part of R. auditory tube
Pharyngeal orifice of L. auditory tube
Tensor veli palatini m.
Levator veli palatini m.
Prevertebral fascia
Retropharyngeal space
Palatoglossus m. (cut)
Medial pterygoid m.
Hypoglossal n. [CN XII]

Sup. nasal concha (portion removed)
Infundibulum
Nasal septum (cut off)
Semilunar hiatus
Middle nasal concha (portion removed)
R. inf. nasal concha (portion removed)
Opening of nasolacrimal duct
L. nasal vestibule
Hard palate
Greater ant. palatine n.
L. central incisor tooth
Gingiva
Mandibular symphysis (median sectioned)

Submandibular ganglion
L. lingual n.
Mylohyoid m. (cut)

PLATE 7.71 ORBIT—SUPERFICIAL

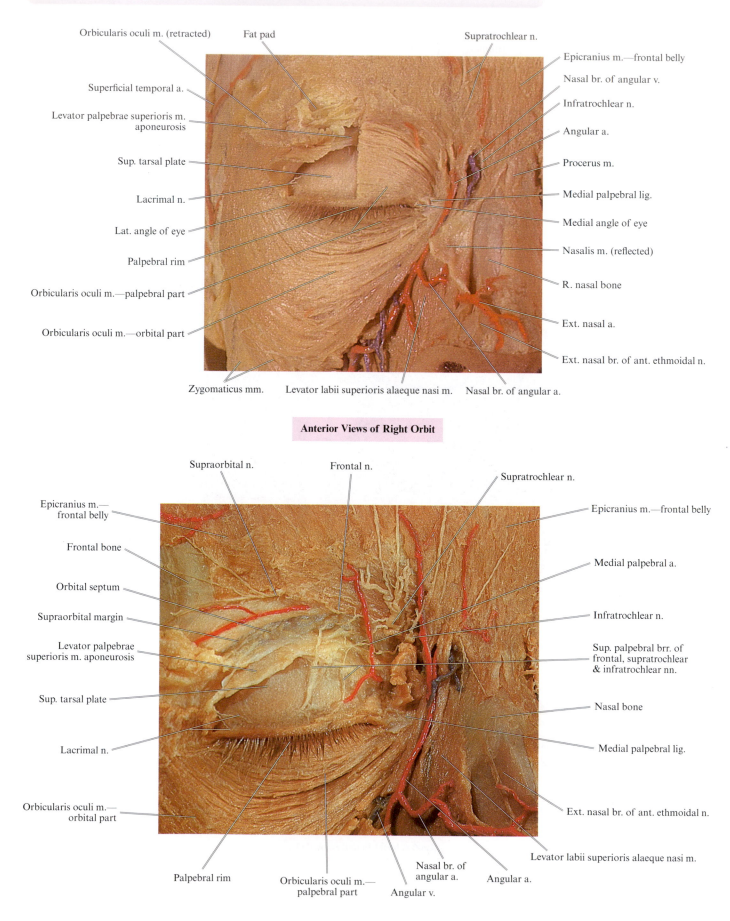

Orbicularis oculi m. (retracted)
Fat pad
Supratrochlear n.
Epicranius m.—frontal belly
Nasal br. of angular v.
Superficial temporal a.
Infratrochlear n.
Levator palpebrae superioris m. aponeurosis
Angular a.
Sup. tarsal plate
Procerus m.
Lacrimal n.
Medial palpebral lig.
Lat. angle of eye
Medial angle of eye
Palpebral rim
Nasalis m. (reflected)
Orbicularis oculi m.—palpebral part
R. nasal bone
Orbicularis oculi m.—orbital part
Ext. nasal a.
Ext. nasal br. of ant. ethmoidal n.
Zygomaticus mm.
Levator labii superioris alaeque nasi m.
Nasal br. of angular a.

Anterior Views of Right Orbit

Supraorbital n.
Frontal n.
Supratrochlear n.
Epicranius m.—frontal belly
Epicranius m.—frontal belly
Frontal bone
Medial palpebral a.
Orbital septum
Infratrochlear n.
Supraorbital margin
Sup. palpebral brr. of frontal, supratrochlear & infratrochlear nn.
Levator palpebrae superioris m. aponeurosis
Nasal bone
Sup. tarsal plate
Medial palpebral lig.
Lacrimal n.
Ext. nasal br. of ant. ethmoidal n.
Orbicularis oculi m.—orbital part
Levator labii superioris alaeque nasi m.
Palpebral rim
Orbicularis oculi m.—palpebral part
Nasal br. of angular a.
Angular a.
Angular v.

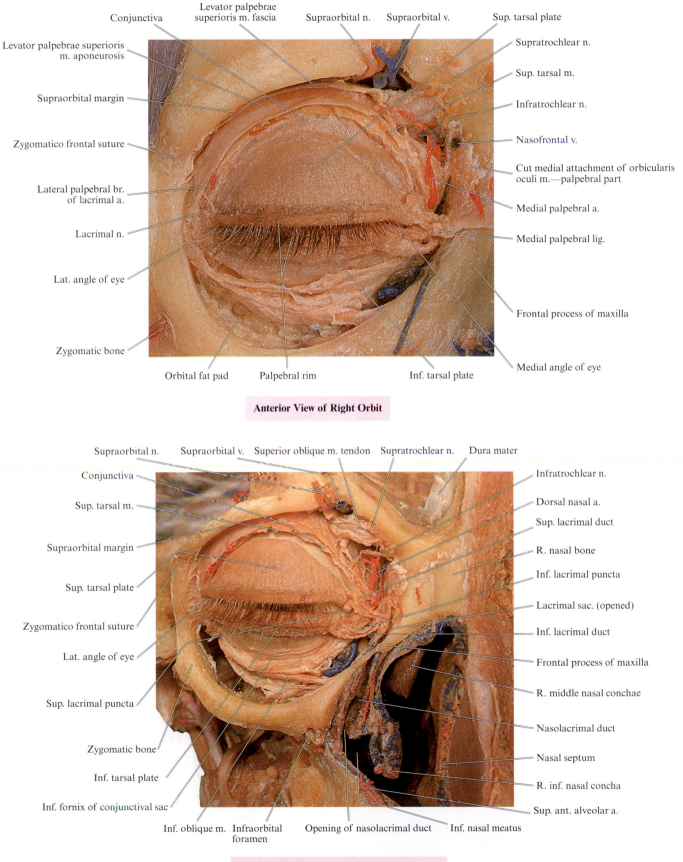

Conjunctiva

Levator palpebrae superioris m. fascia

Supraorbital n.

Supraorbital v.

Sup. tarsal plate

Levator palpebrae superioris m. aponeurosis

Supraorbital margin

Zygomatico frontal suture

Lateral palpebral br. of lacrimal a.

Lacrimal n.

Lat. angle of eye

Zygomatic bone

Supratrochlear n.

Sup. tarsal m.

Infratrochlear n.

Nasofrontal v.

Cut medial attachment of orbicularis oculi m.—palpebral part

Medial palpebral a.

Medial palpebral lig.

Frontal process of maxilla

Medial angle of eye

Orbital fat pad

Palpebral rim

Inf. tarsal plate

Anterior View of Right Orbit

Supraorbital n.

Supraorbital v.

Superior oblique m. tendon

Supratrochlear n.

Dura mater

Conjunctiva

Sup. tarsal m.

Supraorbital margin

Sup. tarsal plate

Zygomatico frontal suture

Lat. angle of eye

Sup. lacrimal puncta

Zygomatic bone

Inf. tarsal plate

Inf. fornix of conjunctival sac

Infratrochlear n.

Dorsal nasal a.

Sup. lacrimal duct

R. nasal bone

Inf. lacrimal puncta

Lacrimal sac. (opened)

Inf. lacrimal duct

Frontal process of maxilla

R. middle nasal conchae

Nasolacrimal duct

Nasal septum

R. inf. nasal concha

Sup. ant. alveolar a.

Inf. oblique m.

Infraorbital foramen

Opening of nasolacrimal duct

Inf. nasal meatus

Anterior View of Right Orbit & Nasal Cavity

PLATE 7.75   ORBIT—LATERAL

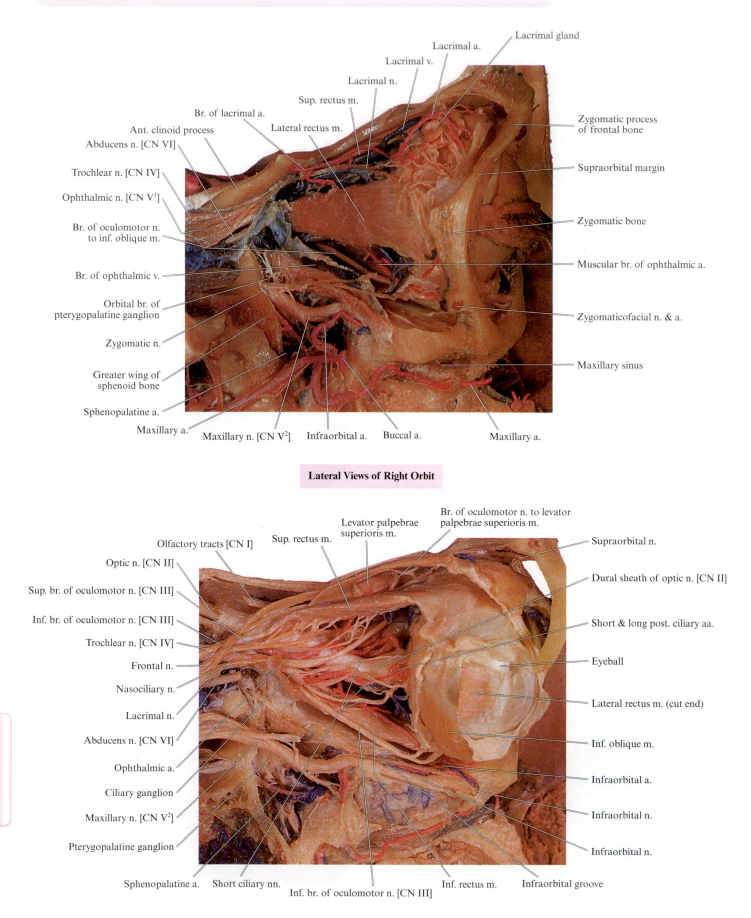

Lacrimal gland
Lacrimal a.
Lacrimal v.
Lacrimal n.
Sup. rectus m.
Br. of lacrimal a.
Lateral rectus m.
Ant. clinoid process
Abducens n. [CN VI]
Trochlear n. [CN IV]
Ophthalmic n. [CN V¹]
Br. of oculomotor n.
to inf. oblique m.
Br. of ophthalmic v.
Orbital br. of
pterygopalatine ganglion
Zygomatic n.
Greater wing of
sphenoid bone
Sphenopalatine a.
Maxillary a.
Maxillary n. [CN V²]
Infraorbital a.
Buccal a.

Zygomatic process
of frontal bone
Supraorbital margin
Zygomatic bone
Muscular br. of ophthalmic a.
Zygomaticofacial n. & a.
Maxillary sinus
Maxillary a.

Lateral Views of Right Orbit

Levator palpebrae
superioris m.
Br. of oculomotor n. to levator
palpebrae superioris m.
Olfactory tracts [CN I]
Sup. rectus m.
Optic n. [CN II]
Sup. br. of oculomotor n. [CN III]
Inf. br. of oculomotor n. [CN III]
Trochlear n. [CN IV]
Frontal n.
Nasociliary n.
Lacrimal n.
Abducens n. [CN VI]
Ophthalmic a.
Ciliary ganglion
Maxillary n. [CN V²]
Pterygopalatine ganglion
Sphenopalatine a.
Short ciliary nn.
Inf. br. of oculomotor n. [CN III]
Inf. rectus m.

Supraorbital n.
Dural sheath of optic n. [CN II]
Short & long post. ciliary aa.
Eyeball
Lateral rectus m. (cut end)
Inf. oblique m.
Infraorbital a.
Infraorbital n.
Infraorbital n.
Infraorbital groove

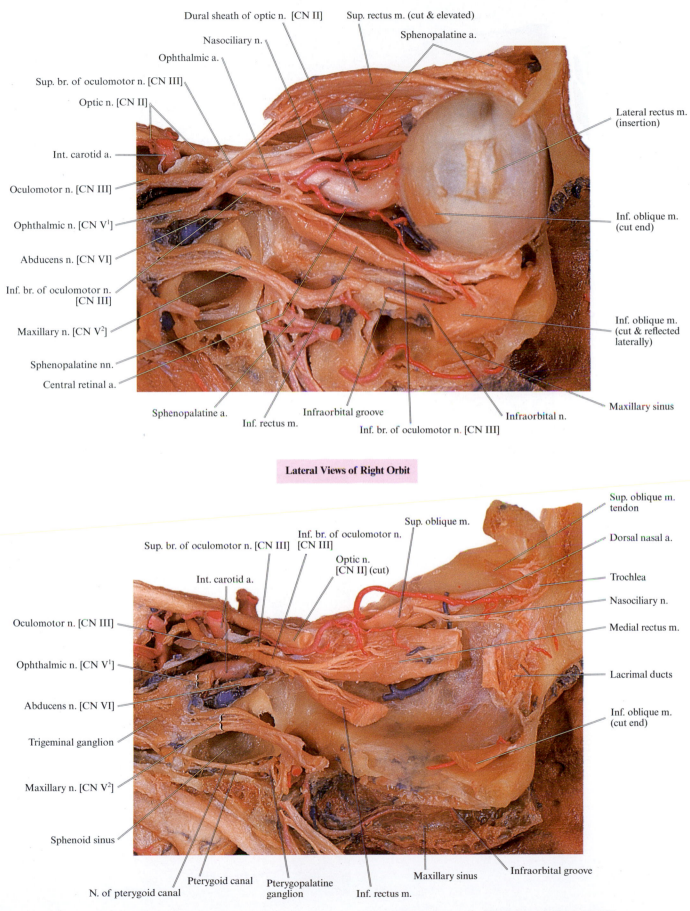

Dural sheath of optic n. [CN II]

Nasociliary n.

Sup. rectus m. (cut & elevated)

Sphenopalatine a.

Ophthalmic a.

Sup. br. of oculomotor n. [CN III]

Optic n. [CN II]

Int. carotid a.

Oculomotor n. [CN III]

Ophthalmic n. [CN V¹]

Abducens n. [CN VI]

Inf. br. of oculomotor n. [CN III]

Maxillary n. [CN V²]

Sphenopalatine nn.

Central retinal a.

Lateral rectus m. (insertion)

Inf. oblique m. (cut end)

Inf. oblique m. (cut & reflected laterally)

Sphenopalatine a.

Inf. rectus m.

Infraorbital groove

Inf. br. of oculomotor n. [CN III]

Infraorbital n.

Maxillary sinus

Lateral Views of Right Orbit

Sup. br. of oculomotor n. [CN III]

Inf. br. of oculomotor n. [CN III]

Sup. oblique m.

Optic n. [CN II] (cut)

Int. carotid a.

Oculomotor n. [CN III]

Ophthalmic n. [CN V¹]

Abducens n. [CN VI]

Trigeminal ganglion

Maxillary n. [CN V²]

Sphenoid sinus

N. of pterygoid canal

Pterygoid canal

Pterygopalatine ganglion

Inf. rectus m.

Maxillary sinus

Infraorbital groove

Sup. oblique m. tendon

Dorsal nasal a.

Trochlea

Nasociliary n.

Medial rectus m.

Lacrimal ducts

Inf. oblique m. (cut end)

PLATE 7.77   ORBIT—SUPERIOR

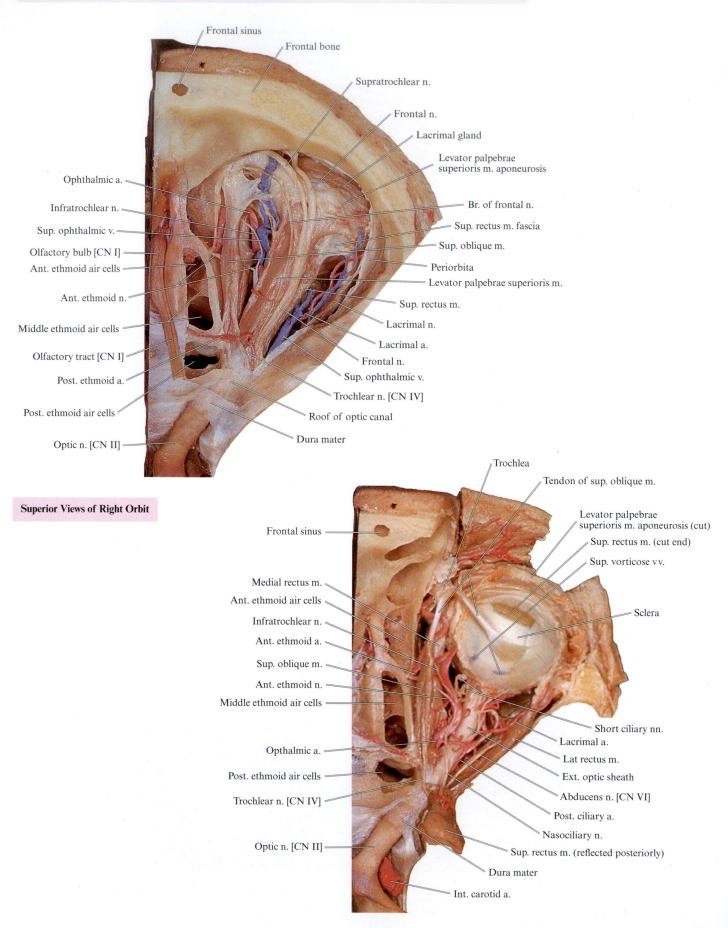

Superior Views of Right Orbit

Frontal sinus
Frontal bone
Supratrochlear n.
Frontal n.
Lacrimal gland
Levator palpebrae superioris m. aponeurosis

Ophthalmic a.
Infratrochlear n.
Sup. ophthalmic v.
Olfactory bulb [CN I]
Ant. ethmoid air cells
Ant. ethmoid n.
Middle ethmoid air cells
Olfactory tract [CN I]
Post. ethmoid a.
Post. ethmoid air cells
Optic n. [CN II]

Br. of frontal n.
Sup. rectus m. fascia
Sup. oblique m.
Periorbita
Levator palpebrae superioris m.
Sup. rectus m.
Lacrimal n.
Lacrimal a.
Frontal n.
Sup. ophthalmic v.
Trochlear n. [CN IV]
Roof of optic canal
Dura mater

Trochlea
Tendon of sup. oblique m.
Levator palpebrae superioris m. aponeurosis (cut)
Sup. rectus m. (cut end)
Sup. vorticose v v.

Frontal sinus

Medial rectus m.
Ant. ethmoid air cells
Infratrochlear n.
Ant. ethmoid a.
Sup. oblique m.
Ant. ethmoid n.
Middle ethmoid air cells

Sclera

Opthalmic a.
Post. ethmoid air cells
Trochlear n. [CN IV]

Optic n. [CN II]

Short ciliary nn.
Lacrimal a.
Lat rectus m.
Ext. optic sheath
Abducens n. [CN VI]
Post. ciliary a.
Nasociliary n.
Sup. rectus m. (reflected posteriorly)
Dura mater
Int. carotid a.

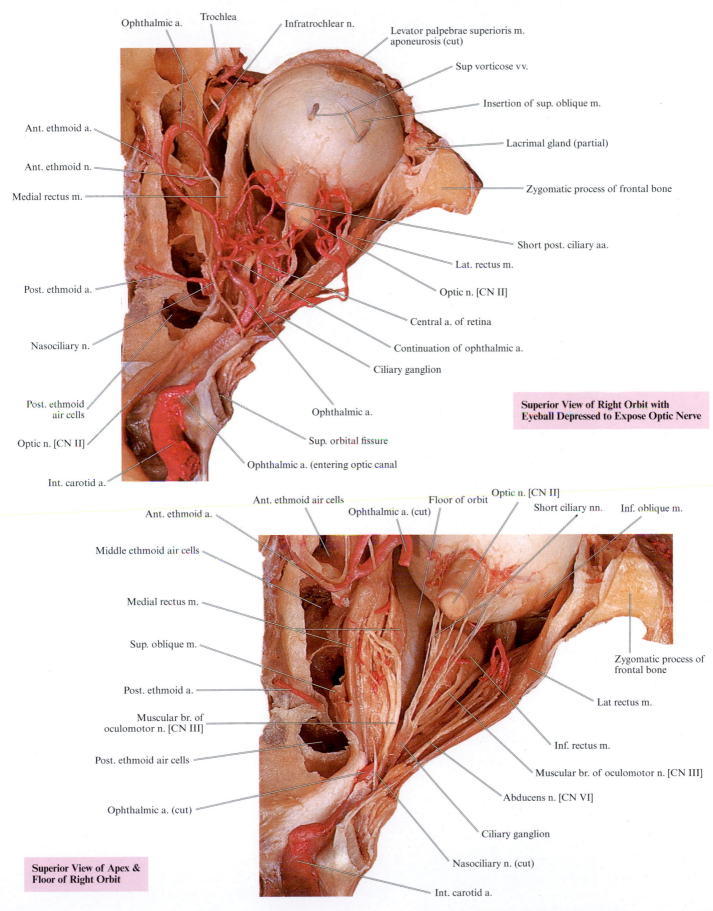

Ophthalmic a.

Trochlea

Infratrochlear n.

Levator palpebrae superioris m. aponeurosis (cut)

Sup vorticose vv.

Insertion of sup. oblique m.

Lacrimal gland (partial)

Zygomatic process of frontal bone

Ant. ethmoid a.

Ant. ethmoid n.

Medial rectus m.

Short post. ciliary aa.

Lat. rectus m.

Optic n. [CN II]

Post. ethmoid a.

Central a. of retina

Continuation of ophthalmic a.

Ciliary ganglion

Nasociliary n.

Post. ethmoid air cells

Optic n. [CN II]

Ophthalmic a.

Sup. orbital fissure

Int. carotid a.

Ophthalmic a. (entering optic canal

Superior View of Right Orbit with Eyeball Depressed to Expose Optic Nerve

Ant. ethmoid air cells

Ophthalmic a. (cut)

Floor of orbit

Optic n. [CN II]

Short ciliary nn.

Inf. oblique m.

Ant. ethmoid a.

Middle ethmoid air cells

Medial rectus m.

Sup. oblique m.

Post. ethmoid a.

Muscular br. of oculomotor n. [CN III]

Post. ethmoid air cells

Ophthalmic a. (cut)

Zygomatic process of frontal bone

Lat rectus m.

Inf. rectus m.

Muscular br. of oculomotor n. [CN III]

Abducens n. [CN VI]

Ciliary ganglion

Nasociliary n. (cut)

Int. carotid a.

Superior View of Apex & Floor of Right Orbit

PLATE 7.79   INFRATEMPORAL FOSSA

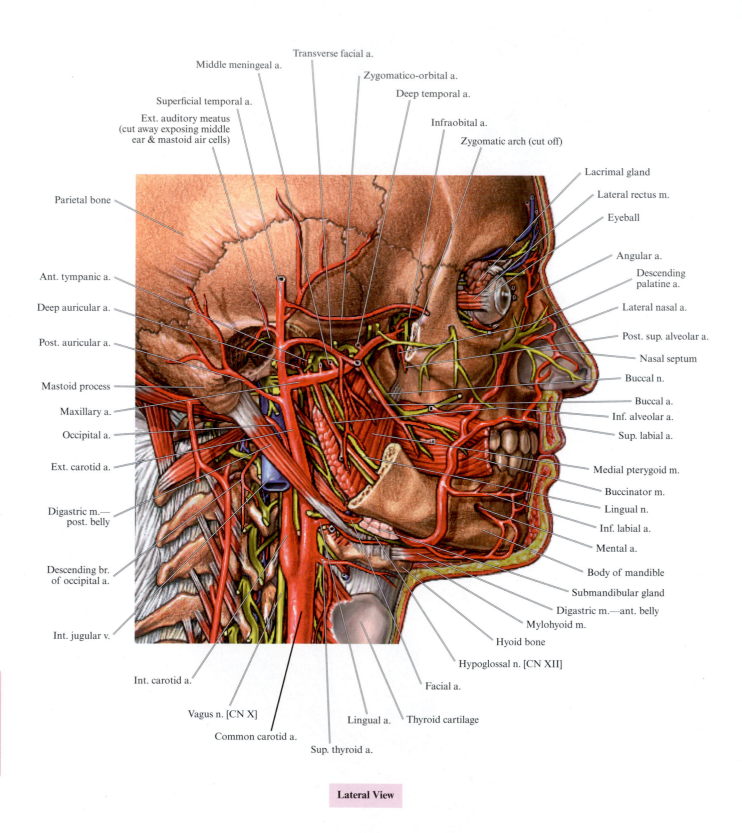

Transverse facial a.

Middle meningeal a.

Zygomatico-orbital a.

Superficial temporal a.

Deep temporal a.

Ext. auditory meatus
(cut away exposing middle
ear & mastoid air cells)

Infraobital a.

Zygomatic arch (cut off)

Parietal bone

Lacrimal gland

Lateral rectus m.

Eyeball

Ant. tympanic a.

Angular a.

Descending
palatine a.

Deep auricular a.

Lateral nasal a.

Post. auricular a.

Post. sup. alveolar a.

Nasal septum

Mastoid process

Buccal n.

Maxillary a.

Buccal a.

Inf. alveolar a.

Occipital a.

Sup. labial a.

Ext. carotid a.

Medial pterygoid m.

Buccinator m.

Digastric m.—
post. belly

Lingual n.

Inf. labial a.

Mental a.

Descending br.
of occipital a.

Body of mandible

Submandibular gland

Digastric m.—ant. belly

Int. jugular v.

Mylohyoid m.

Hyoid bone

Int. carotid a.

Hypoglossal n. [CN XII]

Vagus n. [CN X]

Facial a.

Lingual a.

Thyroid cartilage

Common carotid a.

Sup. thyroid a.

Lateral View

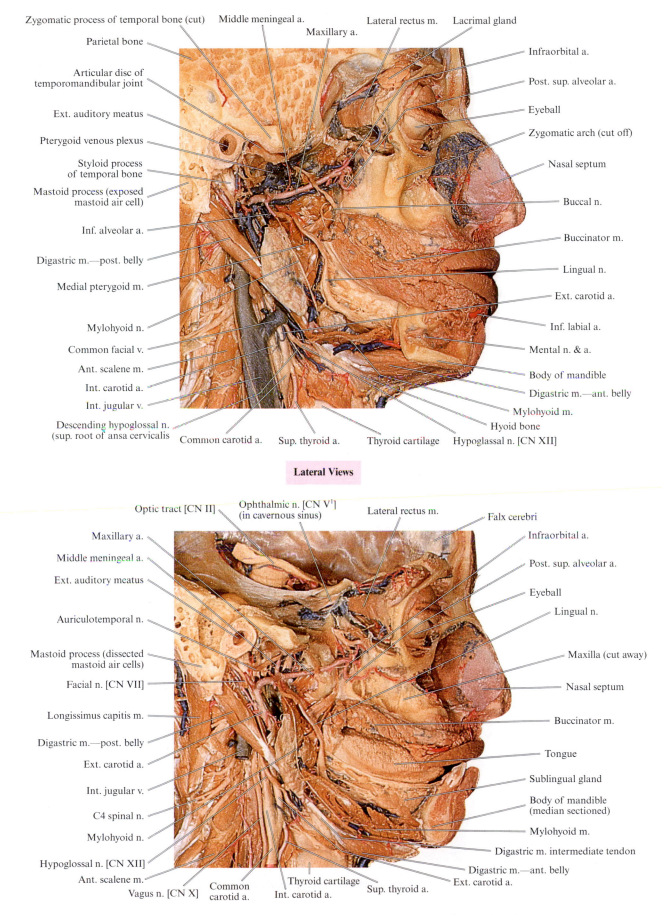

Zygomatic process of temporal bone (cut)
Parietal bone
Articular disc of temporomandibular joint
Ext. auditory meatus
Pterygoid venous plexus
Styloid process of temporal bone
Mastoid process (exposed mastoid air cell)
Inf. alveolar a.
Digastric m.—post. belly
Medial pterygoid m.
Mylohyoid n.
Common facial v.
Ant. scalene m.
Int. carotid a.
Int. jugular v.
Descending hypoglossal n. (sup. root of ansa cervicalis)

Middle meningeal a.
Maxillary a.

Lateral rectus m.   Lacrimal gland

Infraorbital a.
Post. sup. alveolar a.
Eyeball
Zygomatic arch (cut off)
Nasal septum
Buccal n.
Buccinator m.
Lingual n.
Ext. carotid a.
Inf. labial a.
Mental n. & a.
Body of mandible
Digastric m.—ant. belly
Mylohyoid m.
Hyoid bone

Common carotid a.   Sup. thyroid a.   Thyroid cartilage   Hypoglossal n. [CN XII]

Lateral Views

Optic tract [CN II]
Ophthalmic n. [CN V¹] (in cavernous sinus)
Lateral rectus m.
Falx cerebri

Maxillary a.
Middle meningeal a.
Ext. auditory meatus
Auriculotemporal n.
Mastoid process (dissected mastoid air cells)
Facial n. [CN VII]
Longissimus capitis m.
Digastric m.—post. belly
Ext. carotid a.
Int. jugular v.
C4 spinal n.
Mylohyoid n.
Hypoglossal n. [CN XII]
Ant. scalene m.

Infraorbital a.
Post. sup. alveolar a.
Eyeball
Lingual n.
Maxilla (cut away)
Nasal septum
Buccinator m.
Tongue
Sublingual gland
Body of mandible (median sectioned)
Mylohyoid m.
Digastric m. intermediate tendon
Digastric m.—ant. belly
Ext. carotid a.

Vagus n. [CN X]   Common carotid a.   Thyroid cartilage   Int. carotid a.   Sup. thyroid a.

8 CRANIAL AND AUTONOMIC NERVES

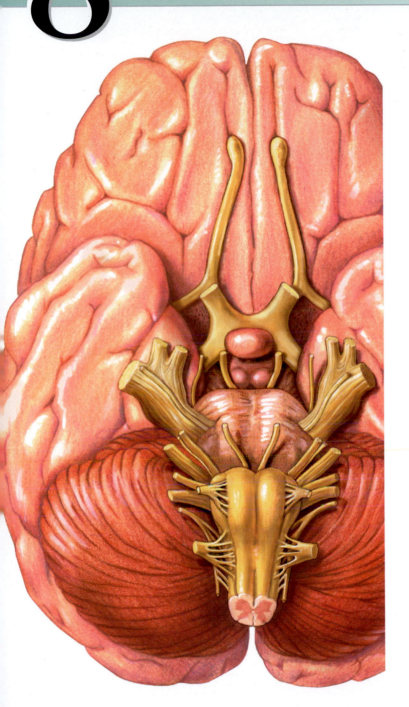

TABLE 8.1   CRANIAL NERVE FUNCTIONS

Overview of Cranial Nerves

Nerve	Efferent or Motor		Afferent or Sensory		
	Striated Muscles	**Smooth & Cardiac Muscles & Glands**	**Skin**	**Mucous Membranes & Organs**	**Special Senses**
CN I					Olfaction or sensation of smell
CN II					Vision or sight
CN III	Supplies all muscles of eyeball except lat. rectus & sup. oblique mm.	Parasympathetic to ciliary m. (lens) & sphincter pupillae m.		Proprioceptive fibers from eye mm.	
CN IV	Supplies sup. oblique m. of eyeball			Proprioceptive fibers from sup. oblique m.	
CN V	Supplies muscles of mastication, tensor tympani, tensor veli palatini, mylohyoid m. & ant. belly of digastric m.	Carries parasympathetic preganglionic nerve fibers of CN III, VII & IX	Face & ant. part of scalp	Teeth, mucous membrane of mouth, nose & eye, general sensory from anterior two-thirds of tongue	Taste (fibers from chorda tympani) from ant. two-thirds of tongue
CN VI	Supplies lat. rectus m. of eyeball			Proprioceptive fibers from lat. rectus m.	
CN VII	Supplies muscles of facial expression, stapedius m., stylohyoid m., & post. belly of digastric m.	Parasympathetic nervus intermedius; glands of mouth, nose & palate; lacrimal gland; submandibular & sublingual glands	Ext. ear	Proprioceptive fibers from muscles of facial expression	Nervus intermedius, taste from ant. two-thirds of tongue
CN VIII					Hearing & equilibrium
CN IX	Supplies stylopharyngeus m.	Parasympathetic to parotid gland		Internal surface of tympanic membrane, middle ear, auditory tube, upper pharynx & general sensory from tongue (post. one-third)	Taste from post. one-third of tongue
CN X	Supplies muscles of soft palate (except tensor veli palatini m.), pharynx (except stylopharyngeus m.), larynx, & palatoglossus m.	Parasympathetic to organs in neck, thorax & abdomen	Ext. acoustic meatus & tympanic membrane	Organs in neck, thorax & abdomen, general sensory from root of tongue	Taste, epiglottis
CN XI	Supplies sternocleidomastoid & trapezius mm.				
CN XII	Supplies extrinsic & intrinsic mm. of tongue except palatoglossus m.				

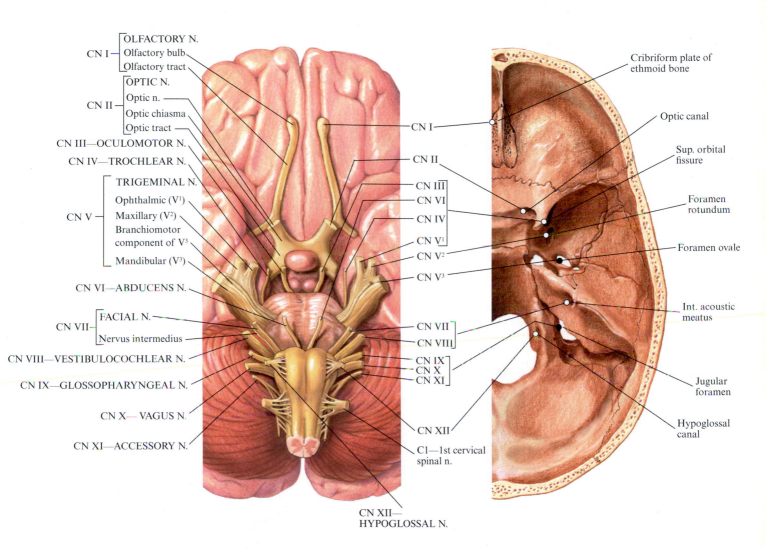

CN I — { OLFACTORY N.
Olfactory bulb
Olfactory tract

CN II — { OPTIC N.
Optic n.
Optic chiasma
Optic tract

CN III—OCULOMOTOR N.

CN IV—TROCHLEAR N.

CN V — { TRIGEMINAL N.
Ophthalmic (V¹)
Maxillary (V²)
Branchiomotor component of V³
Mandibular (V³)

CN VI—ABDUCENS N.

CN VII — { FACIAL N.
Nervus intermedius

CN VIII—VESTIBULOCOCHLEAR N.

CN IX—GLOSSOPHARYNGEAL N.

CN X— VAGUS N.

CN XI—ACCESSORY N.

CN I

CN II

CN III

CN VI

CN IV

CN V¹

CN V²

CN V³

CN VII

CN VIII

CN IX
CN X
CN XI

CN XII

C1—1st cervical spinal n.

CN XII—HYPOGLOSSAL N.

Cribriform plate of ethmoid bone

Optic canal

Sup. orbital fissure

Foramen rotundum

Foramen ovale

Int. acoustic meatus

Jugular foramen

Hypoglossal canal

PLATE 8.2   OLFACTORY NERVE—CN I

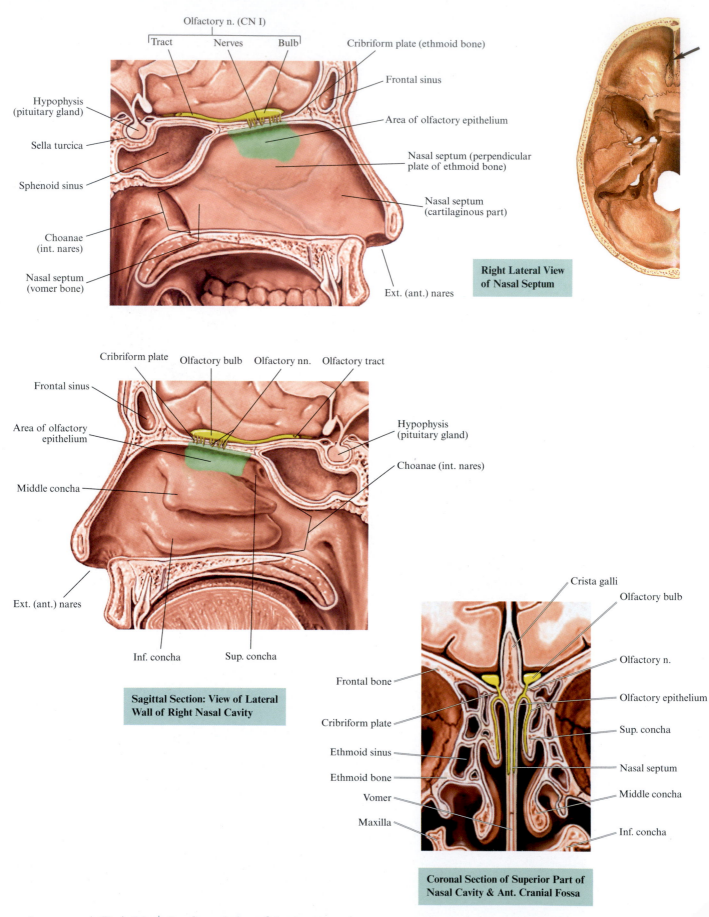

Olfactory n. (CN I)
Tract   Nerves   Bulb

Cribriform plate (ethmoid bone)

Frontal sinus

Hypophysis (pituitary gland)

Sella turcica

Sphenoid sinus

Choanae (int. nares)

Nasal septum (vomer bone)

Area of olfactory epithelium

Nasal septum (perpendicular plate of ethmoid bone)

Nasal septum (cartilaginous part)

Ext. (ant.) nares

Right Lateral View of Nasal Septum

Cribriform plate   Olfactory bulb   Olfactory nn.   Olfactory tract

Frontal sinus

Area of olfactory epithelium

Middle concha

Ext. (ant.) nares

Inf. concha   Sup. concha

Hypophysis (pituitary gland)

Choanae (int. nares)

Sagittal Section: View of Lateral Wall of Right Nasal Cavity

Crista galli

Olfactory bulb

Frontal bone

Cribriform plate

Ethmoid sinus

Ethmoid bone

Vomer

Maxilla

Olfactory n.

Olfactory epithelium

Sup. concha

Nasal septum

Middle concha

Inf. concha

Coronal Section of Superior Part of Nasal Cavity & Ant. Cranial Fossa

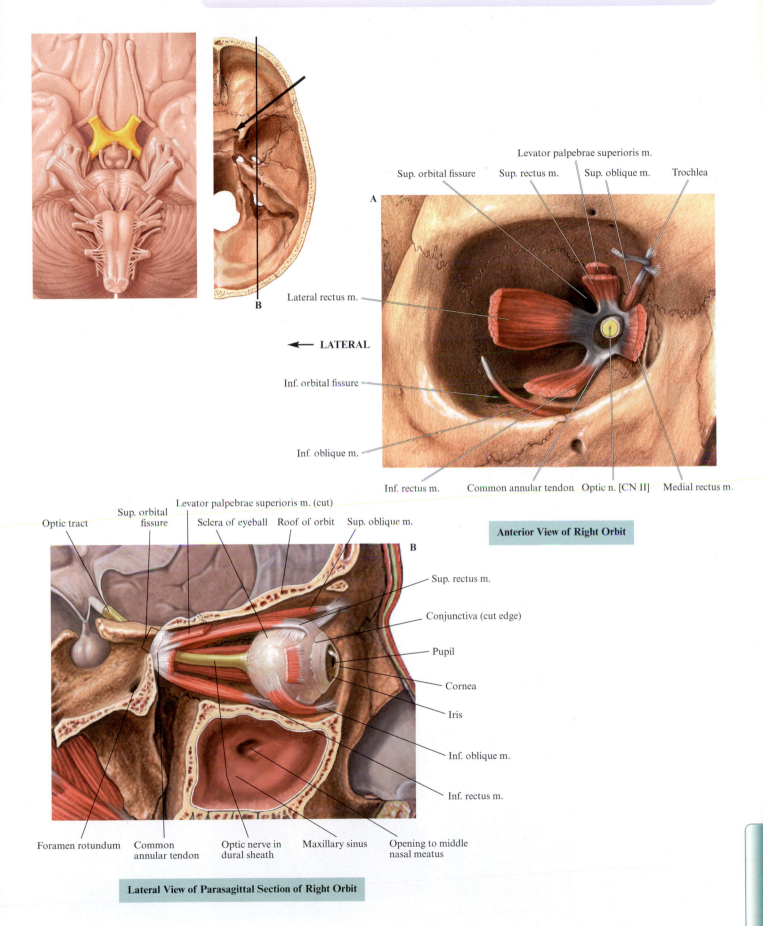

Levator palpebrae superioris m.

Sup. orbital fissure   Sup. rectus m.   Sup. oblique m.   Trochlea

A

Lateral rectus m.

← LATERAL

Inf. orbital fissure

Inf. oblique m.

Inf. rectus m.   Common annular tendon   Optic n. [CN II]   Medial rectus m.

Anterior View of Right Orbit

Optic tract   Sup. orbital fissure   Levator palpebrae superioris m. (cut)   Sclera of eyeball   Roof of orbit   Sup. oblique m.

B

Sup. rectus m.

Conjunctiva (cut edge)

Pupil

Cornea

Iris

Inf. oblique m.

Inf. rectus m.

Foramen rotundum   Common annular tendon   Optic nerve in dural sheath   Maxillary sinus   Opening to middle nasal meatus

Lateral View of Parasagittal Section of Right Orbit

CHAPTER 8 | CRANIAL AND AUTONOMIC NERVES   449

PLATE 8.4   OCULOMOTOR NERVE—CN III

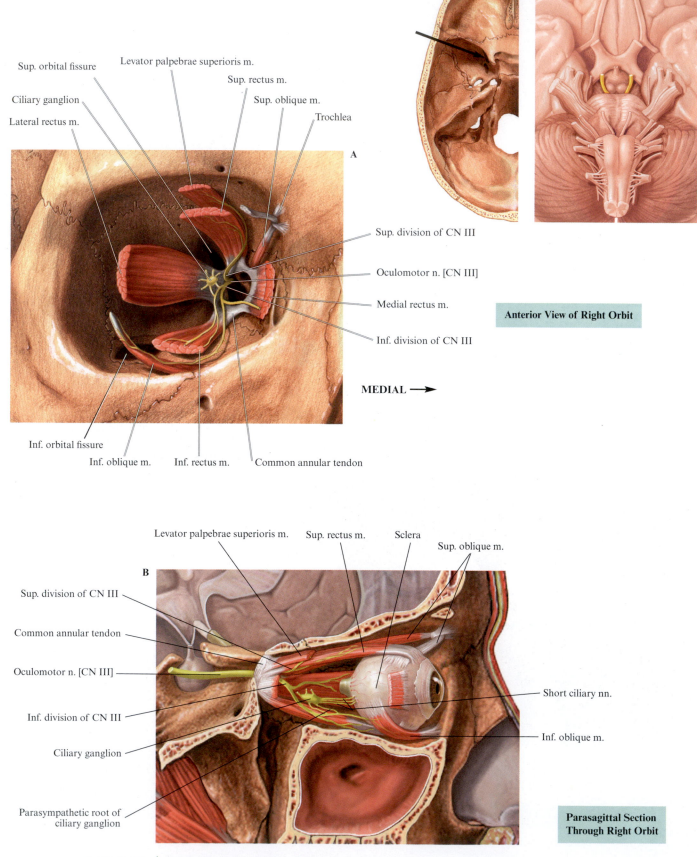

Sup. orbital fissure

Ciliary ganglion

Lateral rectus m.

Levator palpebrae superioris m.

Sup. rectus m.

Sup. oblique m.

Trochlea

A

Sup. division of CN III

Oculomotor n. [CN III]

Medial rectus m.

Inf. division of CN III

Anterior View of Right Orbit

MEDIAL ➔

Inf. orbital fissure

Inf. oblique m.   Inf. rectus m.   Common annular tendon

Levator palpebrae superioris m.   Sup. rectus m.   Sclera   Sup. oblique m.

B

Sup. division of CN III

Common annular tendon

Oculomotor n. [CN III]

Inf. division of CN III

Ciliary ganglion

Parasympathetic root of
ciliary ganglion

Short ciliary nn.

Inf. oblique m.

**Parasagittal Section
Through Right Orbit**

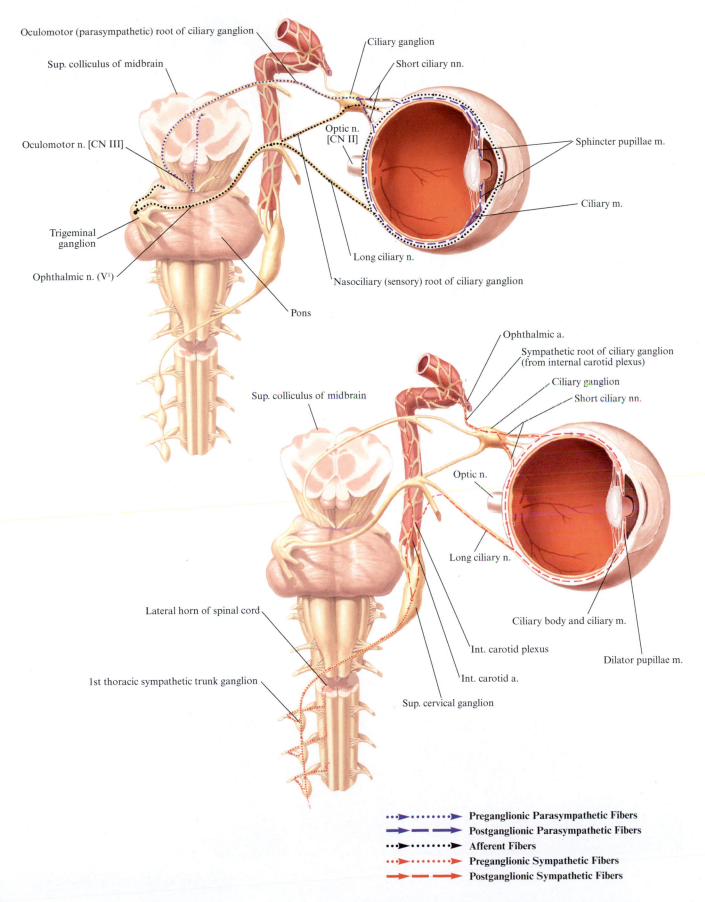

Oculomotor (parasympathetic) root of ciliary ganglion

Sup. colliculus of midbrain

Oculomotor n. [CN III]

Trigeminal ganglion

Ophthalmic n. (V¹)

Pons

Ciliary ganglion

Short ciliary nn.

Optic n. [CN II]

Sphincter pupillae m.

Ciliary m.

Long ciliary n.

Nasociliary (sensory) root of ciliary ganglion

Sup. colliculus of midbrain

Ophthalmic a.

Sympathetic root of ciliary ganglion (from internal carotid plexus)

Ciliary ganglion

Short ciliary nn.

Optic n.

Long ciliary n.

Lateral horn of spinal cord

1st thoracic sympathetic trunk ganglion

Int. carotid plexus

Int. carotid a.

Sup. cervical ganglion

Ciliary body and ciliary m.

Dilator pupillae m.

•••▶•••••••▶ Preganglionic Parasympathetic Fibers
━━▶━ ━ ━▶ Postganglionic Parasympathetic Fibers
•••▶•••••••▶ Afferent Fibers
•••▶•••••••▶ Preganglionic Sympathetic Fibers
━━▶━ ━ ━▶ Postganglionic Sympathetic Fibers

PLATE 8.6   TROCHLEAR NERVE—CN IV

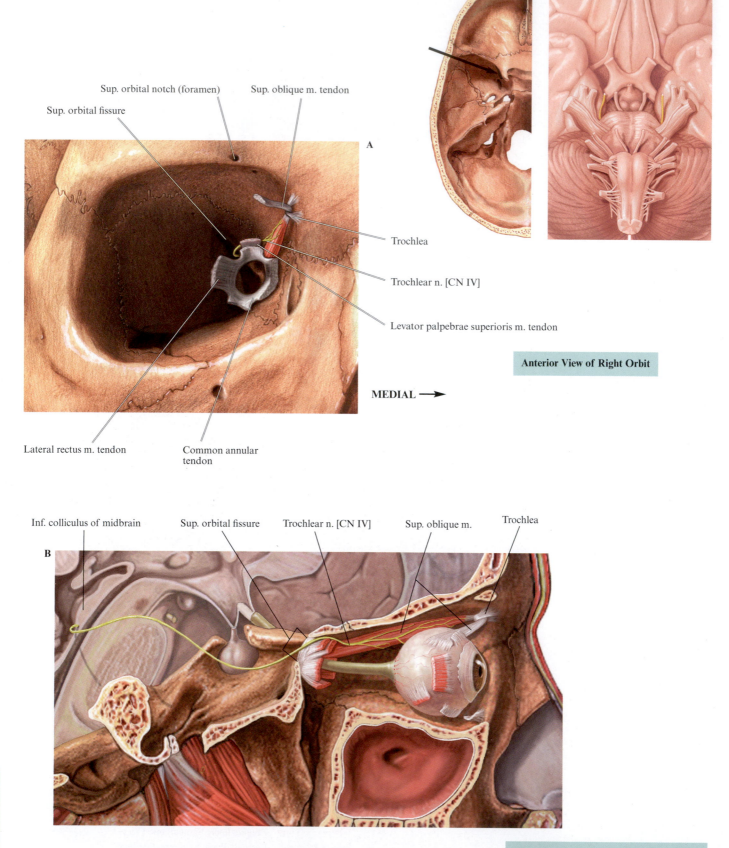

Sup. orbital notch (foramen)

Sup. oblique m. tendon

Sup. orbital fissure

A

Trochlea

Trochlear n. [CN IV]

Levator palpebrae superioris m. tendon

Anterior View of Right Orbit

MEDIAL ⟶

Lateral rectus m. tendon

Common annular tendon

Inf. colliculus of midbrain

Sup. orbital fissure

Trochlear n. [CN IV]

Sup. oblique m.

Trochlea

B

Parasagittal Section Through Right Orbit

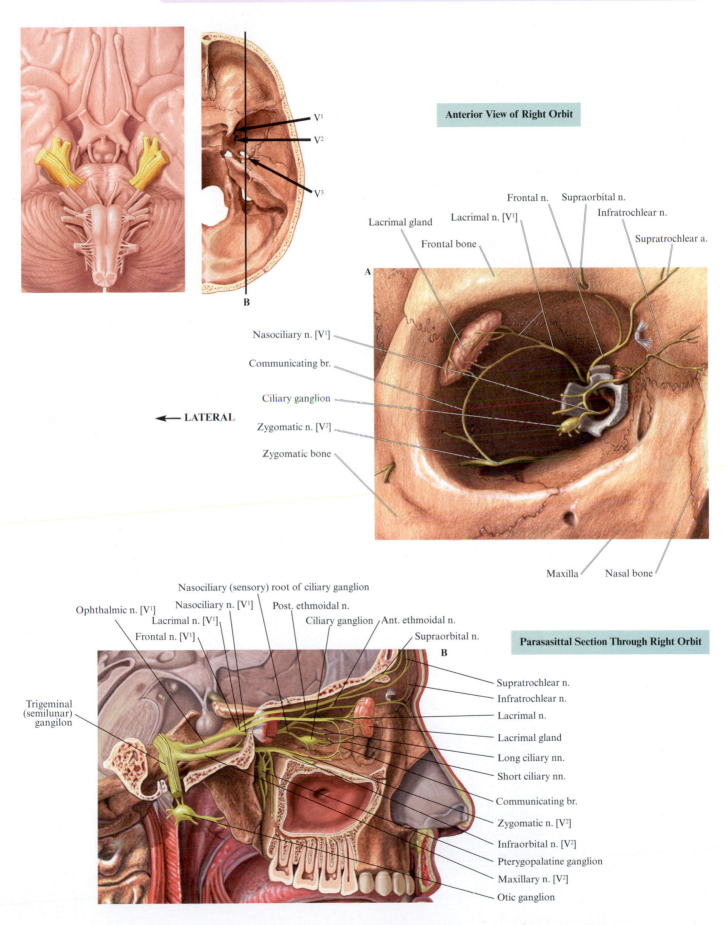

V¹
V²
V³

B

Anterior View of Right Orbit

Frontal n.   Supraorbital n.
Lacrimal n. [V¹]   Infratrochlear n.
Lacrimal gland   Supratrochlear a.
Frontal bone

A

Nasociliary n. [V¹]
Communicating br.
Ciliary ganglion
← LATERAL
Zygomatic n. [V²]
Zygomatic bone

Maxilla   Nasal bone

Nasociliary (sensory) root of ciliary ganglion
Ophthalmic n. [V¹]   Nasociliary n. [V¹]   Post. ethmoidal n.
Lacrimal n. [V¹]   Ciliary ganglion   Ant. ethmoidal n.
Frontal n. [V¹]   Supraorbital n.

B

Parasasittal Section Through Right Orbit

Trigeminal
(semilunar)
ganglion

Supratrochlear n.
Infratrochlear n.
Lacrimal n.
Lacrimal gland
Long ciliary nn.
Short ciliary nn.
Communicating br.
Zygomatic n. [V²]
Infraorbital n. [V²]
Pterygopalatine ganglion
Maxillary n. [V²]
Otic ganglion

PLATE 8.8   TRIGEMINAL NERVE—CN V² MAXILLARY DIVISION

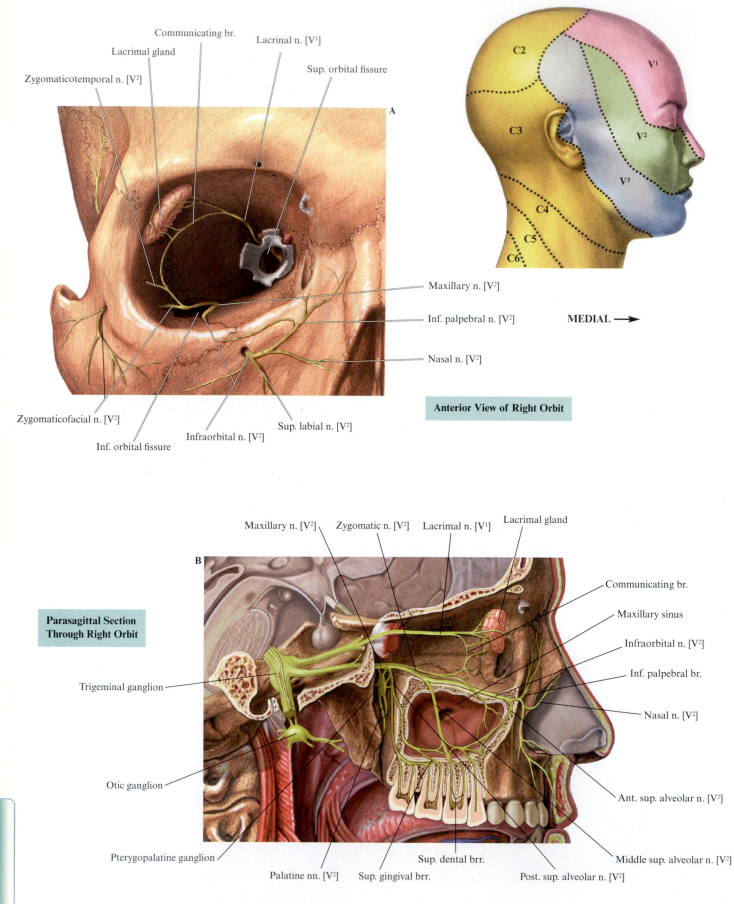

A

Zygomaticotemporal n. [V²]
Lacrimal gland
Communicating br.
Lacrinal n. [V¹]
Sup. orbital fissure

Maxillary n. [V²]

Inf. palpebral n. [V²]

Nasal n. [V²]

Zygomaticofacial n. [V²]

Inf. orbital fissure

Infraorbital n. [V²]

Sup. labial n. [V²]

C2
C3
C4
C5
C6
V¹
V²
V³

MEDIAL ⟶

Anterior View of Right Orbit

Parasagittal Section Through Right Orbit

B

Maxillary n. [V²]
Zygomatic n. [V²]
Lacrimal n. [V¹]
Lacrimal gland

Communicating br.
Maxillary sinus
Infraorbital n. [V²]
Inf. palpebral br.
Nasal n. [V²]
Ant. sup. alveolar n. [V²]
Middle sup. alveolar n. [V²]

Trigeminal ganglion

Otic ganglion

Pterygopalatine ganglion

Palatine nn. [V²]
Sup. gingival brr.
Sup. dental brr.
Post. sup. alveolar n. [V²]

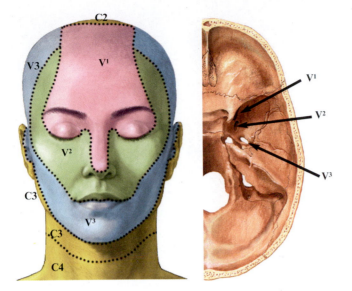

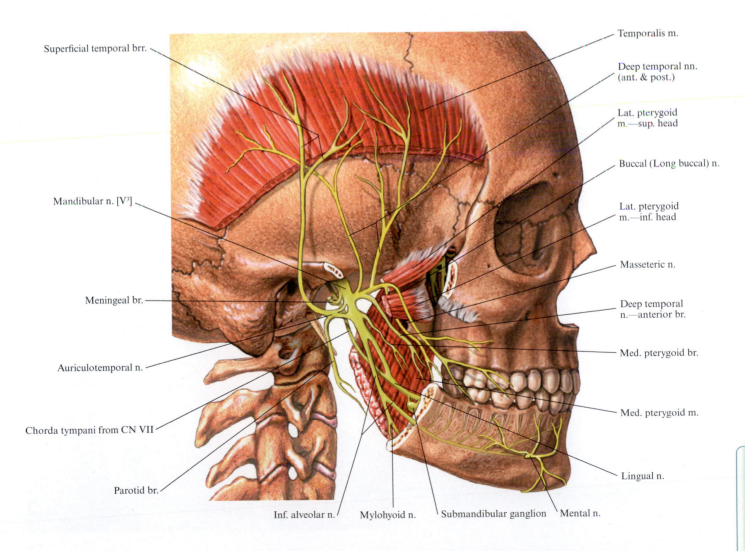

Superficial temporal brr.

Mandibular n. [V³]

Meningeal br.

Auriculotemporal n.

Chorda tympani from CN VII

Parotid br.

Inf. alveolar n.   Mylohyoid n.   Submandibular ganglion   Mental n.

Temporalis m.

Deep temporal nn.
(ant. & post.)

Lat. pterygoid
m.—sup. head

Buccal (Long buccal) n.

Lat. pterygoid
m.—inf. head

Masseteric n.

Deep temporal
n.—anterior br.

Med. pterygoid br.

Med. pterygoid m.

Lingual n.

PLATE 8.10   ABDUCENS NERVE—CN VI

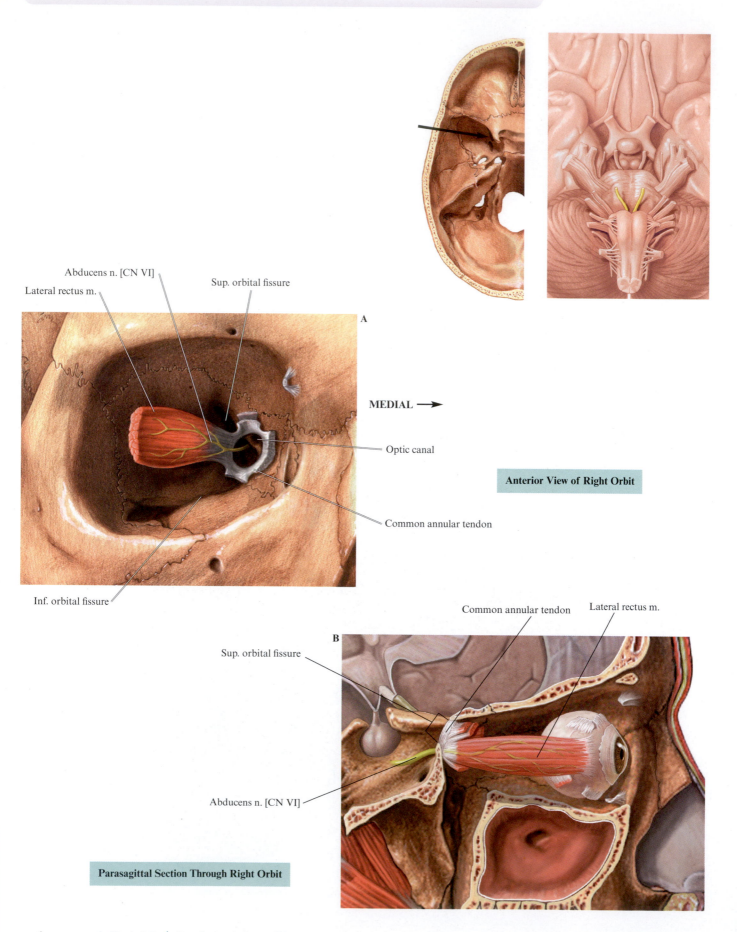

Abducens n. [CN VI]

Lateral rectus m.

Sup. orbital fissure

A

MEDIAL ➜

Optic canal

Anterior View of Right Orbit

Common annular tendon

Inf. orbital fissure

Common annular tendon

Lateral rectus m.

B

Sup. orbital fissure

Abducens n. [CN VI]

Parasagittal Section Through Right Orbit

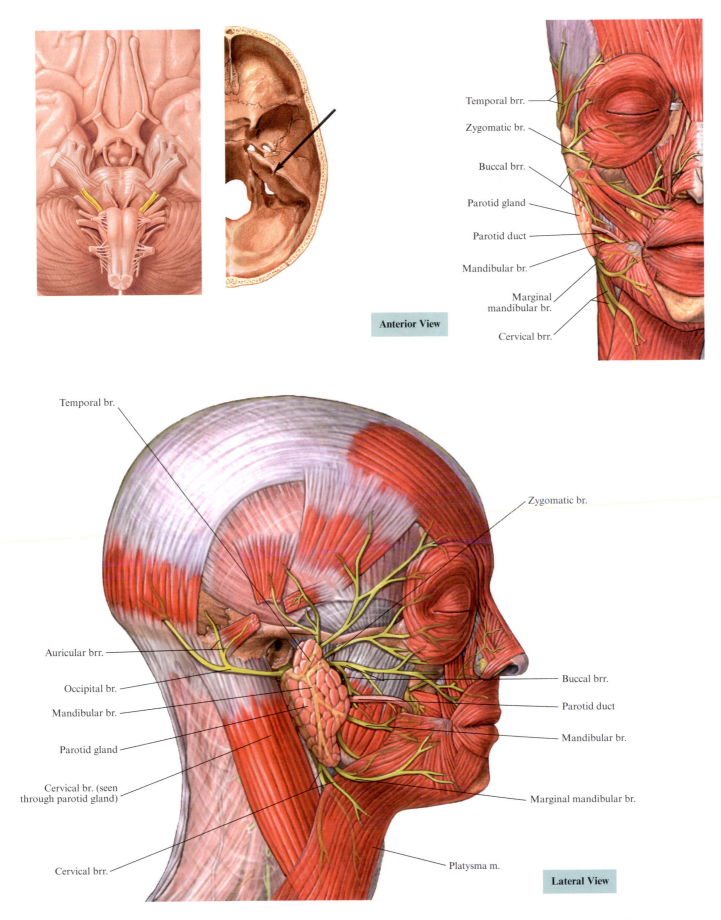

Temporal brr.

Zygomatic br.

Buccal brr.

Parotid gland

Parotid duct

Mandibular br.

Marginal
mandibular br.

Cervical brr.

Anterior View

Temporal br.

Zygomatic br.

Auricular brr.

Occipital br.

Mandibular br.

Parotid gland

Cervical br. (seen
through parotid gland)

Cervical brr.

Buccal brr.

Parotid duct

Mandibular br.

Marginal mandibular br.

Platysma m.

Lateral View

PLATE 8.16   GLOSSOPHARYNGEAL NERVE—CN IX

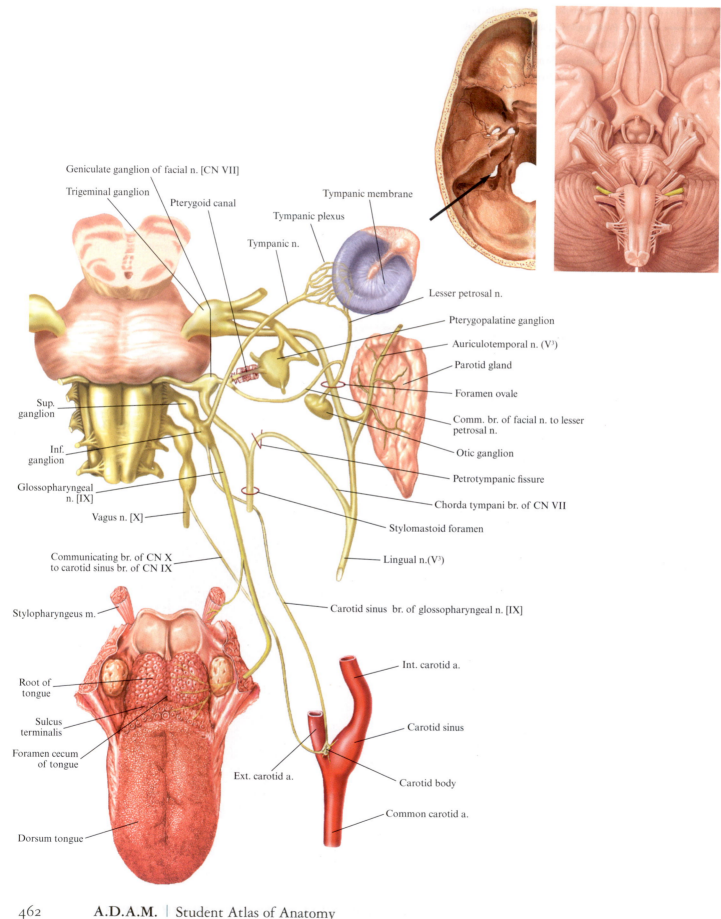

Geniculate ganglion of facial n. [CN VII]

Trigeminal ganglion

Pterygoid canal

Tympanic membrane

Tympanic plexus

Tympanic n.

Lesser petrosal n.

Pterygopalatine ganglion

Auriculotemporal n. (V³)

Parotid gland

Foramen ovale

Comm. br. of facial n. to lesser petrosal n.

Otic ganglion

Petrotympanic fissure

Chorda tympani br. of CN VII

Stylomastoid foramen

Lingual n.(V³)

Sup. ganglion

Inf. ganglion

Glossopharyngeal n. [IX]

Vagus n. [X]

Communicating br. of CN X to carotid sinus br. of CN IX

Carotid sinus br. of glossopharyngeal n. [IX]

Stylopharyngeus m.

Int. carotid a.

Root of tongue

Carotid sinus

Sulcus terminalis

Foramen cecum of tongue

Ext. carotid a.

Carotid body

Common carotid a.

Dorsum tongue

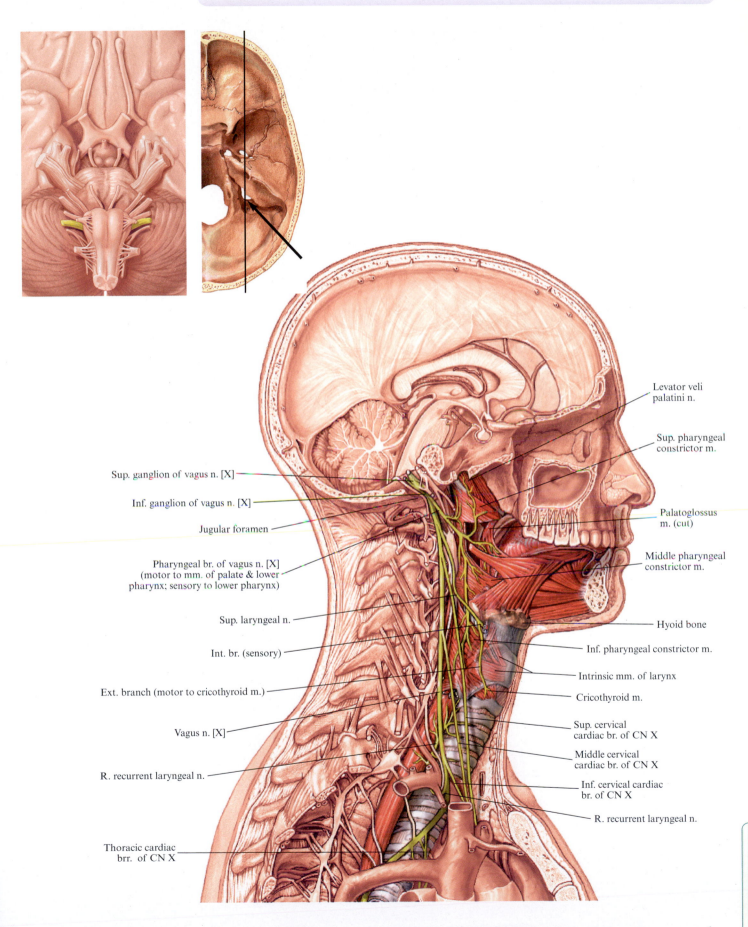

Sup. ganglion of vagus n. [X]

Inf. ganglion of vagus n. [X]

Jugular foramen

Pharyngeal br. of vagus n. [X]
(motor to mm. of palate & lower
pharynx; sensory to lower pharynx)

Sup. laryngeal n.

Int. br. (sensory)

Ext. branch (motor to cricothyroid m.)

Vagus n. [X]

R. recurrent laryngeal n.

Thoracic cardiac
brr. of CN X

Levator veli
palatini n.

Sup. pharyngeal
constrictor m.

Palatoglossus
m. (cut)

Middle pharyngeal
constrictor m.

Hyoid bone

Inf. pharyngeal constrictor m.

Intrinsic mm. of larynx

Cricothyroid m.

Sup. cervical
cardiac br. of CN X

Middle cervical
cardiac br. of CN X

Inf. cervical cardiac
br. of CN X

R. recurrent laryngeal n.

PLATE 8.18   VAGUS NERVE—CN X THORACO-ABDOMINAL BRANCHES

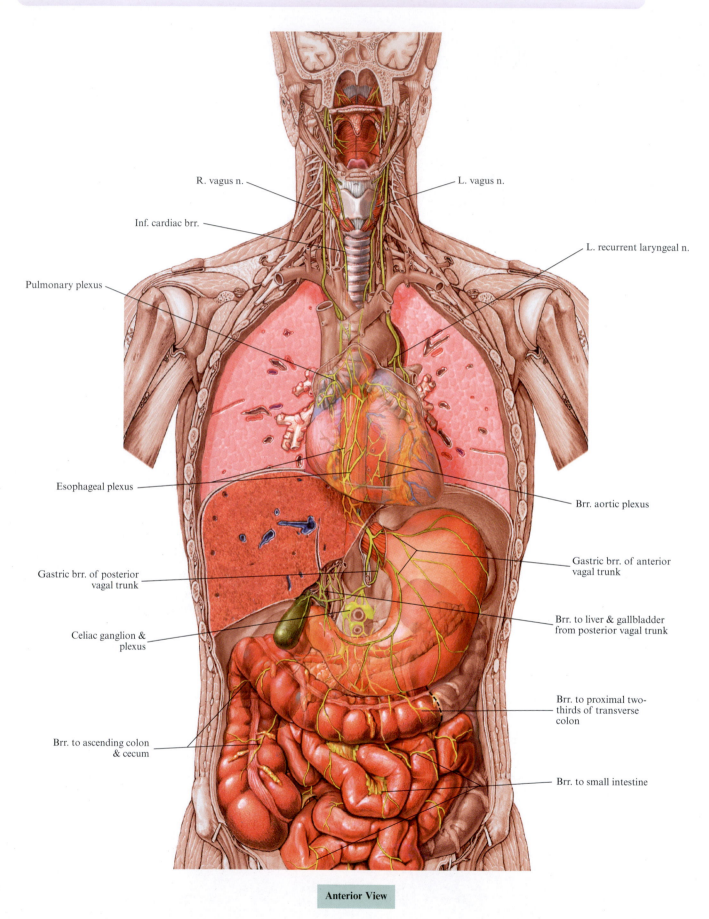

R. vagus n.

Inf. cardiac brr.

Pulmonary plexus

Esophageal plexus

Gastric brr. of posterior
vagal trunk

Celiac ganglion &
plexus

Brr. to ascending colon
& cecum

L. vagus n.

L. recurrent laryngeal n.

Brr. aortic plexus

Gastric brr. of anterior
vagal trunk

Brr. to liver & gallbladder
from posterior vagal trunk

Brr. to proximal two-
thirds of transverse
colon

Brr. to small intestine

Anterior View

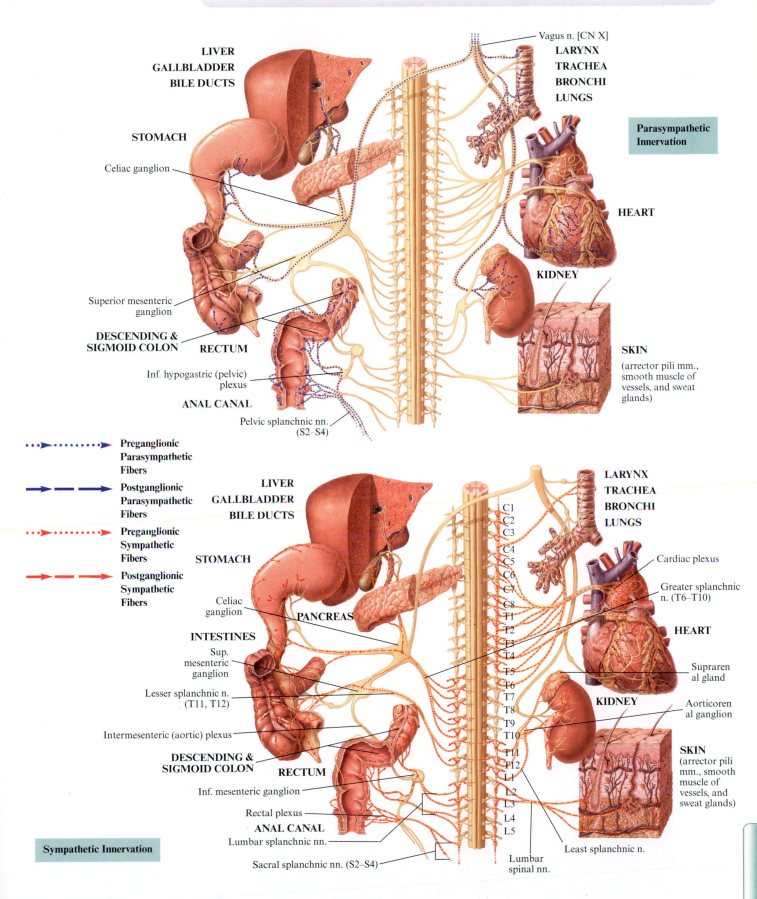

Vagus n. [CN X]

LIVER
GALLBLADDER
BILE DUCTS

LARYNX
TRACHEA
BRONCHI
LUNGS

STOMACH

Parasympathetic
Innervation

Celiac ganglion

HEART

KIDNEY

Superior mesenteric
ganglion

DESCENDING &
SIGMOID COLON

RECTUM

SKIN
(arrector pili mm.,
smooth muscle of
vessels, and sweat
glands)

Inf. hypogastric (pelvic)
plexus

ANAL CANAL

Pelvic splanchnic nn.
(S2–S4)

Preganglionic
Parasympathetic
Fibers

Postganglionic
Parasympathetic
Fibers

Preganglionic
Sympathetic
Fibers

Postganglionic
Sympathetic
Fibers

LIVER
GALLBLADDER
BILE DUCTS

LARYNX
TRACHEA
BRONCHI
LUNGS

C1
C2
C3
C4
C5
C6
C7
C8
T1
T2
T3
T4
T5
T6
T7
T8
T9
T10
T11
T12
L1
L2
L3
L4
L5

Cardiac plexus

Greater splanchnic
n. (T6–T10)

STOMACH

Celiac
ganglion

PANCREAS

INTESTINES

HEART

Sup.
mesenteric
ganglion

Suprarenal gland

Lesser splanchnic n.
(T11, T12)

KIDNEY

Aorticorenal ganglion

Intermesenteric (aortic) plexus

DESCENDING &
SIGMOID COLON

RECTUM

SKIN
(arrector pili
mm., smooth
muscle of
vessels, and
sweat glands)

Inf. mesenteric ganglion

Rectal plexus

ANAL CANAL

Lumbar splanchnic nn.

Least splanchnic n.

Sympathetic Innervation

Sacral splanchnic nn. (S2–S4)

Lumbar
spinal nn.

PLATE 8.20   PELVIC AUTONOMIC NERVES—FEMALE

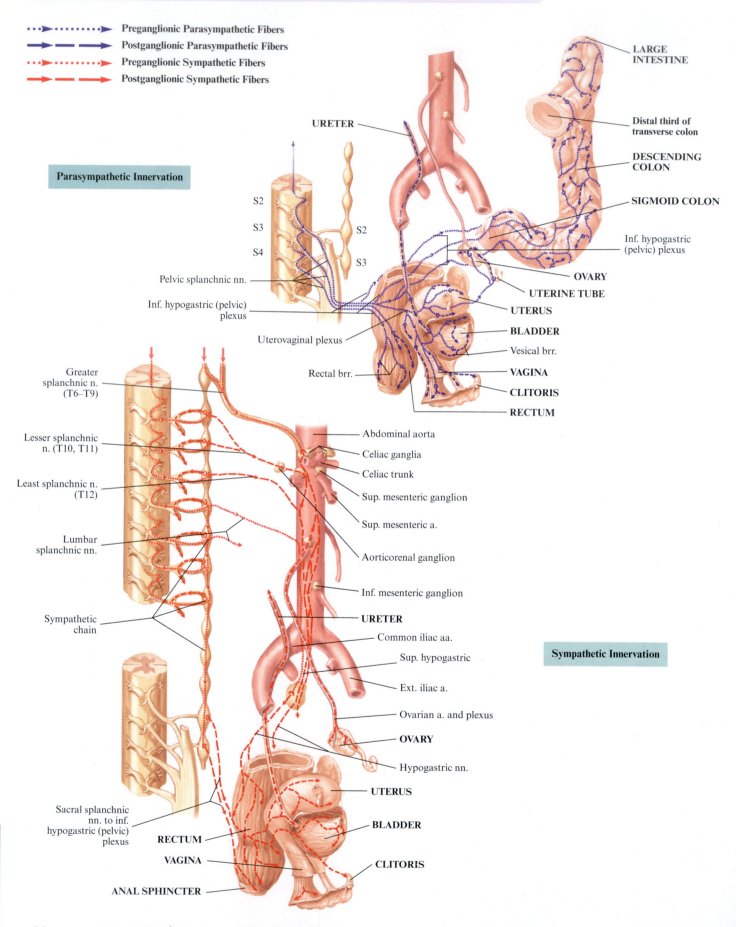

Preganglionic Parasympathetic Fibers
Postganglionic Parasympathetic Fibers
Preganglionic Sympathetic Fibers
Postganglionic Sympathetic Fibers

Parasympathetic Innervation

LARGE INTESTINE

URETER

Distal third of transverse colon

DESCENDING COLON

S2
S3
S4

S2
S3

SIGMOID COLON

Inf. hypogastric (pelvic) plexus

Pelvic splanchnic nn.

Inf. hypogastric (pelvic) plexus

OVARY
UTERINE TUBE
UTERUS

Uterovaginal plexus

BLADDER
Vesical brr.

Rectal brr.

VAGINA
CLITORIS
RECTUM

Greater splanchnic n. (T6–T9)

Abdominal aorta
Celiac ganglia
Celiac trunk

Lesser splanchnic n. (T10, T11)

Sup. mesenteric ganglion
Sup. mesenteric a.

Least splanchnic n. (T12)

Aorticorenal ganglion

Lumbar splanchnic nn.

Inf. mesenteric ganglion

URETER

Sympathetic chain

Common iliac aa.
Sup. hypogastric

Ext. iliac a.

Sympathetic Innervation

Ovarian a. and plexus

OVARY

Hypogastric nn.

UTERUS

Sacral splanchnic nn. to inf. hypogastric (pelvic) plexus

BLADDER

RECTUM

VAGINA

CLITORIS

ANAL SPHINCTER

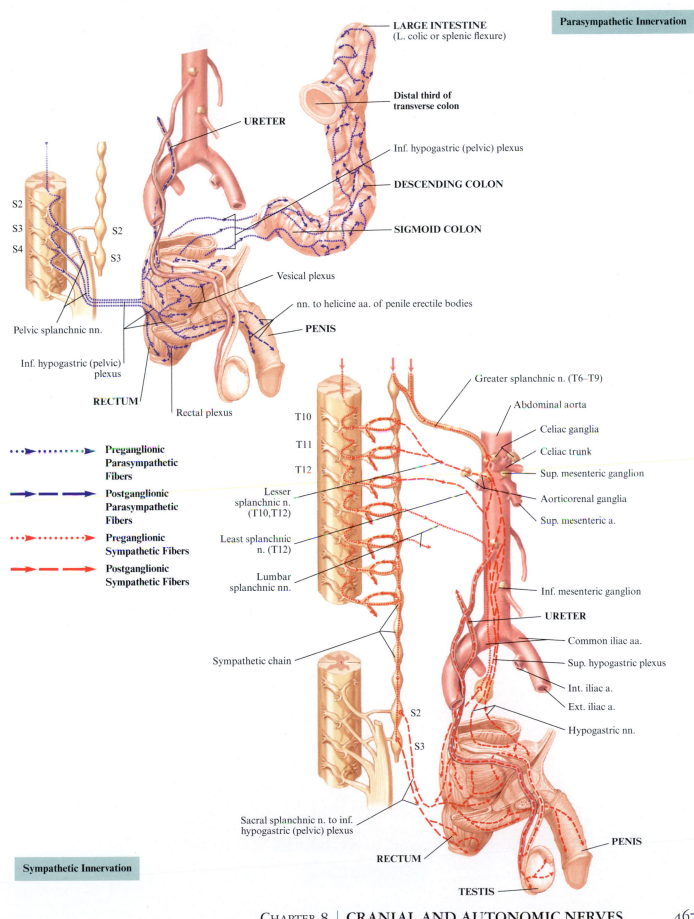

LARGE INTESTINE
(L. colic or splenic flexure)

Distal third of
transverse colon

URETER

Inf. hypogastric (pelvic) plexus

DESCENDING COLON

SIGMOID COLON

S2
S3
S4

S2
S3

Vesical plexus

nn. to helicine aa. of penile erectile bodies

PENIS

Pelvic splanchnic nn.

Inf. hypogastric (pelvic)
plexus

RECTUM

Rectal plexus

- ·····►············► Preganglionic
  Parasympathetic
  Fibers

- ─ ── ── ──► Postganglionic
  Parasympathetic
  Fibers

- ·····►············► Preganglionic
  Sympathetic Fibers

- ─ ── ── ──► Postganglionic
  Sympathetic Fibers

Greater splanchnic n. (T6–T9)

Abdominal aorta

Celiac ganglia

Celiac trunk

Sup. mesenteric ganglion

Aorticorenal ganglia

Sup. mesenteric a.

T10

T11

T12

Lesser
splanchnic n.
(T10, T12)

Least splanchnic
n. (T12)

Lumbar
splanchnic nn.

Inf. mesenteric ganglion

URETER

Common iliac aa.

Sup. hypogastric plexus

Int. iliac a.

Ext. iliac a.

Hypogastric nn.

Sympathetic chain

S2

S3

Sacral splanchnic n. to inf.
hypogastric (pelvic) plexus

RECTUM

PENIS

TESTIS

PLATE 8.22   ACCESSORY NERVE—CN XI

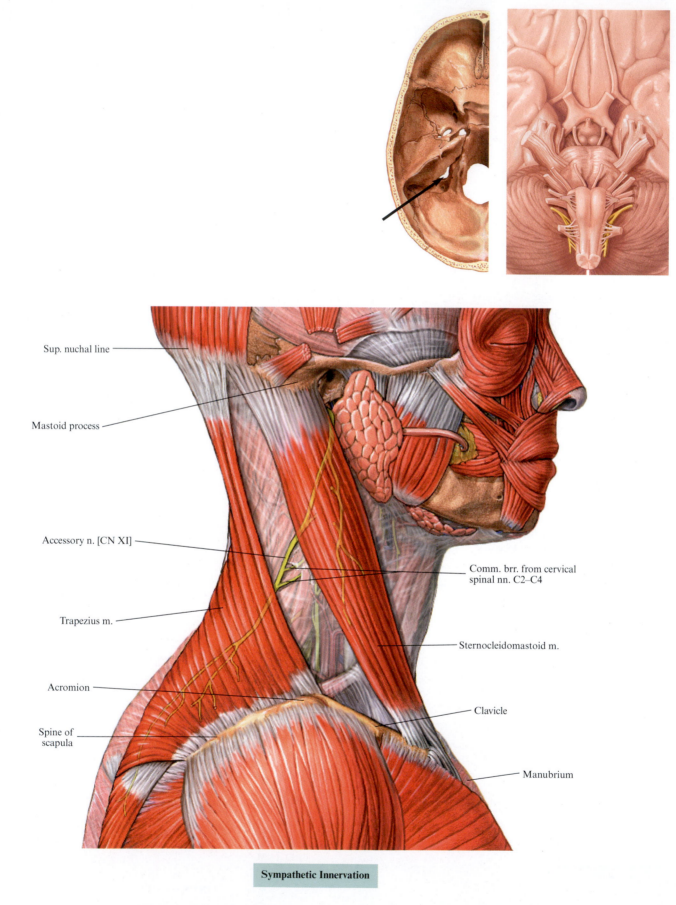

Sup. nuchal line

Mastoid process

Accessory n. [CN XI]

Comm. brr. from cervical
spinal nn. C2–C4

Trapezius m.

Sternocleidomastoid m.

Acromion

Clavicle

Spine of
scapula

Manubrium

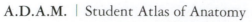

Sympathetic Innervation

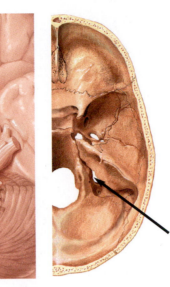

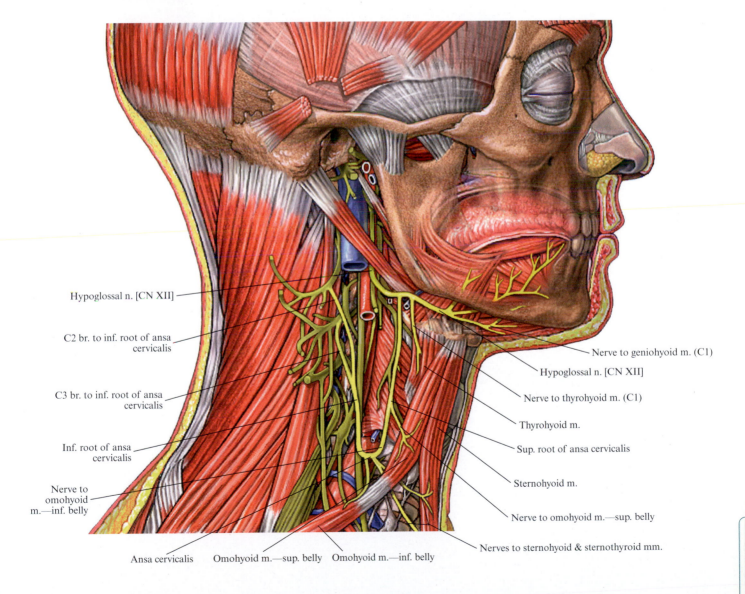

Hypoglossal n. [CN XII]

C2 br. to inf. root of ansa cervicalis

C3 br. to inf. root of ansa cervicalis

Inf. root of ansa cervicalis

Nerve to omohyoid m.—inf. belly

Ansa cervicalis

Omohyoid m.—sup. belly

Omohyoid m.—inf. belly

Nerve to geniohyoid m. (C1)

Hypoglossal n. [CN XII]

Nerve to thyrohyoid m. (C1)

Thyrohyoid m.

Sup. root of ansa cervicalis

Sternohyoid m.

Nerve to omohyoid m.—sup. belly

Nerves to sternohyoid & sternothyroid mm.

PLATE 8.24   CERVICAL PLEXUS

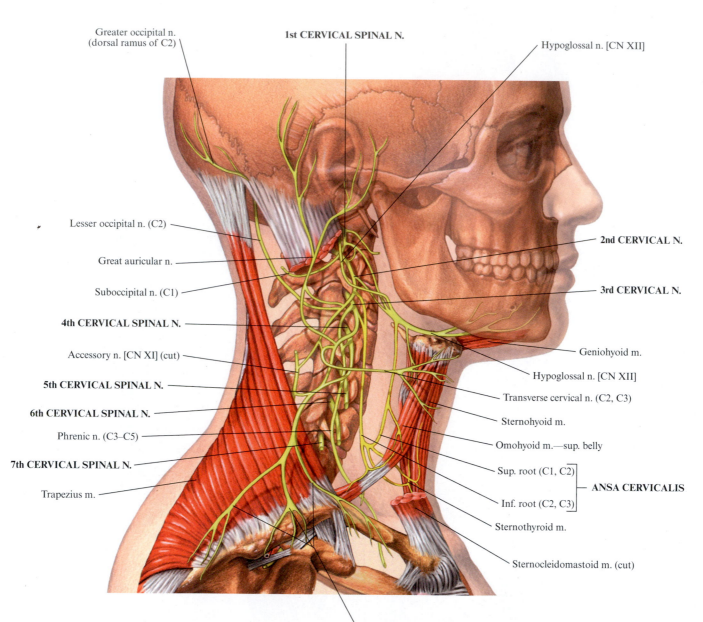

Greater occipital n.
(dorsal ramus of C2)

1st CERVICAL SPINAL N.

Hypoglossal n. [CN XII]

Lesser occipital n. (C2)

Great auricular n.

Suboccipital n. (C1)

4th CERVICAL SPINAL N.

Accessory n. [CN XI] (cut)

5th CERVICAL SPINAL N.

6th CERVICAL SPINAL N.

Phrenic n. (C3–C5)

7th CERVICAL SPINAL N.

Trapezius m.

2nd CERVICAL N.

3rd CERVICAL N.

Geniohyoid m.

Hypoglossal n. [CN XII]

Transverse cervical n. (C2, C3)

Sternohyoid m.

Omohyoid m.—sup. belly

Sup. root (C1, C2)

Inf. root (C2, C3)

ANSA CERVICALIS

Sternothyroid m.

Sternocleidomastoid m. (cut)

Supraclavicular nn. (C3, C4)

Veins, named
jugular—*continued*
external, 30–31, 42–43, 72, 385, 390–391, 400
internal, 30–31, 72–73, 78, 102, 309, 390–391, 401–402, 436–439
labial
inferior, 390
posterior, 167
superior, 390–391
laryngeal, superior, 415–416
lumbar, 30–32
maxillary, 390
mesenteric
inferior, 121–125, 138–139, 166–167, 207
superior, 121–125, 129, 138, 141
metacarpal, dorsal, 298
musculophrenic, 30–31, 97
nasofrontal, 429
obturator, 166–167, 254
occipital, 390–391, 400
ophthalmic, 391, 432, 434
ovarian, 167
palmar digital, 298–299, 336
palmar superficial, 299
pampiniform plexus, 57, 166, 175
pancreaticoduodenal
anterior inferior, 138
anterior superior, 138
paraumbilical, 48, 124
perforating/anastomosing, 232–233, 250–251
pericardiacophrenic, 81, 94–96, 102, 104
perineal superficial, 161
peroneal, 263
phrenic
inferior, 32, 138, 140–142
pial plexus, 34–35
plantar
lateral, 232, 270
medial, 232, 270
network, 232–233
plexus, posterior internal, 33, 35
popliteal, 232, 250–251, 267
portal, 120–121, 123–126, 129
profunda brachii, 298–299, 316, 320
proper digital, 270–271
proper dorsal digital, 298–299
prostatic plexus, 166, 170
pterygoid plexus, 391, 419, 437
pudendal, 52, 232–233
pulmonary
left, 82, 83, 90–92, 94–95, 100, 102
right, 82, 83, 88, 90, 96–97, 100, 102
radial, 298–299, 327–328, 338, 341
rectal
inferior, 166–167, 192, 194–195
interior, 207
middle, 166–167, 207
perimuscular plexus, 207
superior, 138, 141, 166–167, 207
rectal plexus, 163, 167, 207–208
communication, interior/external, 207
external, 163, 207–208
rectosigmoid, 138
renal, 144
left, 30, 32, 142–143, 146–147
right, 30, 32, 142, 146

retromandibular, 391, 404–405
anterior branch, 390, 409, 412, 423
posterior branch, 390
sacral
lateral, 207, 254
middle, 32, 138, 175, 207
saphenous
accessory, 174, 233
great, 30–31, 52–54, 232–233, 244, 248–249, 265–268
small, 232–233, 236, 250–251, 265
scapular
dorsal, 60, 298, 316–317, 332–333, 413
transverse, 312–313
scrotal
left, 164
left posterior, 164
posterior, 166
sigmoid, 138–139, 141, 207
spinal posterior, 35
splenic, 122–125, 138
subclavian, 43, 72, 298–299, 322, 390
left, 72, 94–95
right, 30–31, 97
subcostal, 30–32, 44
subscapular, 30, 298–299
superior vorticose, 435
supraorbital, 429
suprarenal, 32, 140, 146–147
suprascapular, 30–31, 298, 312, 332–333, 390
supreme (highest), 30, 32, 391
temporal, superficial, 390, 400, 404–405
testicular, 48, 248
thigh
anterior, 246–247
cross section, 255–256
medial/lateral, 254
overview, 257
posterior, 250–251
thoracic
internal, 31–33, 44–49, 81–82, 103–104, 207
lateral, 30, 298, 312–313
superficial, 298
thoracoacromial, 30, 298
thoracodorsal, 60, 298–299
thoracoepigastric, 42, 46–47, 52
thymic, 32, 82, 87
thyroid
inferior, 32, 72, 103, 385
superior, 385, 412–413, 416
tibial
anterior, 246–247, 260, 263, 266, 268
posterior, 232, 262–263
tibialis anterior, 232
tibial recurrent, anterior, 265
ulnar, 289, 298–299, 327
ulnar collateral, 323, 332–333
ulnar recurrent, 332–333
upper limb, 298–299
uterine, 167, 207
uterovaginal plexus, 167
vaginal, 167, 207
vena cava
inferior, 30–32, 82–83, 96, 118–123, 126, 129–130, 140–143, 207
superior, 30–32, 81–83, 87–89, 96–97
ventricular posterior, 83
vertebral, 30–32, 385, 391

left, 82, 87
right, 103
vesical
inferior, 166
superior, 166–167, 207
vesical plexus, 166–167, 170–172, 467
vorticose
inferior, 431
superior, 431, 434
zygomaticoorbital, 404–405
Vena caval foramen, 106–107
Vena digiti minimi, 299
Venae comitantes, 33
Ventral division of S2, 243
Vermiform appendix, 49, 111, 136–138, 178
Vertebrae
cervical (*See* Cervical vertebrae)
column, 79
intercostal, 95
ligament attachments, 19
lumbar (*See* Lumbar vertebrae)
muscle attachments, 4–7
paravertebral structures, 98–99
sacral (*See* Sacral vertebrae)
spinous process, 35
thoracic (*See* Thoracic vertebrae)
Vertebral venous plexus, 391
Vertebra prominens. *See under* Cervical vertebrae
Vertebrocostal trigone, 106–107
Vesical venous plexus, 166–167, 170–172, 467
Vesicouterine pouch, 112, 178–181, 190
Vestibular (false vocal) fold, 416
Vestibular ganglion, 443, 460
Vestibular gland, greater, 196
Vestibulocochlear nerve (CN VIII), 392, 396, 443, 460
functions, 471
overview, 446–447, 460
Visceral layer, 191
Visceral pericardium, 81, 93
Visceral peritoneum, 113, 190–191, 208
Vocal fold, 416

W

White ramus communicans, 40–41, 96–97, 102
Wrist
bones of, 344
cross section, 341
joint, 328
radiograph, 329, 345

X

Xiphisternal joint, 18
Xiphoid process, 2, 4, 18, 68, 93

Z

Zona orbicularis, 152, 258
Zygapophyseal joint, 19
Zygomatic arch, 348–349, 356, 404–405, 412, 436–437
Zygomatic bone, 348–349, 352–353, 356–357, 359, 432
frontal process, 440
orbital surface, 364
temporal process, 440
Zygomaticofacial foramen, 352, 356, 358
Zygomatico frontal suture, 429
Zygomatic process, 352–353, 356, 365

**Sidney Silverman Library
and Learning Resource Center
Bergen Community College
400 Paramus Road
Paramus, NJ 07652-1595**

www.bergen.edu
Return Postage Guaranteed